W9-DDC-435

FERGUSON

CAREER RESOURCE GUIDE FOR

PEOPLE

WITH

DISABILITIES

Third Edition

VOLUME 2

Ferguson

An imprint of Infobase Publishing

Ferguson Career Resource Guide for People with Disabilities, Third Edition

Copyright © 2006 by Infobase Publishing

Ferguson
An imprint of Infobase Publishing
132 West 31st Street
New York NY 10001

Library of Congress Cataloging-in-Publication
Ferguson career resource guide for people with disabilities. — 3rd ed.
    p. cm.
   Rev. ed. of: Ferguson's guide for people with disabilities. 2nd ed. c2001.
   Includes bibliographical references and index.
   ISBN 0-8160-6127-0 (set) (hc : alk. paper)
   ISBN 0-8160-6128-9 (vol. 1)— ISBN 0-8160-6129-7 (vol. 2)
1. People with disabilities—Services for—United States—Directories.   2. People with disabilities—Services for—United States—Finance—Directories.   3. Self-help devices for people with disabilities—United States—Directories.   4. People with disabilities—Vocational guidance—United States.   I. J. G. Ferguson Publishing Company.   II. Resources for people with disabilities.
   HV1553.F47 2006
   362.4'04802973—dc22

Ferguson books are available at special discounts when purchased in bulk quantities for businesses, associations, institutions, or sales promotions. Please call our Special Sales Department in New York at (212) 967-8800 or (800) 322-8755.

You can find Ferguson on the World Wide Web at http://www.fergpubco.com

Text design by David Strelecky
Cover design by Salvatore Luongo

Printed in the United States of America

VB FOF 10 9 8 7 6 5 4 3 2 1

This book is printed on acid-free paper.

CONTENTS

PART IV: INDEXES

PART III
DIRECTORY

LIBRARIES AND
RESEARCH CENTERS

LIBRARIES AND RESEARCH CENTERS

Some of these library resources for people with visual impairments and physical disabilities are private. Many are administered by the National Library Service for the Blind and Physically Handicapped, Library of Congress, and provide free services.

ALABAMA

Alabama Institute for Deaf and Blind
Library and Instructional Resource Center for the Blind
412 Cherry Street, PO Box 698
Talladega, AL 35161
256-761-3288, 800-848-4722
Lacy.Teresa@aidb.state.al.us
http://www.aidb.org/asb/aircb.asp
Disability Served: hearing, vision

Alabama Institute for Deaf and Blind
Library and Instructional Resource Center for the Blind
705 South Street, PO Box 698
Talladega, AL 35160
205-761-3287, 800-848-4722
http://www.aidb.org/asb/aircb.asp
Disability Served: hearing, vision

Alabama Public Library Service
Alabama Regional Library for the Blind and Physically
    Handicapped
6030 Monticello Drive
Montgomery, AL 36130-6000
334-213-3906, 800-392-5671
fzaleski@apls.state.al.us
http://www.apls.state.al.us/webpages/services/BPH/
    BPHServices.htm
Disability Served: physically disabled, vision

Alabama Radio Reading Service Network
650 11th Street South
Birmingham, AL 35294
205-934-6576
Disability Served: physically disabled, vision

Birmingham Brailling Group
10 Monte Vallo Lane
Birmingham, AL 35213
205-879-3963
Disability Served: vision

Houston-Love Memorial Library
Department of the Blind and Physically Handicapped
PO Box 1369
Dothan, AL 36302
334-793-9767, 334-793-9767(TDD)
http://www.houstonlovelibrary.org/DBPH.HTM
Disability Served: physically disabled, vision

**Huntsville Subregional Library for the Blind
    and Physically Handicapped**
915 Monroe Street
Huntsville, AL 35801
256-532-5940
jwelch@hpl.lib.al.us
http://www.hpl.lib.al.us/departments/bph
Disability Served: physically disabled, vision

Public Library of Anniston and Calhoun County
Library for the Blind and Handicapped
PO Box 308
Anniston, AL 36202
205-237-8501, 800-392-5671
bandph@anniston.lib.al.us
http://www.anniston.lib.al.us/bandph.htm
Disability Served: various

Tuscaloosa Public Library
Tuscaloosa Subregional Library for the Blind
    and Physically Handicapped
1801 Jack Warner Parkway
Tuscaloosa, AL 35401
205-758-8291
bjbj@tuscaloosa-library.org
http://www.tuscaloosa-library.org/departments/
    extension-services/handicapped
Disability Served: physically disabled, vision

ALASKA

Alaska State Library
Talking Book Center
344 West Third Avenue, Suite 125
Anchorage, AK 99501
907-269-6575, 800-776-6566
Patience_Frederiksen@eed.state.ak.us
http://www.library.state.ak.us/dev/tbc.html
Disability Served: physically disabled, vision

ARIZONA

Arizona State Library
Braille and Talking Books Division
1030 North 32nd Street
Phoenix, AZ 85008
602-255-5578, 800-255-5578
btbl@lib.az.us
http://www.dlapr.lib.az.us/braille
Disability Served: physically disabled, vision

Desert Volunteer Braille Guild
The Foundation for Blind Children
1235 East Harmont Drive
Phoenix, AZ 85020
602-331-1470, 602-678-5810
http://www.the-fbc.org
Disability Served: vision

Flagstaff City-Coconino County Public Library
Services To The Blind, Deaf And Physically Disabled
300 West Aspen Avenue
Flagstaff, AZ 86001
928-779-7670
kwhitake@fpl.lib.az.us
http://www.flagstaffpubliclibrary.org/specialservices.
   htm
Disability Served: hearing, physically disabled, vision

Phoenix Public Library
Special Needs Center
1221 North Central Avenue
Phoenix, AZ 85004
602-261-8690, 602-254-8205 (TTY)
http://www.phoenixpubliclibrary.org/snc.jsp
Disability Served: various

Prescott Public Library
Talking Book Center
215 East Goodwin Street
Prescott, AZ 86303
928-777-1500
toni.kaus@cityofprescott.net
http://www.prescottlibrary.info
Disability Served: physically disabled, vision

Recorded Recreational Reading for the Blind
9447 North 99th Avenue
Peoria, AZ 85345
623-933-0985
Disability Served: vision

Recording for the Blind and Dyslexic
Recording Studio-Phoenix
3627 East Indian School Road, Suite 108
Phoenix, AZ 85018
602-468-9144
http://www.rfbd.org/Arizona_Unit.htm
Disability Served: dyslexic, vision

Recording for the Blind and Dyslexic
Recording Studio-Sun Cities
9449 North 99th Avenue
Peoria, AZ 85345
602-977-6020
imead@rfbd.org
http://www.rfbd.org/Arizona_Unit.htm
Disability Served: dyslexic, vision

ARKANSAS

Arkansas State Library
Arkansas Library for the Blind and Physically
   Handicapped
One Capitol Mall
Little Rock, AR 72201
501-682-1155, 866-660-0885, 501-682-1002 (TDD)
nlsbooks@asl.lib.ar.us
http://www.asl.lib.ar.us/ASL_LBPH.htm
Disability Served: physically disabled, vision

Educational Services for the Visually Impaired
2402 Wildwood, Suite 112
Sherwood, AR 72120
501-835-5448
angylnf@esvi.org
http://www.esvi.org
Disability Served: vision

Library for the Blind and Handicapped, Southwest
220 East Main Street, PO Box 668
Magnolia, AR 71754
870-234-0399, 866-234-8273
lbph@hotmail.com
Disability Served: physically disabled, vision

CALIFORNIA

American Red Cross Braille Service
10771 San Pablo Avenue
El Cerrito, CA 94530
510-526-7206
Disability Served: vision

Beach Cities Braille Guild Inc.
PO Box 712
Huntington Beach, CA 94237
714-536-9666, 800-952-5666
Disability Served: vision

Books Aloud Inc.
PO Box 5731
San Jose, CA 95150-5731
408-808-2613
info@booksaloud.org
http://www.booksaloud.org
Disability Served: physically disabled, vision

Braille Transcribers of Humboldt
PO Box 6363
Eureka, CA 95502
707-442-4048
http://www.members.tripod.com/~Whipkey
Disability Served: vision

California State Library
Braille and Talking Book Library
PO Box 942837
Sacramento, CA 95814
916-654-0640, 800-952-5666
btbl@library.ca.gov
http://www.library.ca.gov/html/pubser05.cfm
Disability Served: physically disabled, vision

California State Library
Braille Institute Library Services
741 North Vermont Avenue
Los Angeles, CA 90029
323-660-3880, 800-808-2555
bils@braillelibrary.org
http://www.brailleinstitute.org
Disability Served: vision

Contra Costa Braille Transcribers
2823 Wiswall Drive
Richmond, CA 94806
510-682-4734
PatBiasca@aol.com
Disability Served: vision

Fresno County Public Library
Talking Book Library for the Blind, Ted Wills
    Community Center
770 North San Pablo Avenue

Fresno, CA 93728
209-488-3217, 800-742-1011, 559-488-1642 (TDD)
wendy.eisenberg@fresnolibrary.org
http://www.fresnolibrary.org
Disability Served: physically disabled, vision

Golden Gate Braille Transcribers Inc.
1466 44th Avenue
San Francisco, CA 94122
415-566-1641
Disability Served: vision

Lutheran Braille Workers Inc.
PO Box 5000
Yucaipa, CA 92399
909-795-8977
lbw@lbwinc.org
http://www.lbwinc.org
Disability Served: vision

Monterey County Braille Transcribers Inc.
225 Laurel Avenue
Pacific Grove, CA 93950
831-394-2033
http://www.ittatc.org/technical/providers
Disability Served: vision

National Association for Visually Handicapped-West
3201 Balboa Street
San Francisco, CA 94121
415-221-3201
staffca@navh.org
http://www.navh.org
Disability Served: vision

Ontario City Library
120 East D Street
Ontario, CA 91764
909-395-2004
http://www.ci.ontario.ca.us/index.cfm/6752/6307
Disability Served: vision

Recording for the Blind and Dyslexic
Recording Studio-Hollywood
5022 Hollywood Boulevard
Los Angeles, CA 90027
323-664-5525, 800-732-8398
los_angeles@rfbd.org
http://www.rfbdla.org
Disability Served: dyslexic, vision

Recording for the Blind and Dyslexic
Recording Studio-Northern California Unit
488 West Charleston Road
Palo Alto, CA 94306
650-493-3717, 866-493-3717
http://www.rfbd.org
Disability Served: dyslexic, vision

Recording for the Blind and Dyslexic
Recording Studio-Orange County
2021 East Fourth Street, Suite 114
Santa Ana, CA 92705
714-547-4171
http://www.rfbd.org
Disability Served: dyslexic, vision

Recording for the Blind and Dyslexic
Recording Studio-San Fernando Valley
6860 Canby Avenue, Suite 111
Reseda, CA 91335
818-654-2747
http://www.rfbd.org
Disability Served: dyslexic, vision

Recording for the Blind and Dyslexic
Recording Studio-Santa Barbara Unit
5638 Hollister Avenue, Suite 210
Goleta, CA 93117
805-681-0531
http://www.rfbd.org
Disability Served: dyslexic, vision

Recording for the Blind and Dyslexic
Recording Studio-South Bay
1310 Kingsdale Avenue
Redondo Beach, CA 90278
310-371-9969
http://www.rfbd.org
Disability Served: dyslexic, vision

Sacramento Braille Transcribers Inc.
2791 24th Street, Room 7
Sacramento, CA 95818
916-455-9121
Disability Served: vision

San Fernando Valley Braille Transcribers Guild
4784 Park Encino Lane, #303
Encino, CA 91436

818-905-1256
Disability Served: vision

San Francisco Public Library, Civic Center
Library for the Blind and Print Disabled
100 Larkin Street
San Francisco, CA 94102
415-557-4253
lbpd@sfpl.org
http://sfpl.lib.ca.us/librarylocations/accessservices/lbpd.
    htm
Disability Served: various

Sequoia Braille Transcribers
2730 West Seeger Avenue
Visalia, CA 93277
559-732-1912
Disability Served: vision

Sonoma County Braille Transcribers Guild
PO Box 502
Santa Rosa, CA 95402
707-579-2544
Disability Served: vision

Transcribers of Orange County
10982 Paddock Lane
Santa Ana, CA 92705
714-731-5899
Disability Served: vision

Transcribing Mariners
PO Box 4232
San Rafael, CA 94913
415-883-3083
peggys@juno.com
Disability Served: vision

Volunteers of Vacaville-Blind Project
1600 California Drive, PO Box 670
Vacaville, CA 95696-0670
707-448-6841, ext. 2044
VOVacaville@yahoo.com
Disability Served: vision

Volunteer Transcribing Services
205 East Third Avenue
San Mateo, CA 94401-4077
650-344-8664
Disability Served: vision

COLORADO

Boulder Public Library
Special Services Department
1000 Canyon Boulevard
Boulder, CO 80302
303-441-3100
http://www.boulder.lib.co.us/special/braille.html
Disability Served: various

Colorado Department of Education
Colorado Talking Book Library
180 Sheridan Boulevard
Denver, CO 80226
303-727-9277, 800-685-2136
ctbl.info@cde.state.co.us
http://www.cde.state.co.us/ctbl
Disability Served: physically disabled, vision

Recording for the Blind and Dyslexic
Recording Studio-Rocky Mountain Unit
1355 South Colorado Boulevard, Suite C-406
Denver, CO 80222
303-757-0787
http://www.rfbd.org
Disability Served: dyslexic, vision

Volunteer Transcribers for the Visually Impaired
833 East Platte Avenue
Colorado Springs, CO 80903
719-632-2299
Disability Served: vision

CONNECTICUT

Connecticut Braille Association Inc.
Large Type Division
664 Oakwood Avenue
West Hartford, CT 06110
860-953-9692
Disability Served: vision

Connecticut State Library
Library for the Blind and Physically Handicapped
198 West Street
Rocky Hill, CT 06067
860-566-2151, 800-842-4516
lbph@cslib.org
http://www.cslib.org/lbph.htm
Disability Served: physically disabled, vision

Connecticut Volunteer Services for the Blind and Handicapped Inc.
Oliver Wolcott Library
160 South Street
Litchfield, CT 06759
860-567-8578
http://www.cslib.org/cvsbh
Disability Served: physically disabled, vision

Prevent Blindness Tri-State
984 Southford Road
Middlebury, CT 06762
800-850-2020
info@preventblindnessct.org
http://www.preventblindnessct.org
Disability Served: vision

Recording for the Blind and Dyslexic-Connecticut Unit
209 Orange Street
New Haven, CT 06510-2014
203-624-4334
http://www.rfbd.org
Disability Served: dyslexic, vision

DELAWARE

Delaware Association for the Blind
800 West Street
Wilmington, DE 19801
302-655-2111
Disability Served: vision

Delaware Division of Libraries
Library for the Blind and Physically Handicapped
43 South DuPont Highway
Dover, DE 19901
302-739-4748, 800-282-8676
jphillos@lib.de.us
Disability Served: physically disabled, vision

DISTRICT OF COLUMBIA

District of Columbia Public Library
Library for the Blind and Physically Handicapped
901 G Street, NW, Room 215
Washington, DC 20001
202-727-2142, 202-727-2145 (TDD)
lbph.dcpl@dc.gov

http://dclibrary.org/lbph
Disability Served: physically disabled, vision

Library of Congress
National Library Service for the Blind and Physically
    Handicapped
1291 Taylor Street, NW
Washington, DC 20542
202-707-5100, 800-424-8567, 202-707-0744 (TDD)
nlsm@loc.gov
http://www.loc.gov/nls
Disability Served: physically disabled, vision

Recording for the Blind and Dyslexic
Metropolitan Washington, DC, Unit
5225 Wisconsin Avenue, NW, Suite 312
Washington, DC 20015
202-244-8990
washingtondc@rfbd.org
http://www.rfbd.org
Disability Served: dyslexic, vision

Volunteer Braille Services
3935 Macomb Street, NW
Washington, DC 20016
202-966-5880
Disability Served: vision

FLORIDA

Braille Association of Mid-Florida Inc.
1500 Falcon Drive
Orlando, FL 32803
407-897-3367
Disability Served: vision

**Brevard Association for the Advancement
    of the Blind**
674 South Patrick Drive
Satellite Beach, FL 32937
407-773-7222
Disability Served: vision

Brevard County Libraries
Talking Books Library
308 Forrest Avenue
Cocoa, FL 32922-7781
321-633-1810, 321-633-1811 (TDD)
kbriley@brev.org
http://www.brev.org/about_bcl/disabled_services.htm
Disability Served: physically disabled, vision

Broward County Talking Book Library
100 South Andrews Avenue
Ft Lauderdale, FL 33301
954-357-7555, 954-357-7413, 954-357-7528 (TDD)
wforbes@browardlibrary.org
Disability Served: physically disabled, vision

Florida Division of Blind Services
Florida Bureau of Braille and Talking Book Library
    Services
420 Platt Street
Daytona Beach, FL 32114-2804
386-239-6000, 800-226-6075
mike_gunde@dbs.doe.state.fl.us
http://www.state.fl.us/dbs/library/index.shtml
Disability Served: physically disabled, vision

**Florida Instructional Materials Center for the
    Visually Impaired**
4210 West Bay Villa Avenue
Tampa, FL 33611
813-837-7826
http://www.fimcvi.org
Disability Served: vision

Hillsborough County Public Library Cooperative
Hillsborough Talking Book Library
3910 South Manhattan Avenue
Tampa, FL 33611
813-272-6070, 813-272-6305 (TDD)
myerslj@hillsboroughcounty.org
http://www.hcplc.org/hcplc/liblocales/tbl
Disability Served: physically disabled, vision

Jacksonville Public Libraries
Talking Books Library
1755 Edgewood Avenue West, Suite 1
Jacksonville, FL 32208
904-765-5588, 904-768-7822 (TDD)
jerryr@coj.net
http://jpl.coj.net/library/tbl.html
Disability Served: physically disabled, vision

Lee County Library System
Lee County Talking Books Library
13240 North Cleveland Avenue, #5-6
North Ft. Myers, FL 33903
239-995-2665, 800-854-8195, 239-995-2665 (TDD)
kmcleish@leegov.com

http://www.lee-county.com/library/progserv/ssvcs/tb.htm
Disability Served: physically disabled, vision

Manatee County Public Library System

Manatee Talking Book Library
6081 26th Street West
Bradenton, FL 34207
813-742-5914
patricia.schubert@co.manatee.fl.us
Disability Served: physically disabled, vision

Miami-Dade Public Library System

Talking Book Library of Dade and Monroe Counties
2455 Northwest 183rd Street
Miami, FL 33056
305-751-8687, 800-451-9544, 305-474-7258 (TDD)
moyerb@mdpls.org
http://www.mdpls.org/services/outreach/talk_books.asp
Disability Served: physically disabled, vision

Orange County Library System

Talking Book Section
101 East Central Boulevard
Orlando, FL 32801
407-835-7323, 407-835-7641 (TDD)
bruton.marcia@ocls.info
http://www.ocls.info/Locations/talking_books.asp
Disability Served: physically disabled, vision

Palm Beach County Library Annex

Talking Books
4639 Lake Worth Road, Mil-Lake Plaza
Lake Worth, FL 33463
888-780-5151
talkingbooks@pbclibrary.org
http://www.pbclibrary.org/outreach-talkingbooks.htm
Disability Served: physically disabled, vision

Pinellas Braille Group Inc.

c/o Temple Beth-El
400 Pasadena Avenue South
St. Petersburg, FL 33707
813-347-6136
Disability Served: vision

Pinellas Talking Book Library

1330 Cleveland Street
Clearwater, FL 33773-2629
727-441-9958, 727-441-3168 (TDD)

mstevenson@pplc.us
http://www.pplc.us/tbl
Disability Served: physically disabled, vision

Recording for the Blind and Dyslexic

Recording Studio-Miami
6704 Southwest 80th Street
Miami, FL 33143
305-666-0552
cmccarthy@rfbd.org
http://www.rfbd.org
Disability Served: dyslexic, vision

Recording for the Blind and Dyslexic

Recording Studio-Palm Beach County
Florida Atlantic University
Gladys Davis Pavilion, Building 49
777 Glades Road
Boca Raton, FL 33431
561-297-4444
http://www.rfbd.org
Disability Served: dyslexic, vision

Sarasota County Braille Transcribers

1519 Blue Heron Drive
Sarasota, FL 34239
813-366-3410
Disability Served: vision

Visual Aid Volunteers of Florida Inc.

c/o Florida Instructional Materials Center
4210 West Bay Villa Avenue
Tampa, FL 33611
813-837-7826
http://www.fimcvi.org
Disability Served: vision

Volunteer Braille Services Inc.

c/o Royal Palm School
6650 Lawrence Road
Lantana, FL 33462
581-649-6850
http://www.palmbeach.k12.fl.us/RoyalPalmSchool
Disability Served: vision

West Florida Regional Library

Subregional Talking Book Library
200 West Gregory Street
Pensacola, FL 32502

850-436-5060, 850-435-1763 (TDD)
http://www.wfrl.lib.fl.us/talkingbooks.asp
Disability Served: physically disabled, vision

GEORGIA

Brunswick-Glynn County Regional Library
Talking Book Center
606 O Street
Brunswick, GA 31523-0901
912-267-1212
Disability Served: physically disabled, vision

Chattahoochee Valley Regional Library System
Columbus Library for Accessible Services
3000 Macon Road
Columbus, GA 31906-2201
706-243-2688, 800-652-0782 (TDD)
sbarnes@cvrls.net
http://www.thecolumbuslibrary.org/class.html
Disability Served: various

Cherokee Regional Library
North Georgia Talking Book Center
305 South Duke Street
LaFayette, GA 30728
706-638-1958, 888-506-0509
cstubblefield@chrl.org
http://www.walker.public.lib.ga.us/tbc/tbc1.htm
Disability Served: physically disabled, vision

Dougherty County Public Library
Albany Library for the Blind and Physically
    Handicapped
300 Pine Avenue
Albany, GA 31701
912-431-2920, 800-337-6251
lbph@docolib.org
http://www.docolib.org/LFTB.html
Disability Served: physically disabled, vision

East Central Georgia Regional Library
Library for the Blind and Physically Handicapped
425 9th Street
Augusta, GA 30901
706-821-2625
talkbook@ecgrl.org
http://www.ecgrl.public.lib.ga.us/lbph.htm
Disability Served: physically disabled, vision

Georgia Library for Accessible Services
Georgia Regional Library for the Blind and Physically
    Handicapped
1150 Murphy Avenue, SW
Atlanta, GA 30310
404-756-4619, 800-248-6701
glass@georgialibraries.org
http://www.georgialibraries.org/public/glass.html
Disability Served: physically disabled, vision

Hall County Library System
East Hall Branch and Special Needs Library
2434 Old Cornelia Highway
Gainesville, GA 30507
770-531-2500, 770-531-2530 (TDD)
amixson@hallcountylibrary.org
http://www.hallcountylibrary.org/ehmap.htm
Disability Served: various

Live Oak Public Libraries
Library for the Blind and Physically Handicapped
2708 Mechanics Avenue
Thunderbolt GA 31404
912-354-5864
stokesl@liveoakpl.org
http://www.liveoakpl.org/Thunderbolt.htm
Disability Served: physically disabled, vision

**Macon Library for the Blind and Physically
    Handicapped**
Washington Memorial Library
1180 Washington Avenue
Macon, GA 31201
478-744-0877, 800-805-7613, 478-744-0877 (TDD)
andersoj@mail.bibb.public.lib.ga.us
Disability Served: physically disabled, vision

Oconee Regional Library
Library for the Blind and Physically Handicapped
801 Bellevue Avenue, PO Box 100
Dublin, GA 31040
478-275-5382, 800-453-5541, 478-275-3821 (TDD)
arenfroe-warren@ocrl.org
http://www.laurens.public.lib.ga.us/index.pl/special_
    service_center
Disability Served: physically disabled, vision

Recording for the Blind and Dyslexic
Recording Studio-Athens Unit
120 Florida Avenue

Athens, GA 30605
706-549-1313
lmartin@rfbd.org
http://www.rfbd.org
Disability Served: dyslexic, vision

Sara Hightower Regional Library
Rome Subregional Library for People With
    Disabilities
205 Riverside Parkway, NE
Rome, GA 30161
706-236-4618, 888-263-0769, 706-236-4618 (TDD)
dhickman@rome-lpd.org
http://www.rome-lpd.org
Disability Served: various

South Georgia Regional Library
Valdosta Talking Book Center
300 Woodrow Wilson Drive
Valdosta, GA 31602
229-333-7658, 800-246-6515
djernigan@sgrl.org
Disability Served: physically disabled, vision

Southwest Georgia Regional Library
Bainbridge Subregional Library for the Blind
    and Physically Handicapped
301 South Monroe Street
Bainbridge, GA 31717
912-248-2680, 800-795-2680, 229-248-2665 (TDD)
lbph@mail.decatur.public.lib.ga.us
http://www.swgrl.org/local/lbph/LBPH1.HTM
Disability Served: physically disabled, vision

Special Needs Library of Northeast Georgia
2025 Baxter Street
Athens, GA 30606
706-613-3655, 800-531-2063, 706-613-3655 (TDD)
specialneedslibrary@athenslibrary.org
http://www.clarke.public.lib.ga.us/main/
    specialneedslibrary/specialneedslibrary.html
Disability Served: dyslexic, physically disabled, vision

HAWAII
Hawaii State Public Library System
Hawaii State Library for the Blind and Physically
    Handicapped
402 Kapahulu Avenue

Honolulu, HI 96815
808-733-8444, 800-559-4096, 808-733-8444 (TDD)
olbcirc@librarieshawaii.org
http://www.librarieshawaii.org/locations/oahu/lbph.
    htm
Disability Served: physically disabled, vision

IDAHO
Idaho State Library
Talking Book Library
325 West State Street
Boise, ID 83702
208-334-2117, 800-458-3271
tblbooks@isl.state.id.us
http://www.lili.org/tbs
Disability Served: physically disabled, vision

ILLINOIS
Chicago Public Library
Talking Book Center
400 South State Street, Fifth Floor North
Chicago, IL 60605
312-747-1616, 800-757-4654
tbc@chipublib.org
http://www.chipublib.org/003cpl/irlbph/cpltbc.html
Disability Served: physically disabled, vision

Educational Tape Recording for the Blind
3915 West 103rd Street
Chicago, IL 60655
312-445-3533
Disability Served: vision

Guild for the Blind
180 North Michigan Avenue, Suite 1700
Chicago, IL 60601-7463
312-236-8569
info@guildfortheblind.org
http://www.guildfortheblind.org
Disability Served: vision

Horizons for the Blind Inc.
2 North Williams Street
Crystal Lake, IL 60014
815-444-8800
mail@horizons-blind.org
Disability Served: vision

Illinois Early Childhood Intervention Clearinghouse
830 South Spring Street
Springfield, IL 62704
217-785-1364, 800-852-4302
clearinghouse@eosinc.com
http://www.eiclearinghouse.org
Disability Served: various

Illinois Library for the Blind and Physically Handicapped
1055 West Roosevelt Road
Chicago, IL 60608
312-746-9219, 800-331-2351
Disability Served: physically disabled, vision

Illinois Regional Library for the Blind and Physically Handicapped
300 South Second Street
Springfield, IL 62701
217-782-9435, 800-665-5576, 800-965-0748 (TDD)
http://www.cyberdriveillinois.com/departments/library
Disability Served: physically disabled, vision

Illinois State Library
Talking Book and Braille Service
401 East Washington
Springfield, IL 62701
217-782-9435, 800-665-5576, 888-261-7863 (TDD)
sruda@ilsos.net
http://www.cyberdriveillinois.com/departments/library/
    who_we_are/talking_book_and_braille_service/
    about.html
Disability Served: physically disabled, vision

Johanna Bureau for the Blind and Physically Handicapped Inc.
8 South Michigan Avenue, Suite 300
Chicago, IL 60603-3305
312-332-0780
Disability Served: physically disabled, vision

Mid-Illinois Talking Book Center
600 High Point Lane, Suite 2
East Peoria, IL 61611
309-694-7935, 800-426-0709
lbell@alliancelibrarysystem.com
http://www.mitbc.org
Disability Served: physically disabled, vision

Mid-Illinois Talking Center
Quincy Office Alliance Library System
515 York

Quincy, IL 62301
217-224-6619, 800-537-1274, 217-224-6619 (TDD)
lbell@alliancelibrarysystem.com
http://www.mitbc.org
Disability Served: physically disabled, vision

Naperville Area Transcribing for the Blind
25 South Washington Street, Suite L300
Naperville, IL 60540
630-357-9464, 630-357-2037 (TDD)
Naperville_area_transcribing@altavista.com
Disability Served: vision

Philip H. Cohen Institute for the Visually Handicapped
5200 South Hyde Park Boulevard
Chicago, IL 60615
312-643-9857
Disability Served: vision

Recording for the Blind and Dyslexic
Recording Studio-Chicago
18 South Michigan Avenue, Suite 806
Chicago, IL 60603
312-236-8715
dsmith@rfbd.org
http://www.rfbd.org
Disability Served: dyslexic, vision

Recording for the Blind and Dyslexic
Recording Studio-Naperville
1266 East Chicago Avenue
Naperville, IL 60540
630-420-0722
nleone@rfbd.org
http://www.rfbd.org
Disability Served: dyslexic, vision

Recording for the Blind and Dyslexic
Recording Studio-Orland Park
9612C West 143rd Street
Orland Park, IL 60462
708-349-9356
selhenicky@rfbd.org
http://www.rfbd.org
Disability Served: dyslexic, vision

River Bend Library System
Talking Book Center of Northwest Illinois
PO Box 125
Coal Valley, IL 61240

309-799-3137, 800-747-3137
tbc@rbls.lib.il.us
http://www.rbls.lib.il.us/rbls/tbc.htm
Disability Served: physically disabled, vision

Shawnee Library System
Southern Illinois Talking Book Center
607 South Greenbriar Road
Carterville, IL 62918
618-985-8375, 800-455-2665, 618-985-8375 (TDD)
dbrawley@shawls.lib.il.us
http://www.shawls.lib.il.us/talkingbooks
Disability Served: physically disabled, vision

Voices of Vision
Talking Book Center
127 South First Street
Geneva, IL 60134
630-208-0398, 800-227-0625
kodean@dupagels.lib.il.us
http://www.dupagels.lib.il.us/pages/voices.html
Disability Served: physically disabled, vision

INDIANA
Bartholomew County Public Library
Columbus Subregional for Talking Books
536 Fifth Street
Columbus, IN 47201
812-379-1277
talkingbooks@barth.lib.in.us
http://www.barth.lib.in.us/TBColSub.html
Disability Served: physically disabled, vision

Elkhart Public Library
Blind and Physically Handicapped Services
300 South Second Street
Elkhart, IN 46516
574-294-2619
pciancio@elkhart.lib.in.us
http://www.elkhart.lib.in.us/cgi-bin/index5.pl?&file
   =bph.html
Disability Served: physically disabled, vision

Evansville-Vanderburgh County Public Library
Talking Book Service
200 Southeast Martin Luther King Jr. Boulevard
Evansville, IN 44713
812-428-8235
tbs@evpl.org
http://www.evpl.org/services/tbs
Disability Served: physically disabled, vision

Indiana State Library
Indiana Talking Book and Braille Library
140 North Senate Street
Indianapolis, IN 46204
317-232-3684, 800-622-4970, 317-232-7763 (TDD)
lbph@statelib.lib.in.us
http://www.statelib.lib.in.us/www//isl/lbph/lbphmenu.
   html
Disability Served: physically disabled, vision

Lake County Public Library
Northwest Indiana Subregional Library for the Blind
   and Physically Handicapped
1919 West 81st Street
Merrillville, IN 46410
219-769-3541, 219-769-3541 (TDD)
tbooks@lakeco.lib.in.us
Disability Served: physically disabled, vision

League for the Blind and Disabled
5821 South Anthony Boulevard
Ft Wayne, IN 46807
800-889-3443
http://www.the-league.org
Disability Served: various

IOWA
Anamosa Braille Center
406 North High Street
Anamosa, IA 52205
319-462-3507, ext. 235
Disability Served: vision

Iowa Department for the Blind
Iowa Library for the Blind and Physically Handicapped
524 Fourth Street
Des Moines, IA 50309
515-281-1333, 800-362-2587
Library@blind.state.ia.us
http://www.blind.state.ia.us/library
Disability Served: physically disabled, vision

KANSAS
American Red Cross Braille Service
Midway-Kansas Chapter
1900 East Douglas
Wichita, KS 67214
316-219-4000
http://midwaykansas.redcross.org
Disability Served: vision

Braille Association of Kansas Inc.
PO Box 17032
Wichita, KS 67217
316-265-6504
Disability Served: vision

Central Kansas Library System
Talking Book Service
1409 Williams
Great Bend, KS 67530
316-792-2393, 800-362-2642
jmasden@ckls.org
http://www.ckls.org/bph/bph.html
Disability Served: physically disabled, vision

Kansas State Library-Talking Book Service
Emporia State University, Memorial Union
1200 Commercial, Box 4055
Emporia, KS 66801
316-343-7124, 800-362-0699
tonih@kslib.info
http://www.kslib.info/talking
Disability Served: physically disabled, vision

Manhattan Public Library, North Central Kansas Libraries System
Talking Book Service
629 Poyntz Avenue
Manhattan, KS 66502
785-776-4741, 800-432-2796
annp@manhattan.lib.ks.us
http://www.manhattan.lib.ks.us/bph.html
Disability Served: physically disabled, vision

Northwest Kansas Library System
Western Kansas Talking Books
2 Washington Square, PO Box 446
Norton, KS 67654
913-877-5148, 800-432-2858, 785-877-5148 (TDD)
tbook@ruraltel.net
http://skyways.lib.ks.us/kansas/nwkls/howard/bph.html
Disability Served: physically disabled, vision

South Central Kansas Library System
Talking Book Subregional
321A North Main Street
South Hutchinson, KS 67505
800-234-0529
jarmour@sckls.org
http://www.sckls.info/depts/talking/index.html
Disability Served: physically disabled, vision

Topeka and Shawnee County Public Library
Talking Books Library
1515 Southwest 10th Avenue
Topeka, KS 66604-1374
785-231-0574, 800-432-4400 (KS)
tbooks@mail.tscpl.org
http://www.tscpl.org
Disability Served: physically disabled, vision

Wichita Public Library
Talking Books Section
223 South Main
Wichita, KS 67202
316-262-0611, 800-362-2869, 316-262-3972 (TDD)
breha@wichita.lib.ks.us
Disability Served: physically disabled, vision

KENTUCKY

American Printing House for the Blind Inc.
1839 Frankfort Avenue, PO Box 6085
Louisville, KY 40206-0085
502-895-2405, 800-223-1839
info@aph.org
http://www.aph.org
Disability Served: vision

Kenton County Public Library
Northern Kentucky Talking Book Library
502 Scott Boulevard
Covington, KY 41011
859-962-4095, 866-491-7610
nktbl@kenton.lib.ky.us
http://www.kenton.lib.ky.us/information/talking.html
Disability Served: physically disabled, vision

Kentucky Department for Libraries and Archives
Talking Book Library
300 Coffee Tree Road, PO Box 818
Frankfort, KY 40602
502-564-8300, 800-372-2968
http://www.kdla.ky.gov/collectionsktbl.htm
Disability Served: physically disabled, vision

Kentucky School for the Blind
Kentucky Instructional Materials Resource Center
1867 Frankfort Avenue
Louisville, KY 40206
502-897-1583
http://www.ksb.k12.ky.us/kimrc.html
Disability Served: vision

Louisville Free Public Library
Louisville Talking Book Library
301 West York Street
Louisville, KY 40203
502-574-1625, 502-574-1621 (TDD)
linda.jarboe@lfpl.org
http://www.lfpl.org/tbl.htm
Disability Served: physically disabled, vision

Recording for the Blind and Dyslexic
Recording Studio-Louisville Unit
240 Haldeman Avenue
Louisville, KY 40206
502-895-9068
mbrown@rfbd.org
http://www.rfbd.org
Disability Served: dyslexic, vision

LOUISIANA

Lighthouse for the Blind in New Orleans
123 State Street
New Orleans, LA 70118
504-899-4501, 888-792-0163
clee@lhb.org
http://lhb.org
Disability Served: vision

State Library of Louisiana
Services for the Blind and Physically Handicapped
701 North Fourth Street
Baton Rouge, LA 70802
225-342-4943, 800-543-4702
sbph@state.lib.la.us
http://www.state.lib.la.us/VisImpaired/visimp_dyn_
    templ.cfm?doc_id=103
Disability Served: physically disabled, vision

MAINE

Maine State Library
Library Services for the Blind and Physically
    Handicapped
64 State House Station
Augusta, ME 04333
207-287-5650, 800-762-7106
melora.norman@maine.gov
http://www.maine.gov/msl/outreach
Disability Served: physically disabled, vision

MARYLAND

Blind Industries and Services of Maryland
3345 Washington Boulevard
Baltimore, MD 21227
410-737-2600, 888-322-4567
http://www.bism.com
Disability Served: vision

Epilepsy Foundation of America
National Epilepsy Library
4351 Garden City Drive
Landover, MD 20785
301-459-3700, 800-332-4050
nel@efa.org
http://www.epilepsyfoundation.org/programs/Library.
    cfm
Disability Served: epilepsy

**Maryland State Library for the Blind and
    Physically Handicapped**
415 Park Avenue
Baltimore, MD 21201
410-230-2424, 800-964-9209, 410-333-8679 (TDD)
recept@lbph.lib.md.us
http://www.lbph.lib.md.us
Disability Served: physically disabled, vision

Montgomery County Department of Libraries
Special Needs Library
99 Maryland Avenue
Rockville, MD 20850
240-777-0960, 301-897-2217 (TDD)
http://www.montgomerycountymd.gov/library
Disability Served: various

National Rehabilitation Information Center
4200 Forbes Boulevard, Suite 202
Lanham, MD 20706
301-459-5900, 800-346-2742, 301-459-5984 (TTY)
naricinfo@heitechservices.com
http://www.naric.com/naric
Disability Served: various

Social Security Library
Braille Services Team
6401 Security Boulevard, L1141 West Low Rise Building
Baltimore, MD 21235-7728
410-965-6414, 410-965-6407
http://www.ssa.gov/pubs/alt-pubs.html
Disability Served: vision

MASSACHUSETTS

National Braille Press
88 St. Stephen Street
Boston, MA 02115
617-266-6160, 888-965-8965
http://www.nbp.org
Disability Served: vision

Perkins School for the Blind
Massachusetts Braille and Talking Book Library
175 North Beacon Street
Watertown, MA 02172
617-972-7240, 800-852-3133
library@perkins.org
http://www.perkins.org
Disability Served: vision

Recording for the Blind and Dyslexic
Recording Studio-Boston Unit
58 Charles Street
Cambridge, MA 02141
617-577-1111
traimo@rfbd.org
http://www.rfbd.org
Disability Served: dyslexic, vision

Recording for the Blind and Dyslexic
Recording Studio-Lenox
55 Pittsfield-Lenox Road
Lenox, MA 01240
413-637-0889
berkshire@rfbd.org
http://www.rfbd.org
Disability Served: dyslexic, vision

Recording for the Blind and Dyslexic
Recording Studio-Williamstown
173 Water Street
Williamstown, MA 01267
413-458-3641
http://www.rfbd.org
Disability Served: dyslexic, vision

Worcester Public Library
Talking Book Library
3 Salem Square
Worcester, MA 01603-2362
508-799-1730, 800-762-0085, 508-799-1731 (TDD)
jizatt@cwmars.org
http://www.worcpublib.org/talkingbook
Disability Served: physically disabled, vision

MICHIGAN

Association for the Blind and Visually Impaired
456 Cherry, SE
Grand Rapids, MI 49503
616-458-1187, 800-466-8084
blindser@abvimichigan.org
http://www.abvimichigan.org
Disability Served: vision

Detroit Public Library
Library for the Blind and Physically Handicapped
3666 Grand River Avenue
Detroit, MI 48226
313-833-5494, 313-833-5492 (TDD)
dmiddle@detroit.lib.mi.us
http://www.detroitpubliclibrary.org/lbph/LBPH_index.
   htm
Disability Served: physically disabled, vision

**Grand Traverse Area Library for the Blind and
   Physically Handicapped**
610 Woodmere
Traverse City, MI 49686
231-932-8558, 877-931-8558, 231-932-8507 (TDD)
lbph@tadl.tcnet.org
http://tadl.tcnet.org/index/lbph.htm
Disability Served: physically disabled, vision

**Kent District Library for the Blind and Physically
   Handicapped**
Wyoming Branch Library
3350 Michael Avenue, SW
Wyoming, MI 49509
616-647-3980
lbphstaff@kdl.org
http://www.kdl.org/about_kdl/lbph
Disability Served: physically disabled, vision

Library of Michigan
Service for the Blind and Physically Handicapped
702 West Kalamazoo
Lansing, MI 48909
517-373-5614, 800-992-9012, 517-373-1592 (TDD)
sbph@michigan.gov
http://www.michigan.gov/sbph
Disability Served: physically disabled, vision

**Macomb Library for the Blind and Physically
   Handicapped**
16480 Hall Road
Clinton Township, MI 48038-1132

586-286-1580
macbld@libcoop.net
http://www.libcoop.net/macspe
Disability Served: physically disabled, vision

Michigan Association of Transcribers for the Visually Impaired

HCR4 Box 2746
Lewiston, MI 49756
517-786-5311
Disability Served: vision

Michigan Braille Transcribing Fund

3500 North Elm Road
Jackson, MI 49201
517-780-5096
Disability Served: vision

Mideastern Michigan Talking Book Center

Library for the Blind and Physically Handicapped
G-4195 West Pasadena Avenue
Flint, MI 48504
810-732-1120, 877-732-1120
dking@the gdl.org
http://www.thegdl.org/talkingbooks.htm
Disability Served: physically disabled, vision

Muskegon County Library

Subregional Library for the Blind and Physically
    Handicapped
97 East Apple Avenue
Muskegon, MI 49442
231-724-6257, 877-569-4801, 231-722-4103 (TDD)
mclsm@llcoop.org
http://www.muskcolib.org/lbph.htm
Disability Served: physically disabled, vision

Nardin Park Braille Transcribers

18305 Netaunee
Redford, MI 48240
313-534-3929
Disability Served: vision

Northland Library Cooperative

Northland Library for the Blind and Physically
    Handicapped
316 East Chisholm
Alpena, MI 49707
517-356-1622, 800-446-1580
nlclbph@northland.lib.mi.us

http://nlc.lib.mi.us/library
Disability Served: physically disabled, vision

Oakland County Library for the Visually and Physically Impaired

1200 North Telegraph Road
Pontiac, MI 48341-0482
248-858-5050, 800-774-4542, 248-452-2247 (TDD)
lvpi@co.oakland.mi.us
http://www.co.oakland.mi.us/lvpi
Disability Served: physically disabled, vision

Onlooker Transcribing Group

421 South Fancher
Mt Pleasant, MI 48858
517-772-1745
Disability Served: vision

Readings for the Blind Inc.

29350 Southfield Road, Suite 130
Southfield, MI 48076-2294
248-557-7776, 888-766-1166
rftb@sbcglobal.net
http://readingsfortheblind.org
Disability Served: vision

Recording for the Blind and Dyslexic

Recording Studio-Troy Unit
5600 Rochester Road
Troy, MI 48095
810-879-0101
creeb@rfbd.org
http://www.rfbd.org
Disability Served: dyslexic, vision

Seedlings Braille Books for Children

PO Box 51924
Livonia, MI 48151-5924
734-427-8552, 800-777-8552
info@seedlings.org
http://www.seedlings.org
Disability Served: vision

St. Clair County Library

Special Technologies Alternative Resource
210 McMorran Boulevard
Port Huron, MI 48060
810-982-3600, 800-272-8570
star@sccl.lib.mi.us
http://www.sccl.lib.mi.us/star.html
Disability Served: various

Tri-County Braille Volunteers
17889 Bonstelle
Southfield, MI 48075
248-559-7112
Disability Served: *vision*

Upper Peninsula Library for the Blind and People with Disabilities
1615 Presque Isle Avenue
Marquette, MI 49855
906-228-7697, 800-562-8985, 906-228-7697 (TDD)
uplbph@uproc.lib.mi.us
http://www.uproc.lib.mi.us/uplbph
Disability Served: *physically disabled, vision*

Washtenaw County Library For The Blind and Physically Handicapped
4135 Washtenaw Avenue, PO Box 8645
Ann Arbor, MI 48107
734-973-4350, 888-460-0680
lbpd@eWashtenaw.org
http://www.ewashtenaw.org/government/departments/
    library/li_liblbpd.html?qlink
Disability Served: *physically disabled, vision*

Wayne County Regional Library for the Blind and Physically Handicapped
30555 Michigan Avenue
Westland, MI 48186-5310
734-727-7300, 888-968-2737, 734-727-7330 (TTY)
http://wayneregional.lib.mi.us
Disability Served: *physically disabled, vision*

MINNESOTA
Martha Arney Library for the Blind
3911 Hayes Street, NE
Minneapolis, MN 55421
612-788-0508
meamra@aol.com
http://www.careministries.org/malb.html
Disability Served: *vision*

Minnesota Department of Education
Minnesota Library for the Blind and Physically
    Handicapped
388 Southeast 6th Avenue
Faribault, MN 55021
507-332-3279, 800-722-0550
mn.lbph@state.mn.us

http://www.education.state.mn.us/html/intro_mlbph.
    htm
Disability Served: *physically disabled, vision*

Minnesota State Services for the Blind
2200 University Avenue West, #240
St. Paul, MN 55114-1840
612-642-0508, 800-652-9000
http://www.mnssb.org
Disability Served: *vision*

Volunteer Braille Services of Minnesota
Volunteer Braille and Large Print Services
1710 Douglas Drive
Golden Valley, MN 55422
763-544-2880
vbsmn@vbsmn.org
http://www.vbsmn.org
Disability Served: *vision*

MISSISSIPPI
Mississippi Library Commission
Blind and Physically Handicapped Library Services
1221 Ellis Avenue
Jackson, MS 39209
601-961-4111, 800-446-0892
lbph@mlc.lib.ms.us
http://www.mlc.lib.ms.us/bphls
Disability Served: *physically disabled, vision*

MISSOURI
Assemblies of God National Center for the Blind
Whitney Library for the Blind
1445 Boonville Avenue
Springfield, MO 65802
417-831-1964
Blind@ag.org
http://blind.ag.org/whitney.cfm
Disability Served: *vision*

Lutheran Library for the Blind
7550 Watson Road
St. Louis, MO 63119
888-215-2455
blind.mission@blindmission.org
http://www.blindmission.org
Disability Served: *vision*

Midwestern Braille Volunteers
325 North Kirkwood Road, Suite G-5
St. Louis, MO 63122
314-966-5828
mbvol@sbcglobal.net
http://www.mbvol.org
Disability Served: vision

Talking Tapes Library
16 Sunnen Drive, Suite 162
St. Louis, MO 63143
877-926-0500
Info@talkingtapes.org
http://www.talkingtapes.org
Disability Served: physically disabled, vision

**Wolfner Library for the Blind and Physically
    Handicapped**
PO Box 387
Jefferson City, MO 65102
573-751-8720, 800-392-2614, 800-347-1379 (TDD)
wolfner@sos.mo.gov
http://www.sos.mo.gov/wolfner
Disability Served: physically disabled, vision

MONTANA
Montana State Library
Montana Talking Books Library
1515 East Sixth Avenue, PO Box 201800
Helena, MT 59620
406-444-2064, 800-332-3400
cbriggs@mt.gov
http://msl.state.mt.us/tbl
Disability Served: physically disabled, vision

Montana Transcribers of Braille
1328 Bench
Billings, MT 59105
406-259-2320
Disability Served: vision

NEBRASKA
Christian Record Services Inc.
4444 South 52nd Street
Lincoln, NE 68516
402-488-0981
info@christianrecord.org
http://www.christianrecord.org
Disability Served: vision

Nebraska Library Commission
Talking Book and Braille Service, The Atrium
1200 N Street, Suite 120
Lincoln, NE 68508-2023
402-471-4038, 800-742-7691, 402-471-4038 (TDD)
doertli@nlc.state.ne.us
http://www.nlc.state.ne.us/tbbs/tbbs1.html
Disability Served: physically disabled, vision

Nebraska State Penitentiary
Prose and Cons Braille Unit
PO Box 2500
Lincoln, NE 68502
402-471-3161, ext. 3373
http://www.corrections.state.ne.us/institutions/nsp.
    html
Disability Served: vision

Omaha Volunteer Braille Services
770 North 93rd Street, #5C3
Omaha, NE 68114-2676
402-397-6755
Disability Served: vision

NEVADA
Consolidated Braille Transcribers
Northern Nevada Correctional Center
1721 East Snyder Avenue, PO Box 7000
Carson City, NV 89701
702-882-9203, ext. 220
http://www.doc.nv.gov/nncc
Disability Served: vision

Las Vegas-Clark County Library District
Homebound Services
833 Las Vegas Boulevard North
Las Vegas, NV 89109
702-507-3456
maglios@lvccld.org
http://www.lvccld.lib.nv.us/about/card_services/
    homebound.htm
Disability Served: various

Nevada State Library and Archives
Nevada Talking Book Services
100 North Stewart Street
Carson City, NV 89710
775-684-3354, 800-922-9334, 775-687-8338 (TDD)
keputnam@clan.lib.nv.us

http://dmla.clan.lib.nv.us/docs/nsla/tbooks
Disability Served: physically disabled, vision

Nevada State Library and Archives
Southern Nevada Talking Books Library
1425 South Green Valley Parkway, Suite 110
Henderson, NV 89052
702-733-1925
keputnam@clan.lib.nv.us
http://dmla.clan.lib.nv.us/docs/nsla/tbooks
Disability Served: physically disabled, vision

NEW HAMPSHIRE
New Hampshire State Library
Library Services to Persons with Disabilities-
   Talking Books Program
117 Pleasant Street
Concord, NH 03301
603-271-3429, 800-491-4200
jbarrett@library.state.nh.us
http://www.state.nh.us/nhsl/talkbks
Disability Served: physically disabled, vision

NEW JERSEY
American Red Cross Braille Services
Metropolitan New Jersey Chapter
209 Fairfield Road
Fairfield, NJ 07004-2206
973-797-3300
http://www.redcrossmetronj.org
Disability Served: vision

American Red Cross Braille Service
Montclair Chapter
63 Park Street
Montclair, NJ 07042
973-746-1800
http://montclair.redcross.org
Disability Served: vision

Fair Lawn Braille Unit
17-16 Split Rock Road
Fair Lawn, NJ 07410
201-796-1388
Disability Served: vision

New Jersey State Library
New Jersey Library for the Blind and Handicapped
PO Box 501

Trenton, NJ 08618-3226
609-530-3239, 800-792-8322, 800-882-5593 (TDD)
njlbh@njstatelib.org
http://www.njlbh.org
Disability Served: physically disabled, vision

Ocean County Volunteers for the Blind
415 Linden Avenue
Pine Beach, NJ 08741
732-240-9066
Disability Served: vision

Princeton Braillists
76 Leabrook Lane
Whiting, NJ 08759
732-350-3708
Disability Served: vision

Recording for the Blind and Dyslexic
Recording Studio-New Jersey Unit
69 Mapleton Road
Princeton, NJ 08540
609-750-1830
http://www.rfbd.org
Disability Served: dyslexic, vision

NEW MEXICO
New Mexico School for the Visually Handicapped
1900 North White Sands Boulevard
Alamogordo, NM 88310
800-437-3503
http://www.nmsvh.k12.nm.us
Disability Served: vision

New Mexico State Library
Library for the Blind and Physically Handicapped
1209 Camino Carlos Rey
Santa Fe, NM 87507
505-476-9700, 800-456-5515 (TDD)
lbph@stlib.state.nm.us
http://www.stlib.state.nm.us
Disability Served: physically disabled, vision

NEW YORK
American Foundation for the Blind
11 Penn Plaza, Suite 300
New York, NY 10001
212-502-7600
afbinfo@afb.net

http://www.afb.org
Disability Served: vision

Braille Group of Buffalo
4660 Sheridan Drive
Buffalo, NY 14221
716-633-8877
brlgrp@juno.com
Disability Served: vision

Central Association for the Blind and Visually Impaired
Mohawk Valley Braille Transcribers
507 Kent Street
Utica, NY 13501
315-797-2233
http://www.cabvi.org
Disability Served: physically disabled, vision

Helen Keller Services for the Blind
Helen Keller Braille Library
One Helen Keller Way
Hempstead, NY 11550
516-485-1234
http://www.helenkeller.org
Disability Served: vision

Jewish Braille Institute of America Inc.
110 East 30th Street
New York, NY 10016
212-889-2525, 800-433-1531
admin@jewishbraille.org
http://www.jewishbraille.org
Disability Served: vision

Jewish Guild for the Blind Cassette Library International
15 West 65th Street
New York, NY 10023
212-769-6200, 800-284-4422
info@jgb.org
http://www.jgb.org
Disability Served: vision

Nassau Library System
Long Island Talking Book Library
900 Jerusalem Avenue
Uniondale, NY 11553
866-833-1122
http://www.litbl.org
Disability Served: physically disabled, vision

National Association for Visually Handicapped
22 West 21st Street
New York, NY 10010
212-889-3141
staff@navh.org
http://www.navh.org
Disability Served: vision

National Braille Association Inc.
3 Townline Circle
Rochester, NY 14623-2513
585-427-8260
http://www.nationalbraille.org
Disability Served: vision

New York Public Library
Andrew Heiskell Braille and Talking Book Library
40 West 20th Street
New York, NY 10011
212-206-5400, 212-206-5458 (TDD)
ahlbph@nypl.org
http://www.nypl.org/branch/lb
Disability Served: physically disabled, vision

New York Public Library
Mid-Manhattan Library
455 Fifth Avenue
New York, NY 10016
212-340-0833
http://www.nypl.org
Disability Served: various

New York State Library
Talking Book and Braille Library
Cultural Education Center Basement, Empire State Plaza
Albany, NY 12230
518-474-5935, 800-342-3688
tbbl@mail.nysed.gov
http://www.nysl.nysed.gov/tbbl/index.html
Disability Served: physically disabled, vision

Onondaga Braillists Organization Inc.
PO Box 326
Syracuse, NY 13215-0326
Disability Served: vision

Recording for the Blind and Dyslexic
Recording Studio-New York Unit
545 Fifth Avenue, Suite 1005
New York, NY 10017
212-557-5720

dcrupain@rfbd.org
http://www.rfbd.org
Disability Served: dyslexic, vision

Suffolk Cooperative Library System, Outreach Services

Long Island Talking Book Library
627 North Sunrise Service Road, PO Box 9000
Bellport, NY 11713
631-286-1600, 866-833-1122, 631-286-4546 (TDD)
vlewis@suffolk.lib.ny.us
http://www.litbl.org
Disability Served: physically disabled, vision

United Spinal Association

75-20 Astoria Boulevard
Jackson Heights, NY 11370
718-803-3782
info@unitedspinal.org
http://www.unitedspinal.org
Disability Served: physically disabled

Wallace Memorial Library

Services for Persons with Disabilities
90 Lomb Memorial Drive
Rochester, NY 14623-5604
585-475-2562
http://wally.rit.edu/services/disabled.html
Disability Served: various

Xavier Society for the Blind

154 East 23rd Street
New York, NY 10010-4595
212-473-7800
Disability Served: vision

NORTH CAROLINA

Etowah Lions Braille Service

PO Box 332
Penrose, NC 28766
704-884-7523
Disability Served: vision

Metrolina Association for the Blind

704 Louise Avenue
Charlotte, NC 28204
704-372-3870, 800-926-5466
rscheffel@mab-jlbm.com

http://www.mabnc.org
Disability Served: vision

State Library of North Carolina, Department of Cultural Resources

Library for the Blind and Physically Handicapped
1811 Capital Boulevard
Raleigh, NC 27635-0001
919-733-4376, 888-388-2460, 919-733-1462 (TDD)
nclbph@ncmail.net
http://statelibrary.dcr.state.nc.us/lbph/lbph.htm
Disability Served: physically disabled, vision

NORTH DAKOTA

North Dakota State Library

Talking Book Services
604 East Boulevard Avenue
Bismarck, ND 58505-0800
701-328-2185, 800-843-9948, 800-892-8622 (TDD)
tbooks@state.nd.us
http://ndsl.lib.state.nd.us/DisabilityServices.html
Disability Served: physically disabled, vision

OHIO

Cleveland Public Library

Library for the Blind and Physically Handicapped
17121 Lake Shore Boulevard
Cleveland, OH 44114
216-623-2911, 800-362-1262
nls@loc.gov
http://www.cpl.org/Locations.asp?FormMode=LBPH
Disability Served: physically disabled, vision

Cleveland Sight Center

1909 East 101st Street
Cleveland, OH 44106
216-791-8118
doswald@clevelandsightcenter.org
http://www.clevelandsightcenter.org
Disability Served: vision

De-Lighted Helpers Braille Library

2013 West Third Street, Roosevelt Center, Room 313
Dayton, OH 45417
937-262-2800
Disability Served: vision

Public Library of Cincinnati and Hamilton County
Library for the Blind and Physically Handicapped
800 Vine Street
Cincinnati, OH 45202
513-369-6074, 800-582-0335, 513-369-3372 (TDD)
lfb@cincinnatilibrary.org
http://www.cincinnatilibrary.org/info/main/lb
Disability Served: physically disabled, vision

State Library of Ohio
Talking Book Program
274 East First Avenue
Columbus, OH 43201
614-644-6895, 800-686-1531
http://winslo.state.oh.us
Disability Served: physically disabled, vision

Toledo Society for the Blind
Sight Center
1819 Canton Street
Toledo, OH 43624
419-241-1183, 800-624-8378
mail@sightcentertoledo.org
http://www.sightcentertoledo.org
Disability Served: vision

Vision Center of Central Ohio Inc.
1393 North High Street
Columbus, OH 43201
614-294-5571
http://www.visioncenter.org
Disability Served: vision

OKLAHOMA

Oklahoma Library for the Blind and Physically Handicapped
300 Northeast 18th Street
Oklahoma City, OK 73105
405-521-3514, 800-523-0288, 405-521-4672 (TDD)
library@drs.state.ok.us
http://www.library.state.ok.us
Disability Served: physically disabled, vision

Tulsa City-County Library
Recording Volunteers of Tulsa Inc.
1520 North Hartford
Tulsa, OK 74106
918-596-7280

http://www.tulsalibrary.org
Disability Served: vision

OREGON

Independent Living Resources
2410 Southeast 11th Avenue
Portland, OR 97214
503-232 7411, 503-232 8408 (TDD)
ilrpdx@qwest.net
http://www.ilr.org
Disability Served: various

Oregon State Library
Talking Book and Braille Services
250 Winter Street NE
Salem, OR 97310
503-378-3849, 800-452-0292, 503-378-4334 (TDD)
tbabs@oslmac.osl.state.or.us
http://egov.oregon.gov/OSL/TBABS
Disability Served: physically disabled, vision

PENNSYLVANIA

Bower Hill Braillists Foundation
70 Moffett Street
Pittsburgh, PA 15243-1195
412-561-6470
Disability Served: vision

Carnegie Library of Pittsburgh
Library for the Blind and Physically Handicapped
4724 Baum Boulevard
Pittsburgh, PA 15213-1389
412-687-2440, 800-242-0586
info@carnegielibrary.org
http://www.carnegielibrary.org/lbph
Disability Served: physically disabled, vision

Free Library of Philadelphia
Library for the Blind and Physically Handicapped
919 Walnut Street
Philadelphia, PA 19107
215-925-3213, 800-222-1754
flpblind@library.phila.gov
http://www.library.phila.gov
Disability Served: physically disabled, vision

Lehigh Valley Braille Guild
2227 South First Avenue
Whitehall, PA 18052
610-433-6018, ext.25
Disability Served: vision

Montgomery County Association for the Blind
212 North Main Street, 3rd Floor
North Wales, PA 19454
215-661-9800
mcab@mcab.org
Disability Served: vision

PennTech Production Services
6340 Flank Drive, Suite 600
Harrisburg, PA 17112
717-541-4960, 800-360-7282
Disability Served: vision

Recording for the Blind and Dyslexic
Recording Studio-Philadelphia Unit
215 West Church Road Suite 111
King of Prussia, PA 19046
610-265-8090
Rjbutton@rfbd.org
http://www.rfbd.org
Disability Served: dyslexic, vision

Technical Assistance for Sensory Impaired Programs
150 South Progress Avenue
Harrisburg, PA 17109
717-657-5840, 800-222-7372
Disability Served: vision

RHODE ISLAND
**Rhode Island Regional Library for the Blind
and Physically Handicapped**
Talking Books Plus
One Capitol Hill
Providence, RI 02908
401-222-5800, 800-734-5555 (TDD)
tbplus@lori.state.ri.us
http://www.lori.ri.gov/tbp
Disability Served: physically disabled, vision

SOUTH CAROLINA
South Carolina State Library
Talking Book Services
1430 Senate Street

Columbia, SC 29201
803-734-4611, 800-922-7818
tbsbooks@leo.scsl.state.sc.us
http://www.state.sc.us/scsl/bph/index.html
Disability Served: physically disabled, vision

SOUTH DAKOTA
South Dakota State Library
South Dakota Braille and Talking Book Library
800 Governors Drive
Pierre, SD 57501
605-773-3131, 800-423-6665
dan.boyd@state.sd.us
http://www.state.sd.us/library
Disability Served: physically disabled, vision

TENNESSEE
Recording for the Blind and Dyslexic
Tennessee Unit
205 Badger Road
Oak Ridge, TN 37830
865-482-3496
http://www.rfbd.org
Disability Served: dyslexic, vision

Tennessee State Library and Archives
Tennessee Library for the Blind and Physically
    Handicapped
403 Seventh Avenue North
Nashville, TN 37243-0313
615-741-3915, 800-342-3308
tlbph.tsla@state.tn.us
http://www.tennessee.gov/tsla/lbph/index.htm
Disability Served: physically disabled, vision

TEXAS
Christian Education for the Blind
4200 South Freeway Drive, Suite 702
Fort Worth, TX 76115
817-920-0444
bcoicebm@juno.com
http://www.careministries.org/cefb.html
Disability Served: vision

Dallas Services for Visually Impaired Children
Braille Transcription Service
4242 Office Parkway
Dallas, TX 75204

214-828-9900
Disability Served: vision

Recording for the Blind and Dyslexic
Recording Studio-Texas Unit
1314 West 45th Street
Austin, TX 78756
512-323-9390, 877-246-7321
lil@rfbdtexas.org
http://www.rfbd.org
Disability Served: dyslexic, vision

Taping for the Blind Inc.
3935 Essex Lane
Houston, TX 77027
713-622-2767
http://www.hal-pc.org/~taping
Disability Served: vision

Texas State Library and Archives Commission
Talking Book Program
PO Box 12927
Austin, TX 78711
512-463-5458, 800-252-9605
tbp.services@tsl.state.tx.us
http://www.tsl.state.tx.us/tbp
Disability Served: physically disabled, vision

University of Texas-Austin
Library Services for Users with Disabilities
1 University Station
Austin, TX 78713-8916
512-495-4654
http://www.lib.utexas.edu/services/assistive
Disability Served: various

UTAH
Utah State Library Division
Program for the Blind and Disabled
250 North 1950 West, Suite A
Salt Lake City, UT 84116
801-715-6789, 800-662-5540, 801-715-6721 (TDD)
blind@utah.gov
http://blindlibrary.utah.gov
Disability served: various

VERMONT
Vermont Association for the Blind and Visually Impaired
37 Elmwood Avenue
Burlington, VT 05401

802-863-1358
http://www.vabvi.org
Disability Served: vision

Vermont Department of Libraries
Special Services Department
RD Number 4, Box 1870
Montpelier, VT 05602
802-828-3273, 800-479-1711
ssu@dol.state.vt.us
http://dol.state.vt.us
Disability Served: various

VIRGINIA
Alexandria Library-Beatley Central
Talking Book Service
5005 Duke Street
Alexandria, VA 22314
703-519-5911, 703-519-5918 (TDD)
emccaffrey@alexandria.lib.va.us
http://www.vdbvi.org/lrcsites.htm
Disability Served: physically disabled, vision

Arlington County Sub-Regional Library
Talking Book Service
1015 North Quincy Street
Arlington, VA 22201
703-228-6333, 703-228-6320 (TDD)
talkingbooks@arlingtonva.us
http://www.arlingtonva.us/Departments/Libraries/
    outreach/LibrariesOutreachSpecialNeeds.aspx
Disability Served: physically disabled, vision

Braille Circulating Library for the Blind
2700 Stuart Avenue
Richmond, VA 23220
804-359-3743
Disability Served: vision

Central Rappahannock Regional Library
Talking Books
1201 Caroline Street
Fredericksburg, VA 22401
540-372-1144, 540-371-3165 (TDD)
nbuck@crrl.org
http://www.librarypoint.org
Disability Served: physically disabled, vision

Fairfax County Public Library
Access Services
12000 Government Center Parkway, Suite 123

Fairfax, VA 22035
703-324-8380, 703-324-8365 (TDD)
access@fairfaxcounty.gov
http://www.fairfaxcounty.gov/library/branches/as/
  default.htm
Disability Served: various

**Hampton Subregional Library for the Blind
  and Physically Handicapped**
1 South Mallory Street
Hampton, VA 23663
757-727-1900, 757-727-1149 (TDD)
mwoolard@city.hampton.va.us
Disability Served: physically disabled, vision

Newport News Public Library System
Newport News Subregional Library for the Blind
  and Physically Handicapped
110 Main Street
Newport News, VA 23601
757-591-4858
nnlbph@ci.newport-news.va.us
http://www.newport-news.va.us/library/libsys/locat/
  mainst/outrech/libblind.htm
Disability Served: physically disabled, vision

Recording for the Blind and Dyslexic
Virginias and Carolinas Unit
1021 Millmont Street
Charlottesville, VA 22903
804-293-4797, 866-887-7323
http://www.rfbd.org
Disability Served: dyslexia, vision

Roanoke Public Library
Talking Book Services
2607 Salem Turnpike, NW
Roanoke, VA 24017
540-853-2648, 800-528-2342
branchmelrose@hotmail.com
http://www.roanokegov.com/library/talking.html
Disability Served: physically disabled, vision

Staunton Public Library
Talking Book Center
1 Churchville Avenue
Staunton, VA 24401
540-885-6215, 800-995-6215
rsonjo@ci.staunton.va.us

http://www.staunton.va.us/default.
  asp?pageID=48BD7E6B-787C-49EE-A7C1-
  8DD714653A32
Disability Served: physically disabled, vision

Virginia Autism Resource Center
PO Box 2500
Winchester, VA 22604
540-542-1723, ext. 6405
http://www.varc.org
Disability Served: autism

Virginia Beach Public Library
Special Services Library
936 Independence Boulevard
Virginia Beach, VA 23455
757-460-7575
awicher@vbgov.com
http://www.vbgov.com/dept/library/accessible_services
Disability Served: various

Virginia Department for the Blind and Vision Impaired
Virginia Library and Resource Center
395 Azalea Avenue
Richmond, VA 23227
804-371-3661, 800-552-7015, 804-371-3661 (TDD)
barbara.mccarthy@dbvi.virginia.gov
http://www.vdbvi.org/lrcservices.htm
Disability Served: vision

WASHINGTON

Northwest Braille Services
PO Box 234
Ferndale, WA 98248
360-714-1630
nwbsbeth@cnw.com
http://www.healthsupportcenter.org/nwbs.shtml
Disability Served: vision

Seattle Area Braillists Inc.
13746 Corliss Avenue North
Seattle, WA 98133
206-362-3764
Disability Served: vision

Seattle Public Library
Washington Talking Book Braille Library
2021 Ninth Avenue

Seattle, WA 98121
206-615-0400, 800-542-0866, 206-615-0418 (TTY)
wtbbl@wtbbl.org
http://www.wtbbl.org
Disability Served: physically disabled, vision

WEST VIRGINIA

Cabell County Public Library
Services for the Blind and Physically Handicapped
455 Ninth Street Plaza
Huntington, WV 25701
304-528-5700, 304-528-5694 (TDD)
Disability Served: physically disabled, vision

Huttonsville Correctional Center
West Virginia Braille Program
PO Box 1, Route 250 South
Huttonsville, WV 26273
304-335-2291, ext. 276
Disability Served: vision

Ohio County Public Library
Services for the Blind and Physically Handicapped,
52 16th Street
Wheeling, WV 26003-3696
304-232-0244
http://wheeling.weirton.lib.wv.us
Disability Served: physically disabled, vision

Parkersburg and Wood County Public Library
Services for the Blind and Physically Handicapped
3100 Emerson Avenue
Parkersburg, WV 26104-2414
304-420-4587, 800-642-8674
hickmanm@hp9k.park.lib.wv.us
http://parkersburg.lib.wv.us
Disability Served: physically disabled, vision

**West Virginia Library Commission-Special
  Libraries**
Blind and Physically Handicapped Services,
  Cultural Center
1900 Kanawha Boulevard East
Charleston, WV 25305
304-558-4061, 800-642-8674
calvertd@wvlc.lib.wv.us
http://librarycommission.lib.wv.us
Disability Served: physically disabled, vision

West Virginia School for the Blind Library
301 East Main Street
Romney, WV 26757
304-822-4894
csjohnso@access.k12.wv.us
http://wvsdb.state.k12.wv.us/WVSB.HTM
Disability Served: vision

WISCONSIN

Milwaukee Public Library
Volunteer Services for the Visually Handicapped Inc.
814 West Wells Street
Milwaukee, WI 53233-1436
414-286-3045, 800-722-0550
evalan@mpl.org
http://www.mpl.org
Disability Served: vision

Volunteer Braillists and Tapists Inc.
517 North Segoe Road, Suite 200
Madison, WI 53705-3172
608-233-0222
vbti@juno.com
http://www.vbti.org
Disability Served: vision

Wisconsin Evangelical Lutheran Synod
Mission for the Visually Handicapped
2929 North Mayfair Road
Milwaukee, WI 53222
414-256-3888
http://www.wels.net/cgi-bin/site.pl?
Disability Served: vision

**Wisconsin Regional Library for the Blind
  and Physically Handicapped**
813 West Wells Street
Milwaukee, WI 53233
414-286-3045, 800-242-8822, 414-286-3548 (TDD)
mvalan@mpl.org
http://regionallibrary.wi.gov/lbphinfo.html
Disability Served: physically disabled, vision

WYOMING

Wyoming State Library
2301 Capitol Avenue
Cheyenne, WY 82002-0060

307-777-6333
http://www.wsl.state.wy.us
Disability Served: various

GUAM

Guam Public Library for the Blind and Physically Handicapped
254 Martyr Street
Agana, GU 96910
671-475-4754
Disability Served: physically disabled, vision

PUERTO RICO

Puerto Rico Regional Library for the Blind and Physically Handicapped
520 Ponce de Leon Avenue
San Juan, PR 00901
787-723-2519, 800-981-8008
ienrique@tld.net
Disability Served: physically disabled, vision

VIRGIN ISLANDS

Virgin Islands Regional Library for the Visually and Physically Handicapped
3012 Golden Rock, Christiansted
St. Croix, VI 80977
809-772-2250
ac757@virgin.usci.net
Disability Served: physically disabled, vision

CANADA

Canada National Institute for the Blind Library for the Blind
1929 Bayview Avenue
Toronto, ON M4G 3E8
Canada
416-486-2500
stan.flamers@cnib.ca
http://www.cnib.ca/library
Disability Served: vision

ORGANIZATIONS AND ASSOCIATIONS

AMERICANS WITH DISABILITIES ACT ORGANIZATIONS

These organizations provide information on the Americans with Disabilities Act, including compliance assistance, explanation of regulations, referral services, and more.

American Institute of Architects
1735 New York Avenue, NW
Washington, DC 20006-5292
800-AIA-3837
infocentral@aia.org
http://www.aia.org
Disability Served: various
This professional organization for architects works with government organizations on issues relating to the Americans with Disabilities Act and the Architectural Barriers Act.

Americans with Disabilities Act Document Portal
U.S. Department of Education
National Institute on Disability and Rehabilitation Research
400 Maryland Avenue, SW
Washington, DC 20202-2572
800-949-4232
http://www.adaportal.org
Disability Served: various
This is an electronic repository of more than 7,400 documents relating to the Americans with Disabilities Act. The Web site has nine subsections: communications, general, employment, enforcement, facility access, interpretation letters, private business, state and local government, and transportation.

Americans with Disabilities Act Information Line
U.S. Department of Justice
PO Box 66738
Washington, DC 20035-6738
800-514-0301, 800-514-0383 (TTY)
http://www.usdoj.gov/crt/ada/adahom1.htm
Disability Served: various
The Department of Justice answers questions about the Americans with Disabilities Act (ADA) and provides free publications by mail and fax through the ADA Information Line.

Center for Universal Design
North Carolina State University
College of Design

Campus Box 8613
Raleigh, NC 27695-8613
800-647-6777
cud@ncsu.edu
http://www.design.ncsu.edu:8120/cud
Disability Served: various
This organization evaluates, develops, and promotes universal design.

Equal Employment Opportunity Commission (EEOC)
PO Box 7033
Lawrence, KS 66044
800-669-4000, 800-669-6820 (TTY)
info@ask.eeoc.gov
http://www.eeoc.gov
Disability Served: various
The EEOC investigates complaints regarding possible violations of the Americans with Disabilities Act by private employers, state and local governments, employment agencies, and labor unions.

Federal Communications Commission (FCC)
445 12th Street, SW
Washington, DC 20554
888-2255-5322, 888-835-5322 (TTY)
http://www.fcc.gov/cgb
Disability Served: various
The FCC addresses Americans with Disabilities Act regulations and issues in telecommunications.

Great Lakes Americans with Disabilities Act Accessible Information Technology Center
University of Illinois-Chicago
Department on Disability and Human Development
1640 West Roosevelt Road
Chicago, IL 60608
312-413-1407 (Voice/TTY)
gldbtac@uic.edu
http://www.adagreatlakes.org
Disability Served: various
This is one of 10 regional centers established by the National Institute on Disability and Rehabilitation Research that provides information regarding

the Americans with Disabilities Act and provides assistance to help businesses and organizations reach ADA compliance. This center provides assistance to people in Illinois, Indiana, Michigan, Minnesota, Ohio, and Wisconsin.

Great Plains Americans with Disabilities Act and Information Technology Center
Americans With Disabilities Act Project
University of Missouri-Columbia
100 Corporate Lake Drive
Columbia, MO 65203
573-882-3600 (Voice/TTY)
hamburgl@missouri.edu
http://www.adaproject.org
Disability Served: various
This is one of 10 regional centers established by the National Institute on Disability and Rehabilitation Research that provides information regarding the Americans with Disabilities Act and provides assistance to help businesses and organizations reach ADA compliance. This center provides assistance to people in Iowa, Kansas, Missouri, and Nebraska.

Independent Living Research Utilization Disability Law Resource Project
2323 South Shepherd Boulevard, Suite 1000
Houston, TX 77019
713-520-0232 (Voice/TTY)
dlrp@ilru.org
http://www.dlrp.org
Disability Served: various
This is one of 10 regional centers established by the National Institute on Disability and Rehabilitation Research that provides information regarding the Americans with Disabilities Act and provides assistance to help businesses and organizations reach ADA compliance. This center provides assistance to people in Arizona, Louisiana, New Mexico, Oklahoma, and Texas.

Institute for Building Technology and Safety
505 Huntmar Park Drive, Suite 250
Herndon, VA 20170
703-481-2000
info@ibts.org
http://www.ibts.org
Disability Served: various
This not-for-profit governmental organization assists government and private sector organizations in the following areas: building design review and technical assistance, building inspection, and independent verification and validation of building systems.

Internal Revenue Service
Washington, DC 20044
800-829-4933
http://www.irs.gov/formspubs/article/0,,id=96151,00.html
Disability Served: various
The IRS offers technical assistance on Americans with Disabilities Act tax code provisions.

Mid-Atlantic Region Americans with Disabilities Act and Information Technology Center
TransCen Inc.
451 Hungerford Drive, Suite 607
Rockville, MD 20850
301-217-0124 (Voice/TTY)
adainfo@transcen.org
http://www.adainfo.org
Disability Served: various
This is one of 10 regional centers established by the National Institute on Disability and Rehabilitation Research that provides information regarding the Americans with Disabilities Act and provides assistance to help businesses and organizations reach ADA compliance. This center provides assistance to people in Delaware, the District of Columbia, Maryland, Pennsylvania, Virginia, and West Virginia.

National Center on Accessibility
501 North Morton Street, Suite 109
Bloomington, IN 47404
812-856-4422, 812-856-4421 (TTY)
nca@indiana.edu
http://www.ncaonline.org
Disability Served: various
This organization promotes accessibility in the recreation, parks, and tourism industries.

National Conference of States on Building Codes and Standards
505 Huntmar Park Drive, Suite 210
Herndon, VA 20170
703-437-0100
http://www.ncsbcs.org
Disability Served: various
This organization advocates for Americans with Disabilities Act standards and policy changes.

National Institute of Building Sciences

1090 Vermont Avenue, NW, Suite 700
Washington, DC 20005-4905
202-289-7800
nibs@nibs.org
http://www.nibs.org
Disability Served: various
This organization works to "improve the building
regulatory environment; facilitate the introduction
of new and existing products and technology into
the building process; and disseminates nationally
recognized technical and regulatory information."

National Institute on Disability and Rehabilitation Research

U.S. Department of Education
400 Maryland Avenue, SW
Washington, DC 20202-2572
202-245-7640 (Voice/TTY)
http://www.ed.gov/about/offices/list/osers/nidrr/index.
html?src=mr
Disability Served: various
The NIDRR provides leadership and support for
programs of disability and rehabilitation research and
administers the Technology Related Assistance for
Individuals with Disabilities Act and the 10 Americans
with Disabilities Act technical assistance centers.

New England Americans with Disabilities Act and Accessible Information Technology Center

Adaptive Environments Center Inc.
374 Congress Street, Suite 301
Boston, MA 02210
617-695-0085 (Voice/TTY)
adainfo@newenglandada.org
http://adaptiveenvironments.org/neada/site/home
Disability Served: various
This is one of 10 regional centers established by the
National Institute on Disability and Rehabilitation
Research that provides information regarding
the Americans with Disabilities Act and provides
assistance to help businesses and organizations reach
ADA compliance. This center provides assistance to
people in Connecticut, Maine, Massachusetts, New
Hampshire, Rhode Island, and Vermont.

Northeast Americans with Disabilities Act and Information Technology Center

Cornell University
331 Ives

Ithaca, NY 14853-3901
800-949-4232, 607-255-6686 (TTY)
northeastada@cornell.edu
http://www.ilr.cornell.edu/extension/ped/northeastADA/
index.html
Disability Served: various
This is one of 10 regional centers established by the
National Institute on Disability and Rehabilitation
Research that provides information regarding
the Americans with Disabilities Act and provides
assistance to help businesses and organizations reach
ADA compliance. This center provides assistance to
people in New Jersey, New York, Puerto Rico, and the
Virgin Islands.

Northwest Americans with Disabilities Act and Information Technology Center

PO Box 574
Portland, OR 97207-0574
503-494-4001
nwada@ohsu.edu
http://www.nwada.org
Disability Served: various
This is one of 10 regional centers established by the
National Institute on Disability and Rehabilitation
Research that provides information regarding
the Americans with Disabilities Act and provides
assistance to help businesses and organizations
reach ADA compliance. This center provides
assistance to people in Alaska, Idaho, Oregon, and
Washington.

Pacific Disability and Business Technical Assistance Center ADA and Information Technology Center

555 12th Street, Suite 1030
Oakland, CA 94607-4046
510-285-5600 (Voice/TTY)
adatech@pdbtac.com
http://www.pacdbtac.org
Disability Served: various
This is one of 10 regional centers established by the
National Institute on Disability and Rehabilitation
Research that provides information regarding
the Americans with Disabilities Act and provides
assistance to help businesses and organizations
reach ADA compliance. This center provides
assistance to people in Arizona, California, Hawaii,
and Nevada.

Rocky Mountain Americans with Disabilities Act and Information Technology Center
Meeting the Challenge Inc.
3630 Sinton Road, Suite 103
Colorado Springs, CO 80907
719-444-0268 (Voice/TTY)
rmdbtac@mtc-inc.com
http://www.adainformation.org
Disability Served: various
This is one of 10 regional centers established by the National Institute on Disability and Rehabilitation Research that provides information regarding the Americans with Disabilities Act and provides assistance to help businesses and organizations reach ADA compliance. This center provides assistance to people in Colorado, Montana, North Dakota, South Dakota, Utah, and Wyoming.

Southeast Disability and Business Technical Assistance Center
Center for Assistive Technology and Environmental Access
490 Tenth Street
Atlanta, GA 30318
404-385-0636 (Voice/TTY)
sedbtacproject@coa.gatech.edu
http://www.sedbtac.org
Disability Served: various
This is one of 10 regional centers established by the National Institute on Disability and Rehabilitation Research that provides information regarding the Americans with Disabilities Act and provides assistance to help businesses and organizations reach ADA compliance. This center provides assistance to people in Alabama, Florida, Georgia, Kentucky, Mississippi, North Carolina, South Carolina, and Tennessee.

United States Access Board
1331 F Street, NW, Suite 1000
Washington, DC 20004-1111
202-272-0080, 800-872-2253, 202-272-0082 (TTY)
http://www.access-board.gov
Disability Served: various
The board provides information on Americans with Disabilities Act and the Architectural Barriers Act for designers, building owners, and government agencies.

United States Small Business Administration
Office of Advocacy
409 Third Street, SW
Washington, DC 20416
202-205-6533
advocacy@sba.gov
http://www.sba.gov/advo
Disability Served: various
This office provides information and assistance on Americans with Disabilities Act regulations that affect small businesses.

Usability.gov
U.S. Department of Health and Human Services
200 Independence Avenue, SW, Room 638 E
Washington, DC 20201
202-619-0257, 877-696-6775
http://www.usability.gov
Disability Served: various
This Web site provides comprehensive resources on designing accessible Web sites and user interfaces.

HOSPITALS AND MEDICAL ORGANIZATIONS

Hospitals and medical organizations serve persons with disabilities, injuries, chronic illnesses, and debilitating conditions. The following hospitals and medical organizations were named by US News & World Report *in 2005 as the best hospitals in their respective specialties. The specialties include cancer; digestive disorders; ear, nose, and throat; geriatrics; gynecology; heart and heart surgery; hormonal disorders; kidney disease; neurology and neurosurgery; ophthalmology; orthopedics; pediatrics; psychiatry; rehabilitation; respiratory disorders; rheumatology; and urology. The top 10 hospitals within each specialty are listed here in order from highest to lowest ranked. For detailed information on how these rankings were compiled, visit http://www.usnews.com/usnews/health/best-hospitals/tophosp.htm.*

CANCER

Memorial Sloan-Kettering Cancer Center
1275 York Avenue
New York, NY 10021
212-639-2000
http://www.mskcc.org
Disability Served: cancer patients and survivors

University of Texas, M. D. Anderson Cancer Center
1515 Holcombe Boulevard
Houston, TX 77030
800-392-1611
http://www.mdanderson.org
Disability Served: cancer patients and survivors

Johns Hopkins Hospital
600 North Wolfe Street
Baltimore, MD 21287
410-502-4003
http://www.hopkinsmedicine.org
Disability Served: cancer patients and survivors

Dana-Farber Cancer Institute
44 Binney Street
Boston, MA 02115
866-408-3324
http://www.dana-farber.org
Disability Served: cancer patients and survivors

Mayo Clinic
200 First Street, SW
Rochester, MN 55902
507-284-2511
http://www.mayoclinic.org
Disability Served: cancer patients and survivors

Duke University Medical Center
Erwin Road
Durham, NC 27710
888-275-3853
http://www.dukehealth.org
Disability Served: cancer patients and survivors

University of Chicago Hospitals
5841 South Maryland Avenue
Chicago, IL 60637
773-702-1000, 888-UCH-0200
http://www.uchospitals.edu
Disability Served: cancer patients and survivors

University of California-Los Angeles Medical Center
10833 Le Conte Avenue
Los Angeles, CA 90095
800-UCLA-MD1
http://www.healthcare.ucla.edu
Disability Served: cancer patients and survivors

University of Michigan Medical Center
1500 East Medical Center Drive
Ann Arbor, MI 48109
734-936-4000
http://www.med.umich.edu
Disability Served: cancer patients and survivors

University of Pittsburgh Medical Center
200 Lothrop Street
Pittsburgh, PA 15213
800-533-8762
http://www.upmc.com
Disability Served: cancer patients and survivors

DIGESTIVE DISORDERS

Mayo Clinic
200 First Street, SW
Rochester, MN 55902
507-284-2511
http://www.mayoclinic.org
Disability Served: physically disabled

Cleveland Clinic
9500 Euclid Avenue
Cleveland, OH 44195
800-223-2273
http://www.clevelandclinic.org
Disability Served: physically disabled

Johns Hopkins Hospital
600 North Wolfe Street
Baltimore, MD 21287
410-502-4003
http://www.hopkinsmedicine.org
Disability Served: physically disabled

Massachusetts General Hospital
55 Fruit Street
Boston, MA 02114
617-726-2000
http://www.mgh.harvard.edu
Disability Served: physically disabled

University of California-Los Angeles Medical Center
10833 Le Conte Avenue
Los Angeles, CA 90095
800-UCLA-MD1
http://www.healthcare.ucla.edu
Disability Served: physically disabled

University of Chicago Hospitals
5841 South Maryland Avenue
Chicago, IL 60637
888-UCH-0200
http://www.uchospitals.edu
Disability Served: physically disabled

Mount Sinai Medical Center
One Gustave L. Levy Place
New York, NY 10029
212-241-6500
http://www.mountsinai.org/msh/msh-home.jsp
Disability Served: physically disabled

Duke University Medical Center
Erwin Road
Durham, NC 27710
888-275-3853
http://www.dukehealth.org
Disability Served: physically disabled

University of California, San Francisco Medical Center
505 Parnassus Avenue
San Francisco, CA 94143
888-689-UCSF
http://www.ucsfhealth.org
Disability Served: physically disabled

Brigham and Women's Hospital
75 Francis Street
Boston, MA 02115
617-732-5500
http://www.brighamandwomens.org
Disability Served: physically disabled

EAR, NOSE, AND THROAT

Johns Hopkins Hospital
600 North Wolfe Street
Baltimore, MD 21287
410-502-4003
http://www.hopkinsmedicine.org
Disability Served: physically disabled

Massachusetts Eye and Ear Infirmary
243 Charles Street
Boston, MA 02114
617-523-7900
http://www.meei.harvard.edu
Disability Served: physically disabled

University of Iowa Hospitals and Clinics
200 Hawkins Drive
Iowa City, IA 52242
800-777-8442
http://www.uihealthcare.com
Disability Served: physically disabled

University of Michigan Medical Center
1500 East Medical Center Drive
Ann Arbor, MI 48109
734-936-4000
http://www.med.umich.edu
Disability Served: physically disabled

Mayo Clinic
200 First Street, SW
Rochester, MN 55902
507-284-2511
http://www.mayoclinic.org
Disability Served: physically disabled

University of Pittsburgh Medical Center
200 Lothrop Street
Pittsburgh, PA 15213
800-533-8762
http://www.upmc.com
Disability Served: physically disabled

Cleveland Clinic
9500 Euclid Avenue
Cleveland, OH 44195
800-223-2273
http://www.clevelandclinic.org
Disability Served: physically disabled

Barnes-Jewish Hospital/Washington University
1 Barnes-Jewish Hospital Plaza
Saint Louis, MO 63110
314-747-3000
http://www.barnesjewish.org
Disability Served: physically disabled

University of California-Los Angeles Medical Center
10833 Le Conte Avenue
Los Angeles, CA 90095
800-UCLA-MD1
http://www.healthcare.ucla.edu
Disability Served: physically disabled

University of Washington Medical Center
1959 Northeast Pacific Street, Box 356151
Seattle, WA 98195
800-852-8546
http://www.uwmedicine.org
Disability Served: physically disabled

GERIATRICS
University of California-Los Angeles Medical Center
10833 Le Conte Avenue
Los Angeles, CA 90095
800-UCLA-MD1
http://www.healthcare.ucla.edu
Disability Served: elderly

Johns Hopkins Hospital
600 North Wolfe Street
Baltimore, MD 21287
410-502-4003
http://www.hopkinsmedicine.org
Disability Served: elderly

Mount Sinai Medical Center
One Gustave L. Levy Place
New York, NY 10029
212-241-6500
http://www.mountsinai.org/msh/msh-home.jsp
Disability Served: elderly

Duke University Medical Center
Erwin Road
Durham, NC 27710
888-275-3853
http://www.dukehealth.org
Disability Served: elderly

Massachusetts General Hospital
55 Fruit Street
Boston, MA 02114
617-726-2000
http://www.mgh.harvard.edu
Disability Served: elderly

Yale-New Haven Hospital
20 York Street
New Haven, CT 06510
203-688-4242
http://www.ynhh.org
Disability Served: elderly

Mayo Clinic
200 First Street, SW
Rochester, MN 55902
507-284-2511
http://www.mayoclinic.org
Disability Served: elderly

St. Louis University Hospital
3635 Vista At Grand Boulevard
Saint Louis, MO 63110
314-577-8000
http://www.sluhospital.com/CWSContent/
    sluhospital
Disability Served: elderly

University of Michigan Medical Center
1500 East Medical Center Drive
Ann Arbor, MI 48109
734-936-4000
http://www.med.umich.edu
Disability Served: elderly

University of Washington Medical Center
1959 Northeast Pacific Street, Box 356151
Seattle, WA 98195
800-852-8546
http://www.uwmedicine.org
Disability Served: elderly

GYNECOLOGY
Johns Hopkins Hospital
600 North Wolfe Street
Baltimore, MD 21287
410-502-4003
http://www.hopkinsmedicine.org
Disability Served: physically disabled

Mayo Clinic
200 First Street, SW
Rochester, MN 55902
507-284-2511
http://www.mayoclinic.org
Disability Served: physically disabled

Brigham and Women's Hospital
75 Francis Street
Boston, MA 02115
617-732-5500
http://www.brighamandwomens.org
Disability Served: physically disabled

Massachusetts General Hospital
55 Fruit Street
Boston, MA 02114
617-726-2000
http://www.mgh.harvard.edu
Disability Served: physically disabled

University of Texas, M. D. Anderson Cancer Center
1515 Holcombe Boulevard
Houston, TX 77030
800-392-1611
http://www.mdanderson.org
Disability Served: physically disabled

Duke University Medical Center
Erwin Road
Durham, NC 27710
888-275-3853
http://www.dukehealth.org
Disability Served: physically disabled

University of California-Los Angeles Medical Center
10833 Le Conte Avenue
Los Angeles, CA 90095
800-UCLA-MD1
http://www.healthcare.ucla.edu
Disability Served: physically disabled

**New York-Presbyterian University Hospital
    of Columbia and Cornell**
525 East 68th Street
New York, NY 10021
877-NYP-WELL
http://www.nyp.org
Disability Served: physically disabled

Cleveland Clinic
9500 Euclid Avenue
Cleveland, OH 44195
800-223-2273
http://www.clevelandclinic.org
Disability Served: physically disabled

Memorial Sloan-Kettering Cancer Center
1275 York Avenue
New York, NY 10021
212-639-2000
http://www.mskcc.org
Disability Served: physically disabled

HEART AND HEART SURGERY
Cleveland Clinic
9500 Euclid Avenue
Cleveland, OH 44195
800-223-2273
http://www.clevelandclinic.org
Disability Served: physically disabled

Mayo Clinic
200 First Street, SW
Rochester, MN 55902
507-284-2511
http://www.mayoclinic.org
Disability Served: physically disabled

Johns Hopkins Hospital
600 North Wolfe Street
Baltimore, MD 21287
410-502-4003
http://www.hopkinsmedicine.org
Disability Served: physically disabled

Duke University Medical Center
Erwin Road
Durham, NC 27710
888-275-3853
http://www.dukehealth.org
Disability Served: physically disabled

Massachusetts General Hospital
55 Fruit Street
Boston, MA 02114
617-726-2000
http://www.mgh.harvard.edu
Disability Served: physically disabled

Brigham and Women's Hospital
75 Francis Street
Boston, MA 02115
617-732-5500
http://www.brighamandwomens.org
Disability Served: physically disabled

**New York-Presbyterian University Hospital
of Columbia and Cornell**
525 East 68th Street
New York, NY 10021
877-NYP-WELL
http://www.nyp.org
Disability Served: physically disabled

**Texas Heart Institute at St. Luke's Episcopal
Hospital**
6720 Bertner Avenue
Houston, TX 77030
800-292-2221
http://www.texasheartinstitute.org
Disability Served: physically disabled

Barnes-Jewish Hospital/Washington University
1 Barnes-Jewish Hospital Plaza
Saint Louis, MO 63110
314-747-3000
http://www.barnesjewish.org
Disability Served: physically disabled

University of Alabama Hospital at Birmingham
619 South 19th Street
Birmingham, AL 35233
205-934-4011
http://www.health.uab.edu
Disability Served: physically disabled

HORMONAL DISORDERS
Mayo Clinic
200 First Street, SW
Rochester, MN 55902
507-284-2511
http://www.mayoclinic.org
Disability Served: physically disabled

Massachusetts General Hospital
55 Fruit Street
Boston, MA 02114
617-726-2000
http://www.mgh.harvard.edu
Disability Served: physically disabled

Johns Hopkins Hospital
600 North Wolfe Street
Baltimore, MD 21287
410-502-4003
http://www.hopkinsmedicine.org
Disability Served: physically disabled

University of California, San Francisco Medical Center
505 Parnassus Avenue
San Francisco, CA 94143
888-689-UCSF
http://www.ucsfhealth.org
Disability Served: physically disabled

Barnes-Jewish Hospital/Washington University
1 Barnes-Jewish Hospital Plaza
Saint Louis, MO 63110
314-747-3000
http://www.barnesjewish.org
Disability Served: physically disabled

University of Virginia Medical Center
1215 Lee Street
Charlottesville, VA 22908
800-251-3627
http://www.healthsystem.virginia.edu/home.html
Disability Served: physically disabled

**New York-Presbyterian University Hospital
    of Columbia and Cornell**
525 East 68th Street
New York, NY 10021
877-NYP-WELL
http://www.nyp.org
Disability Served: physically disabled

Cleveland Clinic
9500 Euclid Avenue
Cleveland, OH 44195
800-223-2273
http://www.clevelandclinic.org
Disability Served: physically disabled

Brigham and Women's Hospital
75 Francis Street
Boston, MA 02115
617-732-5500
http://www.brighamandwomens.org
Disability Served: physically disabled

University of Washington Medical Center
1959 Northeast Pacific Street, Box 356151
Seattle, WA 98195
800-852-8546
http://www.uwmedicine.org
Disability Served: physically disabled

KIDNEY DISEASE
Johns Hopkins Hospital
600 North Wolfe Street
Baltimore, MD 21287
410-502-4003
http://www.hopkinsmedicine.org
Disability Served: kidney disease

Massachusetts General Hospital
55 Fruit Street
Boston, MA 02114
617-726-2000
http://www.mgh.harvard.edu
Disability Served: kidney disease

Mayo Clinic
200 First Street, SW
Rochester, MN 55902
507-284-2511
http://www.mayoclinic.org
Disability Served: kidney disease

**New York-Presbyterian University Hospital
    of Columbia and Cornell**
525 East 68th Street
New York, NY 10021
877-NYP-WELL
http://www.nyp.org
Disability Served: kidney disease

Brigham and Women's Hospital
75 Francis Street
Boston, MA 02115
617-732-5500
http://www.brighamandwomens.org
Disability Served: kidney disease

Cleveland Clinic
9500 Euclid Avenue
Cleveland, OH 44195
800-223-2273
http://www.clevelandclinic.org
Disability Served: kidney disease

Barnes-Jewish Hospital/Washington University
1 Barnes-Jewish Hospital Plaza
Saint Louis, MO 63110
314-747-3000
http://www.barnesjewish.org
Disability Served: kidney disease

University of California-Los Angeles Medical Center
10833 Le Conte Avenue
Los Angeles, CA 90095
800-UCLA-MD1
http://www.healthcare.ucla.edu
Disability Served: kidney disease

Duke University Medical Center
Erwin Road
Durham, NC 27710
888-275-3853
http://www.dukehealth.org
Disability Served: kidney disease

University of Colorado Hospital
4200 East Ninth Avenue
Denver, CO 80262

800-621-7621
http://www.uch.edu
Disability Served: kidney disease

NEUROLOGY AND NEUROSURGERY

Mayo Clinic
200 First Street, SW
Rochester, MN 55902
507-284-2511
http://www.mayoclinic.org
Disability Served: physically disabled

Johns Hopkins Hospital
600 North Wolfe Street
Baltimore, MD 21287
410-502-4003
http://www.hopkinsmedicine.org
Disability Served: physically disabled

**New York-Presbyterian University Hospital
   of Columbia and Cornell**
525 East 68th Street
New York, NY 10021
877-NYP-WELL
http://www.nyp.org
Disability Served: physically disabled

Massachusetts General Hospital
55 Fruit Street
Boston, MA 02114
617-726-2000
http://www.mgh.harvard.edu
Disability Served: physically disabled

**University of California, San Francisco
   Medical Center**
505 Parnassus Avenue
San Francisco, CA 94143
888-689-UCSF
http://www.ucsfhealth.org
Disability Served: physically disabled

Cleveland Clinic
9500 Euclid Avenue
Cleveland, OH 44195
800-223-2273
http://www.clevelandclinic.org
Disability Served: physically disabled

Saint Joseph's Hospital and Medical Center
350 West Thomas Road
Phoenix, AZ 85013
602-406-3000
http://www.ichosestjoes.com
Disability Served: physically disabled

Barnes-Jewish Hospital/Washington University
1 Barnes-Jewish Hospital Plaza
Saint Louis, MO 63110
314-747-3000
http://www.barnesjewish.org
Disability Served: physically disabled

**University of California-Los Angeles Medical
   Center**
10833 Le Conte Avenue
Los Angeles, CA 90095
800-UCLA-MD1
http://www.healthcare.ucla.edu
Disability Served: physically disabled

Methodist Hospital
6565 Fannin Street
Houston, TX 77030
713-790-3333
http://www.methodisthealth.com
Disability Served: physically disabled

OPHTHALMOLOGY

Bascom Palmer Eye Institute
900 Northwest 17th Street
Miami, FL 33136
800-329-7000
http://www.bascompalmer.org/site/default.asp
Disability Served: vision

Johns Hopkins Hospital
600 North Wolfe Street
Baltimore, MD 21287
410-502-4003
http://www.hopkinsmedicine.org
Disability Served: vision

Wills Eye Hospital
840 Walnut Street
Philadelphia, PA 19107
215-928-3000

http://www.atwills.com
Disability Served: vision

Massachusetts Eye and Ear Infirmary
243 Charles Street
Boston, MA 02114
617-523-7900
http://www.meei.harvard.edu
Disability Served: vision

University of California-Los Angeles Medical Center
10833 Le Conte Avenue
Los Angeles, CA 90095
800-UCLA-MD1
http://www.healthcare.ucla.edu
Disability Served: vision

University of Iowa Hospitals and Clinics
200 Hawkins Drive
Iowa City, IA 52242
800-777-8442
http://www.uihealthcare.com
Disability Served: vision

Doheny Eye Institute, University of Southern California University Hospital
1500 San Pablo Street
Los Angeles, CA 90033
323-442-8500
http://www.uscuh.com/CWSContent/uscuh
Disability Served: vision

Duke University Medical Center
Erwin Road
Durham, NC 27710
888-275-3853
http://www.dukehealth.org
Disability Served: vision

New York-Presbyterian University Hospital of Columbia and Cornell
525 East 68th Street
New York, NY 10021
877-NYP-WELL
http://www.nyp.org
Disability Served: vision

University of California, San Francisco Medical Center
505 Parnassus Avenue
San Francisco, CA 94143
888-689-UCSF

http://www.ucsfhealth.org
Disability Served: vision

ORTHOPEDICS
Mayo Clinic
200 First Street, SW
Rochester, MN 55902
507-284-2511
http://www.mayoclinic.org
Disability Served: physically disabled

Hospital for Special Surgery
535 East 70th Street
New York, NY 10021
212-606-1000
http://www.hss.edu
Disability Served: physically disabled

Massachusetts General Hospital
55 Fruit Street
Boston, MA 02114
617-726-2000
http://www.mgh.harvard.edu
Disability Served: physically disabled

Johns Hopkins Hospital
600 North Wolfe Street
Baltimore, MD 21287
410-502-4003
http://www.hopkinsmedicine.org
Disability Served: physically disabled

Cleveland Clinic
9500 Euclid Avenue
Cleveland, OH 44195
800-223-2273
http://www.clevelandclinic.org
Disability Served: physically disabled

University of California-Los Angeles Medical Center
10833 Le Conte Avenue
Los Angeles, CA 90095
800-UCLA-MD1
http://www.healthcare.ucla.edu
Disability Served: physically disabled

University of Iowa Hospitals and Clinics
200 Hawkins Drive
Iowa City, IA 52242
800-777-8442

http://www.uihealthcare.com
Disability Served: physically disabled

Rush University Medical Center
1653 West Congress Parkway
Chicago, IL 60612
312-942-5000
http://www.rush.edu
Disability Served: physically disabled

University of Washington Medical Center
1959 Northeast Pacific Street, Box 356151
Seattle, WA 98195
800-852-8546
http://www.uwmedicine.org
Disability Served: physically disabled

Duke University Medical Center
Erwin Road
Durham, NC 27710
888-275-3853
http://www.dukehealth.org
Disability Served: physically disabled

PEDIATRICS
Children's Hospital of Philadelphia
34th Street and Civic Center Boulevard
Philadelphia, PA 19104
215-590-1000
http://www.chop.edu/consumer/index.jsp
Disability Served: physically disabled

Children's Hospital Boston
300 Longwood Avenue
Boston, MA 02115
617-355-6000
http://www.childrenshospital.org
Disability Served: physically disabled

Johns Hopkins Hospital
600 North Wolfe Street
Baltimore, MD 21287
410-502-4003
http://www.hopkinsmedicine.org
Disability Served: physically disabled

Texas Children's Hospital
6621 Fannin Street
Houston, TX 77030
832-824-1000

http://www.texaschildrenshospital.org
Disability Served: physically disabled

**New York-Presbyterian University Hospital
   of Columbia and Cornell**
525 East 68th Street
New York, NY 10021
877-NYP-WELL
http://www.nyp.org
Disability Served: physically disabled

Rainbow Babies and Children's Hospital
11100 Euclid Avenue
Cleveland, OH 44106
888-844-8447
http://www.uhhs.com
Disability Served: physically disabled

The Children's Hospital
1056 East 19th Avenue
Denver, CO 80218
303-861-8888
http://www.thechildrenshospital.org
Disability Served: physically disabled

Children's Hospital Medical Center
3333 Burnet Avenue
Cincinnati, OH 45229
800-344-2462
http://www.cincinnatichildrens.org
Disability Served: physically disabled

Children's National Medical Center
111 Michigan Avenue, NW
Washington, DC 20010
888-884-2327
http://www.cnmc.org
Disability Served: physically disabled

Lucile Packard Children's Hospital
725 Welch Road
Palo Alto, CA 94304
650-497-8000
http://www.lpch.org
Disability Served: physically disabled

PSYCHIATRY
Massachusetts General Hospital
55 Fruit Street
Boston, MA 02114

617-726-2000
http://www.mgh.harvard.edu
Disability Served: mental health

**New York-Presbyterian University Hospital
    of Columbia and Cornell**
525 East 68th Street
New York, NY 10021
877-NYP-WELL
http://www.nyp.org
Disability Served: mental health

Johns Hopkins Hospital
600 North Wolfe Street
Baltimore, MD 21287
410-502-4003
http://www.hopkinsmedicine.org
Disability Served: mental health

McLean Hospital
115 Mill Street
Belmont, MA 02478
617-855-2000
http://www.mclean.harvard.edu
Disability Served: mental health

**University of California-Los Angeles
    Neuropsychiatric Hospital**
760 Westwood Plaza
Los Angeles, CA 90095
310-825-0511
http://www.npi.ucla.edu
Disability Served: mental health

Yale-New Haven Hospital
20 York Street
New Haven, CT 06510
203-688-4242
http://www.ynhh.org
Disability Served: mental health

Stanford Hospital and Clinics
300 Pasteur Drive
Palo Alto, CA 94304
800-756-9000
http://www.stanfordhospital.com/default
Disability Served: mental health

Duke University Medical Center
Erwin Road
Durham, NC 27710

888-275-3853
http://www.dukehealth.org
Disability Served: mental health

University of Pittsburgh Medical Center
200 Lothrop Street
Pittsburgh, PA 15213
800-533-8762
http://www.upmc.com
Disability Served: mental health

Menninger Clinic
2801 Gessner
Houston, TX 77080
800-351-9058
http://www.menningerclinic.com
Disability Served: mental health

REHABILITATION
Rehabilitation Institute of Chicago
345 East Superior Street
Chicago, IL 60611
312-238-1000
http://www.ric.org
Disability Served: physically disabled

Kessler Institute for Rehabilitation
1199 Pleasant Valley Way
West Orange, NJ 07052
888-KESSLER
http://www.kessler-rehab.com/new/intro.asp
Disability Served: physically disabled

University of Washington Medical Center
1959 Northeast Pacific Street, Box 356151
Seattle, WA 98195
800-852-8546
http://www.uwmedicine.org
Disability Served: physically disabled

Mayo Clinic
200 First Street, SW
Rochester, MN 55902
507-284-2511
http://www.mayoclinic.org
Disability Served: physically disabled

The Institute for Rehabilitation and Research
1333 Moursund
Houston, TX 77030

713-942-6159
http://www.tirr.org
Disability Served: physically disabled

Spaulding Rehabilitation Hospital
125 Nashua Street
Boston, MA 02114
617-573-7000
http://www.spauldingrehab.org
Disability Served: physically disabled

Craig Hospital
3425 South Clarkson Street
Englewood, CO 80113
303-789-8000
http://www.craighospital.org
Disability Served: physically disabled

Rusk Institute, New York University Medical Center
530 First Avenue
New York, NY 10016
212-263-7300
http://www.med.nyu.edu/index.html
Disability Served: physically disabled

Ohio State University Hospital
410 West 10th Avenue
Columbus, OH 43210
800-293-5123
http://www.medicalcenter.osu.edu
Disability Served: physically disabled

MossRehab
1200 West Tabor Road
Philadelphia, PA 19141
215-456-9900
http://www.einstein.edu/facilities/mossrehab/index.html
Disability Served: physically disabled

RESPIRATORY DISORDERS
National Jewish Medical and Research Center
1400 Jackson Street
Denver, CO 80206
303-388-4461
http://www.nationaljewish.org
Disability Served: physically disabled

Mayo Clinic
200 First Street, SW
Rochester, MN 55902

507-284-2511
http://www.mayoclinic.org
Disability Served: physically disabled

Johns Hopkins Hospital
600 North Wolfe Street
Baltimore, MD 21287
410-502-4003
http://www.hopkinsmedicine.org
Disability Served: physically disabled

Barnes-Jewish Hospital/Washington University
1 Barnes-Jewish Hospital Plaza
Saint Louis, MO 63110
314-747-3000
http://www.barnesjewish.org
Disability Served: physically disabled

Massachusetts General Hospital
55 Fruit Street
Boston, MA 02114
617-726-2000
http://www.mgh.harvard.edu
Disability Served: physically disabled

University of Colorado Hospital
4200 East Ninth Avenue
Denver, CO 80262
800-621-7621
http://www.uch.edu
Disability Served: physically disabled

University of California, San Diego Medical Center
200 West Arbor Drive
San Diego, CA 92103
800-926-8273
http://health.ucsd.edu/default.htm
Disability Served: physically disabled

University of California, San Francisco Medical Center
505 Parnassus Avenue
San Francisco, CA 94143
888-689-UCSF
http://www.ucsfhealth.org
Disability Served: physically disabled

Duke University Medical Center
Erwin Road
Durham, NC 27710
888-275-3853

http://www.dukehealth.org
Disability Served: physically disabled

Cleveland Clinic
9500 Euclid Avenue
Cleveland, OH 44195
800-223-2273
http://www.clevelandclinic.org
Disability Served: physically disabled

RHEUMATOLOGY

Johns Hopkins Hospital
600 North Wolfe Street
Baltimore, MD 21287
410-502-4003
http://www.hopkinsmedicine.org
Disability Served: immune deficiency disorders,
physically disabled

Mayo Clinic
200 First Street, SW
Rochester, MN 55902
507-284-2511
http://www.mayoclinic.org
Disability Served: immune deficiency disorders,
physically disabled

Hospital for Special Surgery
535 East 70th Street
New York, NY 10021
212-606-1000
http://www.hss.edu
Disability Served: immune deficiency disorders,
physically disabled

Cleveland Clinic
9500 Euclid Avenue
Cleveland, OH 44195
800-223-2273
http://www.clevelandclinic.org
Disability Served: immune deficiency disorders,
physically disabled

Brigham and Women's Hospital
75 Francis Street
Boston, MA 02115
617-732-5500
http://www.brighamandwomens.org

Disability Served: immune deficiency disorders,
physically disabled

University of Alabama Hospital at Birmingham
619 South 19th Street
Birmingham, AL 35233
205-934-4011
http://www.health.uab.edu
Disability Served: immune deficiency disorders,
physically disabled

University of California-Los Angeles Medical Center
10833 Le Conte Avenue
Los Angeles, CA 90095
800-UCLA-MD1
http://www.healthcare.ucla.edu
Disability Served: immune deficiency disorders,
physically disabled

Massachusetts General Hospital
55 Fruit Street
Boston, MA 02114
617-726-2000
http://www.mgh.harvard.edu
Disability Served: immune deficiency disorders,
physically disabled

Duke University Medical Center
Erwin Road
Durham, NC 27710
888-275-3853
http://www.dukehealth.org
Disability Served: immune deficiency disorders,
physically disabled

University of California, San Francisco Medical Center
505 Parnassus Avenue
San Francisco, CA 94143
888-689-UCSF
http://www.ucsfhealth.org
Disability Served: immune deficiency disorders,
physically disabled

UROLOGY

Johns Hopkins Hospital
600 North Wolfe Street
Baltimore, MD 21287
410-502-4003

http://www.hopkinsmedicine.org
Disability Served: physically disabled

Cleveland Clinic
9500 Euclid Avenue
Cleveland, OH 44195
800-223-2273
http://www.clevelandclinic.org
Disability Served: physically disabled

Mayo Clinic
200 First Street, SW
Rochester, MN 55902
507-284-2511
http://www.mayoclinic.org
Disability Served: physically disabled

University of California-Los Angeles Medical Center
10833 Le Conte Avenue
Los Angeles, CA 90095
800-UCLA-MD1
http://www.healthcare.ucla.edu
Disability Served: physically disabled

**New York-Presbyterian University Hospital
of Columbia and Cornell**
525 East 68th Street
New York, NY 10021
877-NYP-WELL
http://www.nyp.org
Disability Served: physically disabled

Barnes-Jewish Hospital/Washington University
1 Barnes-Jewish Hospital Plaza
Saint Louis, MO 63110
314-747-3000
http://www.barnesjewish.org
Disability Served: physically disabled

Massachusetts General Hospital
55 Fruit Street
Boston, MA 02114
617-726-2000
http://www.mgh.harvard.edu
Disability Served: physically disabled

Memorial Sloan-Kettering Cancer Center
1275 York Avenue
New York, NY 10021
212-639-2000
http://www.mskcc.org
Disability Served: physically disabled

Duke University Medical Center
Erwin Road
Durham, NC 27710
888-275-3853
http://www.dukehealth.org
Disability Served: physically disabled

Stanford Hospital and Clinics
300 Pasteur Drive
Palo Alto, CA 94304
800-756-9000
http://www.stanfordhospital.com/default
Disability Served: physically disabled

INDEPENDENT LIVING CENTERS

Independent living centers provide services to people with disabilities, including information and referral, independent living skills instruction, personal assistant services, advocacy, group and individual counseling, assistive technology resources, and socialization and recreation activities.

ALABAMA

Birmingham Independent Living Center
206 13th Street South
Birmingham, AL 35233
205-251-2223 (Voice/TTY)
bilc@bellsouth.net
http://www.birminghamilc.org
Disability Served: various

Independent Living Center of Mobile
5304 B Overlook Road
Mobile, AL 36618
251-460-0301, 251-460-2872 (TTY)
ilc@ilcmobile.org
http://www.ilcmobile.org
Disability Served: various

ALASKA

Access Alaska Inc.
121 West Fireweed Lane, Suite 105
Anchorage, AK 99503
907-248-4777, 800-770-4488
info@accessalaska.org
http://www.accessalaska.org
Disability Served: various

Hope Community Resources Inc.
540 West International Airport Road, #100
Anchorage, AK 99518
907-561-5335
slesko@hopealaska.org
http://www.hopealaska.org
Disability Served: various

Southeastern Alaska Independent Living Inc.
3225 Hospital Drive, Suite 300
Juneau, AK 99803
907-586-4920, 907-523-5285 (TTY)
info@sailinc.org
http://www.sailinc.org
Disability Served: various

ARIZONA

Arizona Bridge to Independent Living
1229 East Washington Street
Phoenix, AZ 85034
602-256-2245, 800-280-2245
azbridge@abil.org
http://www.abil.org
Disability Served: various

Community Outreach Program for the Deaf
268 West Adams Street
Tucson, AZ 85705
520-792-1906
http://www.angelfire.com/az2/valleyctrofdeaf/copd.
   html
Disability Served: hearing

DIRECT Center for Independence
1023 North Tyndall Avenue
Tucson, AZ 85719
520-624-6452, 800-342-1853
http://www.directilc.org
Disability Served: various

Services Maximizing Independent Living
1929 Sputh Arizona Avenue, Suite 12
Yuma, AZ 85366
928-783-0515
http://www.snap211.com
Disability Served: various

ARKANSAS

Delta Resource Center for Independent Living
400 Main, Suite 118
Pine Bluff, AR 71601
870-535-2222 (Voice/TTY)
deltar@seark.net
Disability Served: various

Mainstream Living
300 South Rodney Parham, Suite 5
Little Rock, AR 72204
501-280-0012

http://www.mainstreamilrc.com
Disability Served: various

Our Way Inc.
10434 West 36th Street
Little Rock, AR 72204
501-225-5030
Disability Served: physically disabled

**Sources for Community Independent
    Living Services**
1918 North Birch Avenue
Fayetteville, AR 72703
479-442-5600, 479-251-1378 (TDD)
http://www.arsources.org
Disability Served: various

Spa Area Independent Living Services Inc.
600 Main
Hot Springs, AR 71913
501-624-7710
sails@direclynx.net
Disability Served: various

CALIFORNIA
Access Center of San Diego
1295 University Avenue, Suite 10
San Diego, CA 92103
619-293-3500, 619-293-7757 (TDD)
http://www.accesscentersd.org
Disability Served: various

Center for Independence of the Disabled
875 O'Neill Avenue
Belmont, CA 94002
650-595-0783, 650-595-0743 (TDD)
info@cidbelmont.org
http://www.cidbelmont.org
Disability Served: various

Center for Independent Living-Berkeley Office
2539 Telegraph Avenue
Berkley, CA 94704
510-841-4776, 510-848-3101 (TDD)
http://www.cilberkeley.org
Disability Served: various∫

Center for Independent Living-Fruitvale Office
1470 Fruitvale Avenue
Oakland, CA 94601
510-536-2271
http://www.cilberkeley.org
Disability Served: various

**Center for Independent Living-East Oakland
    Satellite Office**
7200 Bancroft Avenue, Suite 9A
Oakland, CA 94601
510-635-4920
http://www.cilberkeley.org
Disability Served: various

Center for Independent Living-Oakland Office
610 16th Street, 4th Floor
Oakland, CA 94612
510-763-9999, 510-444-1837 (TDD)
http://www.cilberkeley.org
Disability Served: various

Center for Independent Living of Fresno
3475 West Shaw Avenue, Suite 101
Fresno, CA 93711
559-276-6777, 559-276-6779 (TTY)
publicaffairs@dor.ca.gov
http://www.rehab.cahwnet.gov
Disability Served: various

Center for Independent Living-Visalia Office
122 East Main, Suite 110
Visalia, CA 92277
559-622-9276
http://www.rehab.cahwnet.gov
Disability Served: various

**Central Coast Center for Independent
    Living-Monterey County**
234 Capitol Street, Suites A-B
Salinas, CA 93901
831-757-2968
cccil@cccil.org
http://www.cccil.org
Disability Served: various

**Central Coast Center for Independent Living-
    Santa Cruz County**
1395 41st Avenue, Suite B
Capitola, CA 95010

408-462-8720, 831-462-8729 (TDD)
cccilcap@cccil.org
http://www.cccil.org
Disability Served: various

Community Access Center-Beaumont Senior Center
550 East Sixth Street
Beaumont, CA 92223
909-769-8539
pmgr1@ilcac.org
http://www.communityaccesscenter.org
Disability Served: various

Community Access Center-Indio Office
81-730 Highway 111, Suite 2
Indio, CA 92201
760-347-4888, 760-347-6802 (TTY)
pmgr2@ilcac.org
http://www.communityaccesscenter.org
Disability Served: various

Community Access Center-Perris Office
371 Wilderson Avenue
Perris, CA 92570
909-443-1158 (Voice /TTY)
spmgr@ilcac.org
http://www.communityaccesscenter.org
Disability Served: various

Community Access Center-Riverside Office
6848 Magnolia Avenue, Suite 150
Riverside, CA 92506
909-274-0358, 909-274-0834 (TTY)
execdir@ilcac.org
http://www.communityaccesscenter.org
Disability Served: various

Community Rehabilitation Services
4716 Cesar E. Chavez Avenue
Los Angeles, CA 90022
213-266-0453
Disability Served: various

Community Resources for Independence-Mendocino and Lake Counties
1040 North State Street, Suite E
Ukiah, CA 95482
707-463-8875, 707-462-4498 (TTY)
criukiah@cri-dove.org
http://www.cri-dove.org
Disability Served: various

Community Resources for Independence-Napa County
1040 Main Street, Suite 208
Napa, CA 94558
707-258-0270, 707-257-0274 (TTY)
crinapa@cri-dove.org
http://www.cri-dove.org
Disability Served: various

Community Resources for Independence-Sonoma County
980 Hopper Avenue
Santa Rosa, CA 95403
707-528-2745, 707-528-2151 (TTY)
cri-santarosa@cri-dove.org
http://www.cri-dove.org
Disability Served: various

Community Resources for Independent Living
439 A Street
Hayward, CA 94541
510-881-5743, 510-881-0218 (TTY)
info@cril-online.org
http://www.cril-online.org
Disability Served: various

Dayle McIntosh Center for the Disabled-Garden Grove Office
13272 Garden Grove Boulevard
Garden Grove, CA 92843
714- 621-3300, 714-663-2087 (TTY)
info@daylemc.org
http://daylemc.org
Disability Served: various

Dayle McIntosh Center-South County Office
24012 Calle De La Plata, #210
Laguna Niguel, CA 92653
949-460-7784, 949-855-6749 (TTY)
info@daylemc.org
http://daylemc.org
Disability Served: various

Disabled Resources Center Inc.
2750 East Spring Street, Suite 100
Long Beach, CA 90806
562-427-1000
atprogram@drcinc.org
http://www.drcinc.org
Disability Served: various

FREED-Foundation of Resources for Equality and Employment for the Disabled
154 Hughes Road, Suite 1
Grass Valley, CA 95945
530-272-1732
contact-04@freed.org
http://www.freed.org
Disability Served: various

Humboldt Access Project Inc.
955 Myrtle Avenue
Eureka, CA 95501
707-445-8404, 707-445-8405 (TTY), 877-576-5000
Disability Served: various

Independent Living Center
109 South Spring Street, PO Box 549
Claremont, CA 91711-1296
800-491-6722, 909-445-0726 (TTY)
http://www.ilc-clar.org
Disability Served: various

Independent Living Center of Kern County
1631 30th Street
Bakersfield, CA 93301-4409
661-325-1063, 800-529-9541
davidt@ilcofkerncounty.org
http://ilcofkerncounty.org
Disability Served: various

Independent Living Center of Southern California-Lancaster Office
1505 West Avenue J
Lancaster, CA 93534
661-945-6602, 661-945-6604 (TDD)
Disability Served: various

Independent Living Center of Southern California-Main Office
14407 Gilmore Street
Van Nuys, CA 91401
818-785-6934
ilcsc@ilcsc.org
http://www.ilcsc.org
Disability Served: various

Independent Living Resource
3200 Clayton Road
Concord, CA 94519
925-363-7293

http://www.ilrccc.org
Disability Served: various

Independent Living Resource Center
423 West Victoria
Santa Barbara, CA 93101
805-963-0595, 805-963-8265 (TDD/TTY)
desparza@ilrc-trico.org
http://www.ilrc-trico.org
Disability Served: physically disabled

Independent Living Resource Center San Francisco
649 Mission Street, Third Floor
San Francisco, CA 94105
415-543-6222
info@ilrcsf.org
http://www.ilrcsf.org
Disability Served: various

Independent Living Resource Center-San Luis Obispo County
1150 Laurel Lane, Suite 184
San Luis Obispo, CA 93401
805-593-0667 (Voice/TTD)
http://www.ilrc-trico.org
Disability Served: various

Independent Living Resource Center-Ventura County
1802 Eastman Avenue, Suite 112
Ventura, CA 93003
805-650-5993 (Voice/TTD/TTY)
http://www.ilrc-trico.org
Disability Served: various

Independent Living Services of Northern California-Chico Office
1161 East Avenue
Chico, CA 95926-1847
800-464-8527, 530-893-8527 (Voice/TTY)
ilsnc@sunset.net
http://www.ilsnc.org
Disability Served: various

Independent Living Services of Northern California-Redding Office
1411 Yuba Street
Redding, CA 96001-1010
530-242-8550 (Voice/TTY)
ilsncrdg@sunset.net
http://www.ilsnc.org
Disability Served: various

**Marin Center for Independent Living-
San Rafael Office**
710 Fourth Street
San Rafael, CA 94901
415-459-6245 (Voice/TDD)
http://www.marincil.org
Disability Served: various

Modesto Independent Living Center
221 McHenry Avenue
Modesto, CA 95354
209-521-7260, 209-521-1425 (TDD)
dwight@drail.org
http://www.drail.org
Disability Served: various

Mother Lode Independent Living Center
975 Morning Star, Suite A
Sonora, CA 95370
209-532-0963, 209-532-1280 (TTY)
Disability Served: various

Placer Independent Resource Services
11768 Atwood Road, Suite 29
Auburn, CA 95603
530-885-6100, 800-833-3453, 530-885-0326 (TTY)
administrator@pirs.org
http://www.pirs.org
Disability Served: various

Resources for Independent Living
1211 H Street, Suite B
Sacramento, CA 95814
916-446-3074
monicag@ril-sacramento.org
http://www.ril-sacramento.org
Disability Served: various

Rolling Start Inc.
570 West Fourth Street, #103
San Bernardino, CA 92401-2810
909-884-2129
support@rollingstart.com
http://www.rollingstart.com
Disability Served: various

San Joaquin Independent Living Center
4505 Precissi, Suite A
Stockton, CA 95207
209-477-8143
Disability Served: various

**Service Center for Independent Living-
San Gabriel Valley Branch Office**
963 West Badillo Street
Covina, CA 91722
818-967-0995
scilcovn@tstonramp.com
Disability Served: various

**Silicon Valley Independent Living Center-
Gilroy Office**
7800 Arroyo Circle, Suite A
Gilroy, CA 95020
408-846-1480, 408-842-2591 (TTY)
francesm@svilc.org
http://www.svilc.org
Disability Served: various

**Silicon Valley Independent Living Center-
San Jose Office**
2306 Zanker Road
San Jose, CA 95131
408-894-9041, 408-894-9012 (TTY)
francesm@svilc.org
http://www.svilc.org
Disability Served: various

Southern California Rehabilitation Services
7830 Quill Drive, Suite D
Downey, CA 90242
562-862-6531, 562-869-0931 (TTY)
scrs@scrs-ilc.org
http://www.scrs-ilc.org
Disability Served: various

**Westside Center for Independent Living-
Mar Vista Office**
12901 Venice Boulevard
Los Angeles, CA 90066
310-390-3611, 310-398-9204 (TTY)
WCIL@wcil.org
http://www.wcil.org
Disability Served: various

**Westside Center for Independent Living-
Santa Monica Office**
1527 Fourth Street, Suite 250
Santa Monica, CA 90401
310-394-9871
wcil@wcil.org
http://www.wcil.org
Disability Served: various

COLORADO

Atlantis Community Inc.
201 South Cherokee Street
Denver, CO 80209-3195
303-733-9324, 303-733-0047 (TDD)
http://www.atlantiscom.org
Disability Served: various

Center for Independence
1600 Ute Avenue, Suite 100
Grand Junction, CO 81501
970-241-0315, 800-613-2271
http://www.cfigj.org
Disability Served: various

Center for People with Disabilities
1675 Range Street
Boulder, CO 80301
303-442-8662, 303-449-8158 (TDD)
ddebrohun@cpwd-ilc.org
http://www.cpwd-ilc.org
Disability Served: various

Colorado Springs Independence Center
21 East Las Animas Street
Colorado Springs, CO 80903
719-471-8181
nancycsic@qwest.net
http://www.csicindliving.org
Disability Served: various

Connections for Independent Living
1024 Ninth Avenue, Suite E
Greeley, CO 80631
970-352-8682, 800-887-5828
Disability Served: various

Disabled Resource Services
424 Pine Street, Suite 101
Ft Collins, CO 80524
970-482-2700
drs@fortnet.org
http://www.fortnet.org/drs
Disability Served: various

Greeley Center for Independent Living
2780 28th Avenue
Greeley, CO 80631
970-339-2444, 800-748-1012
gciinc@gci.org
http://www.gci.org
Disability Served: various

Pikes Peak Center on Deafness
225 South Academy Boulevard, #100
Colorado Springs, CO 80910
719-591-2777 (Voice/TTY)
http://www.ppcod.org
Disability Served: hearing

Sangre de Cristo Center for Independent Living
131 South Union
Pueblo, CO 81003-3207
719-546-1271
Disability Served: various

CONNECTICUT

Chapel Haven Inc.
1040 Whalley Avenue
New Haven, CT 06515
203-397-1714
http://www.chapelhaven.org
Disability Served: developmentally disabled

Disabilities Network of Eastern Connecticut
238 West Town Street
Norwich, CT 06360
860-823-1898
rjdeluca@snet.net
http://www.disability-dnec.org
Disability Served: various

Disability Resource Center of Fairfield County
80 Ferry Boulevard
Stratford, CT 06497
203-378-6977
info@drcfc.org
http://www.drcfc.org
Disability Served: various

Independence Northwest Inc.
1183 New Haven Road, Suite 200
Naugatuck, CT 06770
203-729-3299, 203-729-1281 (TDD)
indnw@aol.com
Disability Served: various

DELAWARE
Easter Seal Independent Living Center
24 Read's Way
New Castle, DE 19720-2405
302-324-4488, 302-324-4482 (TTY)
Disability Served: various

DISTRICT OF COLUMBIA
District of Columbia Center for Independent Living
1400 Florida Avenue, NE, Suite 3
Washington, DC 20002
202-388-0033
info@dccil.org
http://www.dccil.org
Disability Served: various

FLORIDA
Ability1st
1823 Buford Court
Tallahassee, FL 32304
850-575-9621
ability1st@ability1st.info
http://www.ability1st.info
Disability Served: various

Briarwood Center for Independent Living
1023 Southeast 4th Avenue, Suite 23
Gainesville, FL 32604
352-378-7474
hamricc@mail.firn.edu
Disability Served: various

Caring and Sharing Center for Independent Living Inc.
12552 Belcher Road South
Largo, FL 33773
http://www.cascil.org
727-577-0065 (Voice/TDD)
cascil@cascil.org
http://www.cascil.org
Disability Served: various

Center for Independent Living in Central Florida Inc.-Lakeland Office
111 North Eastside Drive
Lakeland, FL 33801
863-413-2722, 888-263-6692
dpirozzoli@cilorlando.org
http://www.cilorlando.org
Disability Served: various

Center for Independent Living in Central Florida Inc.-Winter Park Office
720 North Denning Drive
Winter Park, FL 32789
407-623-1070, 407-623-1185 (TDD)

jgassie@cilorlando.org
http://www.cilorlando.org
Disability Served: various

Center for Independent Living of Broward
8857 West McNab Road
Tamarac, FL 33321
954-722-6400 (Voice/TTY)
cilb@cilbroward.org
http://www.cilbroward.org/website
Disability Served: various

Center for Independent Living of North Central Florida-Gainesville Office
720 Northwest 23rd Avenue
Gainesville, FL 32609
352-378-7474, 800-265-5724
admin@cilncf.org
http://www.cilncf.org
Disability Served: various

Center for Independent Living of North Central Florida-Lecanto Office
3774 West Lake to Gulf Highway
Lecanto, FL 34461
352-527-8399, 800-265-5724
admin@cilncf.org
http://www.cilncf.org
Disability Served: various

Center for Independent Living of North Central Florida-Ocala Office
3445 Northeast 24th Street
Ocala, FL 34470
352-368-3788, 800-265-5724
admin@cilncf.org
http://www.cilncf.org
Disability Served: various

Center for Independent Living of Northwest Florida
3600 North Pace Boulevard
Pensacola, FL 32505
850-595-5566, 877-245-2457
cilnwf@cilnwf.org
http://www.cilnwf.org
Disability Served: various

Center for Independent Living of South Florida
6660 Biscayne Boulevard
Miami, FL 33138

305-751-8025 (Voice/TTY), 800-854-7551
Info@soflacil.org
http://www.soflacil.org
Disability Served: various

Center for Independent Living of Southwest Florida
3626 Evans Avenue
Ft Myers, FL 33901
239-277-1447
cilfl@neosmart.com
http://www.cilfl.org
Disability Served: various

Center for Independent Living of the Florida Keys
103400 Overseas Highway, Suite 17
Islamorada, FL 33036
877-335-0187, 305-453-3491
cilofthekeys@aol.com
Disability Served: various

Coalition for Independent Living Options Inc.
6800 Forest Hill Boulevard
West Palm Beach, FL 33413
561-966-4288, 800-683-7337
http://www.cilo.org
Disability Served: various

Coalition for Independent Living Options-
Okeechobee County
One Stop Career Center, 209 Southwest Park Street
Okeechobee, FL 34974
863-462-5350
http://www.cilo.org
Disability Served: various

Coalition for Independent Living Options-
Royal Palm Beach
Harvin Center, 1030 Royal Palm Beach Boulevard
Royal Palm Beach, FL 33411
561-798-7997
http://www.cilo.org
Disability Served: various

Coalition for Independent Living Options-
St. Lucie County
One Stop Career Center, 2415 South 29th Street
Ft. Pierce, FL 34981
772-462-6180
http://www.cilo.org
Disability Served: various

Independent Living Resource Center of Northeast
Florida
2709 Art Museum Drive
Jacksonville, FL 32207
904-399-8484, 888-427-4313, 904-398-6322 (TTY)
mattm@cilj.com
http://www.cilj.com
Disability Served: various

Self-Reliance Inc. Center for Independent Living
8901 North Armenia Avenue
Tampa, FL 33612
813-975-6560, 813-375-3972 (TTY)
http://www.self-reliance.org
Disability Served: various

South Florida Association for Disability Advocacy Inc.
1335 Northwest 14th Street, Suite 200
Miami, FL 33125
305-547-5444
Disability Served: various

Space Coast Center for Independent Living
331 Ramp Road
Cocoa Beach, FL 32931
321-784-9008 (Voice/TTY)
sccil@bellsouth.net
Disability Served: various

Suncoast Center for Independent Living
2989 Fruitville Road
Sarasota, FL 34237
941-351-9545, 941-351-9945 (TDD)
http://www.scil4u.com
Disability Served: various

Watson Center for the Blind and Visually Impaired
6925 112th Circle North, Suite 103
Largo, FL 33773
727-544-4433
http://www.watsoncenter.org
Disability Served: vision

GEORGIA
DisABILITY LINK
755 Commerce Drive, Suite 415
Decatur, GA 30030-2618
404-687-8890, 800-239-2507, 404-687-9175 (TTY)
hilarye@disabilitylink.org

http://www.disabilitylink.org
Disability Served: various

Living Independence For Everyone Inc.
17-21 East Travis Street
Savannah, GA 31406
912-920-2414, 912-920-2419 (TTY)
Disability Served: various

Roosevelt Warm Springs Institute for Rehabilitation
PO Box 1000
Warm Springs, GA 31830
706-655-5000
http://www.rooseveltrehab.org
Disability Served: various

Walton Options for Independent Living-Augusta Office
948 Walton Way
Augusta, GA 30903-0519
706-724-6262 (Voice/TTY)
http://www.waltonoptions.org
Disability Served: various

Walton Options for Independent Living-Warrenton Office
928 East Warrenton Highway
Warrenton, GA 30828
706-465-1148 (Voice/TTY)
http://www.waltonoptions.org
Disability Served: various

Walton Options for Independent Living-Waynesboro Office
808 Davis Road
Waynesboro, GA 30830
706-437-9740 (Voice/TTY)
http://www.waltonoptions.org
Disability Served: various

HAWAII
Big Island Center for Independent Living
1190 Waianuenue Avenue
Hilo, HI 96720
808-935-3777, 808-935-3777 (TDD)
cileh@interpac.net
Disability Served: various

Hawaii Centers for Independent Living
414 Kuwili Street, Suite 102
Honolulu, HI 96817
808-522-5400, 808-522-5415 (TTY/TDD)
http://search.volunteerhawaii.org/org/5779305.html
Disability Served: various

Kailua Kona Center for Independent Living-West Hawaii
81-6627 Mamaloha Highway, Suite B-5
Kealakekua, HI 96750
808-323-2221, 808-323-2262 (TDD)
Disability Served: various

Kauai Center for Independent Living
Lihue United Church, 4340 Nawiliwili Road
Lihue, HI 96766
808-245-4034
kcil@aloha.net
Disability Served: various

Maui Center for Independent Living
220 Imikala Street, Suite 103
Wailuku, HI 96793
808-242-4966, 808-242-4968 (TDD)
mcilogg@gte.net
Disability Served: various

IDAHO
Disability Action Center Northwest-Coeur d'Alene Office
1323 Sherman Avenue, Suite 7
Coeur d'Alene, ID 83814
208-664-9896, 800-854-9500
dac@icehouse.net
Disability Served: various

Disability Action Center Northwest-Moscow Office
124 East Third Street
Moscow, ID 83843
208-883-0523
dac@moscow.com
Disability Served: various

Eastern Idaho Center for Independence
280 North Cedar, PO Box 388
Blackfoot, ID 83221
208-785-5890
Disability Served: various

Idaho Commission for the Blind
341 West Washington Street
Boise, ID 83702
208-334-3220
mblackal@icbvi.state.id.us
http://www.icbvi.state.id.us
Disability Served: vision

Living Independence Network Corporation-
Boise Office
2500 Kootenai
Boise, ID 83705-2408
208-336-3335
info@lincidaho.org
http://www.lincidaho.org
Disability Served: various

Living Independence Network Corporation-
Caldwell Office
2922 East Cleveland, Suite #800
Caldwell, ID 83605
208-454-5511 (Voice/TTY)
http://www.lincidaho.org
Disability Served: various

Living Independence Network Corporation-
Twin Falls Office
132 Main Avenue South
Twin Falls, ID 83301
208-733-1712 (Voice/TTY)
http://www.lincidaho.org
Disability Served: various

Living Independently For Everyone Inc.-
Black Foot Office
67 North Maple
Black Foot, ID 83221
208-785-9648 (Voice/TTY)
lucyn@idlife.org
http://www.idaholifecenter.org
Disability Served: various

Living Independently For Everyone Inc.-Burley Office
2311 Parke Avenue, Suite 7
Burley, ID 83318
208-678-7705 (Voice/TTY)
sandrad@idlife.org
http://www.idaholifecenter.org
Disability Served: various

Living Independently For Everyone Inc.-
Idaho Falls Office
2110 South Rollandet Avenue
Idaho Falls, ID 83402
208-529-8610 (Voice/TTY)
valeriej@idlife.org
http://www.idaholifecenter.org
Disability Served: various

Living Independently For Everyone Inc.-
Main Office
640 Pershing, Suite A
Pocatello, ID 83204
208-232-2747 (Voice/TTY), 800-631-2747
deann@idlife.org
http://www.idaholifecenter.org
Disability Served: various

ILLINOIS
Access Living of Metropolitan Chicago
614 West Roosevelt Road
Chicago, IL 60607
312-253-7000, 312-253-7002
generalinfo@accessliving.org
http://www.accessliving.org
Disability Served: various

Central Illinois Center for Independent Living
614 West Glen
Peoria, IL 61614
309-682-3500, 877-501-9808, 309-682-3567 (TTY)
http://www.cicil.org
Disability Served: various

DuPage Center for Independent Living
739 Roosevelt Road, Building 8, Suite 109
Glen Ellyn, IL 60137
630-469-2300 (Voice/TTY)
dcil@mcs.com
http://www.glen-ellyn.com/dcil
Disability Served: various

Fox River Valley Center for Independent Living
730 West Chicago Street
Elgin, IL 60123
847-695-5818, 847-695-5868 (TTY)
FRVCIL@mail.com
Disability Served: various

GAIL Center for Independent Living
112 West Washington Street, PO Box 486
Effingham, IL 62401
217-342-7110
gailcil@xel.net
Disability Served: various

Illinois Iowa Center for Independent Living
3708 11th Street, PO Box 6156
Rock Island, IL 61231
309-793-0090 (Voice/TTY), 877-541-2505
iicil@iicil.com
http://www.iicil.com
Disability Served: various

Illinois Valley Center for Independent Living
18 Gunia Drive
LaSalle, IL 61301
815-224-3126, 815-224-8271 (TTY)
ivcil@ivcil.com
http://www.ivcil.com
Disability Served: various

IMPACT Inc.
2735 East Broadway
Alton, IL 62002
618-462-1411, 618-474-5333 (TTY)
contarino@impactcil.org
http://www.impactcil.org
Disability Served: various

Jacksonville Area Center for Independent Living
60 East Central Park Plaza
Jacksonville, IL 62650-2090
217-245-8371 (Voice/TTY)
Toll Free: 888-317-3287
info@jacil.org
http://www.jacil.org
Disability Served: various

Lake County Center for Independent Living
377 North Seymour Avenue
Mundelein, IL 60060
847-949-4440, 847-949-4440 (TTY)
lccil@dls.net
http://www.lccil.org
Disability Served: various

LIFE Center for Independent Living
2201 Eastland Drive, Suite #1
Bloomington, IL 61701

309-663-5433, 888-543-3245
lifecil@lifecil.org
http://www.lifecil.org
Disability Served: various

Living Independently Now Center-Main Office
120 East A Street
Belleville, IL 62220-1401
618-235-9988 (Voice/TTY)
info@lincinc.org
http://www.lincinc.org
Disability Served: various

**Living Independently Now Center-
    Monroe Randolph Center**
1514 South Main Street, Suite 4
Red Bud, IL 62278
618-282-3700 (Voice/TTY)
info@lincinc.org
http://www.incil.org
Disability Served: various

Northwestern Illinois Center for Independent Living
229 First Avenue, Suite 2
Rock Falls, IL 61071
815-625-7860, 815-625-6863 (TTY)
nicil@essex1.com
http://www.incil.org/home.asp?id=18
Disability Served: various

Opportunities for Access
4206 Williamson Place, Suite 3
Mt Vernon, IL 62864
618-244-9212, 618-244-9575 (TTY)
info@ofacil.org
http://www.ofacil.org
Disability Served: various

Options Center for Independent Living
61 Meadowview Center
Kankakee, IL 60901
815-936-0100, 815-936-0132 (TTY)
options@daily-journal.com
Disability Served: various

PACE Inc.
1317 East Florida Avenue
Urbana, IL 61801
217-344-5433, 217-344-5024 (TTY)
paceurbana@aol.com

http://www.incil.org/home.asp?id=12
Disability Served: various

Progress Center for Independent Living
7521 Madison Street
Forest Park, IL 60130
708-209-1500, 708-209-1826
info@progresscil.org
http://progresscil.org
Disability Served: various

Regional Access and Mobilization Project Inc.
202 Market Street
Rockford, IL 61107
815-968-7467, 815-968-2401 (TTY)
rampcil@rampcil.org
http://www.rampcil.org
Disability Served: various

Southern Illinois Center for Independent Living
100 North Glenview Drive, PO Box 627
Carbondale, IL 62903
618-457-3318, 618-457-3318 (TTY)
sicil@intrnet.net
http://www.incil.org/home.asp?id=21
Disability Served: various

Soyland Access to Independent Living
2449 Federal Drive
Decatur, IL 62526
217-876-8888 (Voice/TTY), 800-358-8080 (Voice/TTY)
sail@midwest.net
http://www.decatursail.com
Disability Served: various

Springfield Center for Independent Living
330 South Grand Avenue West
Springfield, IL 62702
217-523-2587 (Voice/TTY)
scil@scil.org
http://www.scil.org
Disability Served: various

Stone-Hayes Center for Independent Living
39 North Prairie Street
Galesburg, IL 61410
309-344-1306, 309-344-1269 (TYY)
stonehayes@misslink.net
Disability Served: various

West Central Illinois Center for Independent Living
406 North 24th Street, Suite 3, PO Box 1065
Quincy, IL 62306-1065
217-223-0400, 217-223-0475 (TTY)
wcicil@adams.net
Disability Served: various

Will Grundy Center for Independent Living
2415 #A West Jefferson Street
Joliet, IL 60435
815-729-0162, 815-729-2085 (TTY)
wgcil@sbcglobal.net
http://www.will-grundycil.org
Disability Served: various

INDIANA

ATTIC
1721 Washington Avenue
Vincennes, IN 47591
812-886-0575, 877-96-ATTIC
inattic1@aol.com
http://www.theattic.org
Disability Served: various

Everybody Counts Center for Independent Living
Broadfield Center, 9111 Broadway, Suite A
Merrillville, IN 46410
219-769-5055, 888-769-3636, 219-756-3323 (TTY)
ecounts@netnitco.net
Disability Served: various

Indianapolis Resource Center for Independent Living
1426 West 29th Street, Suite 207
Indianapolis, IN 46250
317-926-1660, 800-860-7181
ircil@netdirect.net
http://www.ircil.org
Disability Served: various

League for the Blind and Disabled Inc.
5821 South Anthony Boulevard
Ft Wayne, IN 46816
260-441-0551 (Voice/TTY), 800-889-3443
http://www.the-league.org
Disability Served: various

Southern Indiana Center for Independent Living-
    Lawrence County Office
3300 West 16th Street
Bedford, IN 47421

800-845-6914
bsrimst@kiva.net
Disability Served: various

Southern Indiana Center for Independent Living-Monroe County Office
516 Hamilton Court
Bloomington, IN 47408
800-845-6914
bsrimst@kiva.net
Disability Served: various

WILL Center
4312 South Seventh Street
Terre Haute, IN 47802
812-298-9455, 877-915-9455
info@thewillcenter.org
http://www.thewillcenter.org
Disability Served: various

IOWA
Central Iowa Center for Independent Living
1024 Walnut Street, Suite 131
Des Moines, IA 50309-3424
515-243-1742, 888-503-2287
cicil@raccoon.com
http://www.raccoon.com/~cicil
Disability Served: various

Evert Conner Rights and Resources Center for Independent Living
20 East Market Street
Iowa City, IA 52240
319-338-3870
Disability Served: various

Hope Haven Inc.
1800 19th Street
Rock Valley, IA 51247
712-476-2737
http://www.hopehaven.org
Disability Served: various

League of Human Dignity
1417-1/2 West Broadway
Council Bluffs, IA 51501
712-323-6863
Cinfo@leagueofhumandignity.com
http://www.leagueofhumandignity.com
Disability Served: various

Three Rivers Independent Living Center
Gordon Recovery Center, 800 5th Street, Suite 131
Sioux City, IA 51101
712-255-1065
trilcbjd@aol.com
Disability Served: various

KANSAS
Coalition for Independence
4911 State Avenue
Kansas City, KS 66102
913-321-5140, 913-321-5216 (TTY)
jnicol@cfi-kc.org
http://www.cfi-kc.org
Disability Served: various

Cowley County Developmental Services
Strother Field, PO Box 133
Arkansas City, KS 67005
316-442-3575, 316-221-6140
Disability Served: developmentally disabled

Independence Inc.
2001 Haskell Avenue
Lawrence, KS 66045
785-841-0333, 888-824-7277, 785-841-1046 (TDD)
http://www.independenceinc.org
Disability Served: various

Independent Living Center of Northeast Kansas
521 Commercial, Suite C
Atchison, KS 66002
913-367-1830 (Voice/TDD), 888-845-2879
ilcnek@journey.com
http://www.ilcnek.org
Disability Served: various

Independent Living Resource Center
3033 West Second Street
Wichita, KS 67203-5415
316-942-6300 (Voice/TDD), 800-479-6861
jclifton@ilrcks.org
http://www.ilrcks.org
Disability Served: various

Kansas Services for the Blind and Visually Impaired
2601 Southwest East Circle Drive North
Topeka, KS 66606
785-296-3311, 800-547-5789

rehab@srskansas.org
http://www.srskansas.org/rehab/text/SBVI.htm
Disability Served: vision

LINK Inc.
2401 East 13th Street
Hays, KS 67601
785-625-6942 (Voice/TDD), 800-569-5926
batwell@eaglecom.net
Disability Served: various

Resource Center for Independent Living
PO Box 257
Osage City, KS 66523
785-528-3105, 785-528-3106 (TTY)
mary@rcilinc.org
http://www.rcilinc.org
Disability Served: various

Three Rivers Inc.-Centralia Office
314 Mulberry, PO Box 236
Centralia, KS 66415-0236
785-857-3515
http://www.threeriversinc.org
Disability Served: various

Three Rivers Inc.-Clay Center Office
308 Court Street, PO Box 33
Clay Center, KS 67432-0033
785-632-6117 (Voice/TDD)
http://www.threeriversinc.org
Disability Served: various

Three Rivers Inc.-Manhattan Office
323 Poyntz, Suite 202
Manhattan, KS 66502
785-537-8985 (Voice/TDD)
http://www.threeriversinc.org
Disability Served: various

Three Rivers Inc.-Topeka Office
PO Box 4152
Topeka, KS 66604-4152
785-273-0249
http://www.threeriversinc.org
Disability Served: various

Three Rivers Inc.-Wamego Office
408 Lincoln Avenue, PO Box 408
Wamego, KS 66547

785-456-9915 (Voice/TDD)
reception@threeriversinc.org
http://www.threeriversinc.org
Disability Served: various

Topeka Independent Living Resource Center
501 Southwest Jackson Street, Suite 100
Topeka, KS 66603
785-233-4572 (Voice/TDD), 785-233-1815 (TTY)
ilrc2@tilrc.org
http://www.tilrc.org
Disability Served: various

Whole Person Inc.-Nortonville Office
PO Box 117
Nortonville, KS 66606
913-886-2615
http://www.thewholeperson.org
Disability Served: various

Whole Person Inc.-Prairie Village Office
7301 Mission Road
Prairie Village, KS 66208
913-262-1294, 913-262-1294 (TTY)
http://www.thewholeperson.org
Disability Served: various

Whole Person Inc.-Tonganoxie Office
1381 South Greenwood Drive
Tonganoxie, KS 66086
913-369-9005
http://www.thewholeperson.org
Disability Served: various

KENTUCKY
Center for Accessible Living-Louisville Office
305 West Broadway, Suite 200
Louisville, KY 40202
502-589-6620, 502-589-6690 (TTY)
jday@calky.org
http://www.calky.org
Disability Served: various

Center for Accessible Living-Murray Office
1051 North 16th Street, Suite C
Murray, KY 42071
270-7589-6620, 888-261-6194
jgallimore@calky.org
http://www.calky.org
Disability Served: various

Community Alternatives Kentucky
859 East Main Street
Frankfort, KY 40601
502-875-5777
Disability Served: various

LOUISIANA

Independent Living Center Inc.
1001 Howard Avenue, Suite 300
New Orleans, LA 70119
504-522-1955
Disability Served: various

New Horizons Inc.-Central Louisiana Office
3400 Jackson Street, Suite A
Alexandria, LA 71301
318-484-3596, 888-361-3596
nhilc@nhilc.org
http://www.nhilc.org
Disability Served: various

New Horizons Inc.-Northeast Louisiana
1900 Lamy Lane, Suite H
Monroe, LA 71201
318-323-4374, 800-428-5505
nhilc@nhilc.org
http://www.nhilc.org
Disability Served: various

New Horizons Inc.-Northwest Louisiana Office
9300 Mansfield Road, Suite 204
Shreveport, LA 71118
318-671-8131, 877-219-7327
nhilc@nhilc.org
http://www.nhilc.org
Disability Served: various

Resources for Independent Living-Baton Rouge Office
11931 Industriplex Boulevard, Suite 200
Baton Rouge, LA 70809
225-753-4772, 225-753-4831 (TTY)
http://www.noril.org
Disability Served: various

Resources for Independent Living-Metairie Office
3616 S I-10 Service Road West, Suite 111
Metairie, LA 70001

504-522-1955, 504-522-1956 (TTY)
http://www.noril.org
Disability Served: various

Southwest Louisiana Independence Center
1202 Kirkman, Suite C
Lake Charles, LA 70607
337-477-7194, 337-477-7196 (TTY)
mitch@slic-la.org
http://www.slic-la.org
Disability Served: various

Volunteers of America Independent Living Program
360 Jordan Street
Shreveport, LA 71101
318-221-2669
lisa@voanorthla.org
http://www.voanorthla.org
Disability Served: vision

MAINE

Maine Independent Living Services
331 State Street
Augusta, ME 04330-6014
207-622-5434
Disability Served: various

Maine Mental Health Connections Inc.
150 Union Street
Bangor, ME 04401
207-941-2907
http://www.mmhcommunityconnection.org
Disability Served: mental health

Motivational Services Inc.
14 Glenridge Drive
Augusta, ME 04330
207-626-3465, 207-621-2542 (TTY)
rweiss@mocomaine.com
http://www.mocomaine.com
Disability Served: various

Shalom House Inc.
106 Gilman Street
Portland, ME 04102
207-874-1080
generalmail@shalomhouseinc.org

http://www.shalomhouseinc.org
Disability Served: mental health

MARYLAND

Freedom Center
Rose Hill Plaza, Unit A-20, 1560 Opossumtown Pike
Frederick, MD 21702
301-846-7811
http://www.thefreedomcenter-md.org
Disability Served: various

Independence Now Inc.-Montgomery County Office
1400 Spring Street, Suite 400
Silver Spring, MD 20910
301-587-4162
independence@innow.org
http://www.innow.org
Disability Served: various

Independence Now Inc.-Prince George County Office
6811 Kenilworth Avenue, #504
Riverdale, MD 20737
301-277-2839
independence@innow.org
http://www.innow.org
Disability Served: various

**Making Choices for Independent Living: Resources
    for Independent Living**
3011 Montebello Terrace
Baltimore, MD 21214
410-444-1400, 800-735-2258 (TTY)
mcil@mcil-md.org
http://www.mcil-md.org
Disability Served: various

Resources for Independence
708 Fayette Street
Cumberland, MD 21502
800-371-1986
http://www.rficil.org
Disability Served: various

MASSACHUSETTS

AD-LIB Inc.
215 North Street
Pittsfield, MA 01201

413-442-7047
jcastellani@adlib.bz
Disability Served: various

Boston Center for Independent Living
95 Berkeley Street, Suite 206
Boston, MA 02116
617-338-6665, 617-338-6662 (TTY)
info@bostoncil.org
http://www.bostoncil.org
Disability Served: various

Cape Organization for the Rights of the Disabled
1019 Iyannough Road, #4
Hyannis, MA 02601
508-775-8300 (Voice/TTY), 800-541-0282 (Voice/TTY)
pburkley@cape.com
http://www.cordonline.org
Disability Served: various

Center for Living and Working Inc.
67 Millbrook Street
Worcester, MA 01606
508-363-1226 (Voice/TTY)
centerlw@centerlw.org
http://www.centerlw.org
Disability Served: various

Independence Associates Inc.
10 Oak Street, Second Floor
Taunton, MA 02780
508-880-5325 (Voice/TTY)
cgallant@iacil.org
http://www.iacil.org
Disability Served: various

**Independent Living Center of the North Shore
    and Cape Ann**
27 Congress Street, Suite 107
Salem, MA 01970
978-741-0077, 978-745-1735 (TTY)
mmmoore@ilcnsca.org
http://www.ilcnsca.org
Disability Served: various

MetroWest Center for Independent Living
280 Irving Street
Framingham, MA 01701
508-875-7853 (Voice/TTY)

pspooner@mwcil.org
http://www.mwcil.org
Disability Served: various

Renaissance Program
21 Branch Street
Lowell, MA 01851
978-454-7944
Disability Served: various

Southeast Center for Independent Living
Merrill Building, 66 Troy Street
Fall River, MA 02721
508-679-9210
scil@choiceonemail.com
http://www.secil.org
Disability Served: various

Stavros Center for Independent Living
691 Southeast Street
Amherst, MA 01002
413-256-0473, 800-442-1185
info@stavros.org
http://www.stavros.org
Disability Served: various

MICHIGAN
Ann Arbor Center for Independent Living
2568 Packard Road, Georgetown Mall
Ann Arbor, MI 48104-6831
734-971-0277
sprobert@aacil.org
http://www.aacil.org
Disability Served: various

ARC Detroit
51 West Hancock
Detroit, MI 48201
313-831-0202
thearcdetroit@aol.com
Disability Served: developmentally disabled, mentally disabled

Blue Water Center for Independent Living
310 Water Street
Port Huron, MI 48060
810-987-9337, 800-527-2167 (TTY)
stclair@bwcil.org
http://www.bwcil.org
Disability Served: various

Capital Area Center for Independent Living
1048 Pierpoint, Suite 9-10
Lansing, MI 48911
517-241-0393, 877-864-9683
cacil@cacil.org
http://www.cacil.org
Disability Served: various

Center for Independent Living of Mid-Michigan
1206 James Savage Road
Midland, MI 48640
517-835-4041
Disability Served: various

Community Connections
133 East Napier, Suite 2
Benton Harbor, MI 49022
269-925-6422
communityconnections@match.org
http://www.cil.match.org
Disability Served: various

Disability Advocates of Kent County
3600 Camelot Drive, SE
Grand Rapids, MI 46546
616-949-1100, 616-949-1100 (TTY)
contact@disabilityadvocates.us
http://www.disabilityadvocates.us
Disability Served: various

Disability Network
3600 South Dort Highway, Suite 54
Flint, MI 48507
810-742-1800, 810-742-7647 (TDD)
tdn@disnetwork.org
http://www.disnetwork.org
Disability Served: various

Disability Resource Center of Southwestern Michigan
517 East Crosstown Parkway
Kalamazoo, MI 49001
269-345-1516, 800-394-7450, 269-345-5925 (TTY)
tveld@drccil.org
http://www.drccil.org
Disability Served: various

Family and Children Services
1608 Lake Street
Kalamazoo, MI 49001
269-344-0202
http://www.fcsource.org
Disability Served: various

Grand Traverse Regional Community Foundation
250 East Front Street, Suite 310
Traverse City, MI 49684
231-935-4066
info@gtrcf.org
http://www.gtrcf.org
Disability Served: various

Great Lakes Center for Independent Living
4 East Alexandrine, Suite 104
Detroit, MI 48201
313-832-3371, 313-832-3372 (TDD)
Disability Served: various

**Jewish Association for Residential Care for Persons
with Developmental Disabilities**
30301 Northwestern Highway, Suite 100
Farmington Hills, MI 48334
248-538-6611 (Voice/TTY)
jarc@jarc.org
http://www.jarc.org
Disability Served: developmentally disabled

Lakeshore Center for Independent Living
426 Century Lane
Holland, MI 49423
616-396-5326 (Voice/TTY)
http://www.lcil.org
Disability Served: various

Oakland/Macomb Center for Independent Living
13213 East 14 Mile Road
Sterling Heights, MI 48312
586-268-4160
info@omcil.org
http://www.omcil.org
Disability Served: various

**Southeastern Michigan Center for Independent
Living**
1200 6th Avenue, 15th Floor
Detroit, MI 48226
313-256-1524
Disability Served: various

MINNESOTA

Accessible Space Inc.
2550 University Avenue West, Suite 330N
St Paul, MN 55114
651-645-7271, 800-466-7722

info@accessiblespace.org
http://www.accessiblespace.org
Disability Served: various

**Center for Independent Living of Northeastern
Minnesota-Aitkin Branch Office**
105 Fourth Street NW
Aitkin, MN 56431
218-927-3748 (Voice/TTY)
brian@accessnorth.net
http://accessnorth.net
Disability Served: various

**Center for Independent Living of Northeastern
Minnesota-Duluth Branch Office**
2016 West Superior Street
Duluth, MN 55806
218-625-1400 (Voice/TTY)
erint@accessnorth.net
http://accessnorth.net
Disability Served: various

**Center for Independent Living of Northeastern
Minnesota -Main Office**
Mesabi Mall, 1101 East 37th Street, Suite 25
Hibbing, MN 55746
218-262-6675 (Voice/TTY)
alice@accessnorth.net
http://accessnorth.net
Disability Served: various

Deaf Blind Services
2344 Nicollet Avenue, #420
Minneapolis, MN 55404
612-871-4788
Disability Served: hearing, vision

**Freedom Resource Center for Independent
Living Inc.**
125 West Lincoln, #17
Fergus Falls, MN 56537
218-998-1799
kerians@freedomrc.org
http://www.freedomrc.org
Disability Served: various

Independence Crossroads Inc.
8932 Old Cedar Avenue South
Bloomington, MN 55425
612-854-8004
Disability Served: various

Independent Lifestyles Inc.
519 Second Street North
Saint Cloud, MN 56303
320-529-9000 (Voice/TTY)
CaraR@IndependentLifestyles.org
http://independentlifestyles.org
Disability Served: various

Metropolitan Center for Independent Living Inc.
1600 University Avenue West, Suite 16
St. Paul, MN 55104
651-646-8342
mcil@mcil-mn.org
 http://frontpage.mcil-mn.org/
Disability Served: various

OPTIONS, Interstate Resource Center for Independent Living
318 Third Street, NW
East Grand Forks, MN 56721
218-773-6100
randy@myoptions.info
 http://www.macil.org/options.html
Disability Served: various

Southeastern Minnesota Center for Independent Living Inc.-Red Wing Office
217 Plum Street
Red Wing, MN 55066
651-388-0466
semcil.uhhc@semcil.org
http://www.semcil.org
Disability Served: various

Southeastern Minnesota Center for Independent Living-Rochester Office
2720 North Broadway
Rochester, MN 55906
507-285-1815, 888-460-1815
semcil.uhhc@semcil.org
http://www.semcil.org
Disability Served: various

Southeastern Minnesota Center for Independent Living Inc.-Winona Office
1790 West Broadway
Winona, MN 55987
507-452-5490
semcil.luminet.net
http://www.semcil.org
Disability Served: various

Southern Minnesota Independent Living Enterprises and Services Inc.
709 South Front Street
Mankato, MN 56001
507-345-7139 (Voice/TTY)
smiles@smilescil.org
http://www.smilescil.org
Disability Served: various

Southwestern Center for Independent Living
109 South Fifth Street, Suite 700
Marshall, MN 56258
507-532-2221, 800-422-1485 (Voice/TTY)
swcil@swcil.com
http://www.swcil.com
Disability Served: various

Vinland Center
PO Box 308
Loretto, MN 55357-0308
763-479-3555
http://www.vinlandcenter.org
Disability Served: various

MISSISSIPPI
Gulf Coast Independent Living Center
18 John M. Taturn Industrial Drive
Hattiesburg, MS 39401
601-544-4860
Disability Served: various

LIFE of Mississippi-Biloxi Office
188 C Main Street
Biloxi, MS 39530
228-435-5433
http://www.lifeofms.com
Disability Served: various

LIFE of Mississippi-Greenwood Office
502-A West Park Avenue
Greenwood, MS 38930
662-453-9940
http://www.lifeofms.com
Disability Served: various

LIFE of Mississippi-Hattiesburg Office
710 Katie Avenue
Hattiesburg, MS 39401
601-583-2108

http://www.lifeofms.com
Disability Served: various

LIFE of Mississippi-Main Office
754 North President Street
Jackson, MS 39202
601-969-4009, 800-748-9398
http://www.lifeofms.com
Disability Served: various

LIFE of Mississippi-McComb Office
PO Box 545
McComb, MS 39649
601-684-3079
http://www.lifeofms.com
Disability Served: various

LIFE of Mississippi-Meridian Office
2440 North Hill Street, Suite 103C
Meridian, MS 39305
601-485-799
http://www.lifeofms.com
Disability Served: various

LIFE of Mississippi-Oxford Office
1914 East University Avenue
Oxford, MS 38655
662-234-7010
http://www.lifeofms.com
Disability Served: various

LIFE of Mississippi-Tupelo Office
1051 Cliff Gookin Boulevard
Tupelo, MS 38801
662-844-6633
http://www.lifeofms.com
Disability Served: various

MISSOURI

Access II Independent Living Center
611 West Johnson
Gallatin, MO 64640
660-663-2423, 660-663-2517 (TTY)
access@accessii.org
http://www.accessii.org
Disability Served: various

Bootheel Area Independent Living Services
900 South Bypass, PO Box 326
Kennett, MO 63857

573-888-0036 (Voice/TTY)
tshaw@bails.org
http://www.bails.org
Disability Served: various

Disability Resource Association
420B South Truman Boulevard
Crystal City, MO 63019
636-931-7696
dra@resourceassoiation.org
http://www.disabilityresourceassociation.org
Disability Served: various

Independent Living Center Inc.
1001 East 32nd
Joplin, MO 64804
417-659-8086 (Voice/TTY)
tilc@ilcenter.org
http://www.ilcenter.org
Disability Served: various

Independent Living Resource Center
3620 West Truman Boulevard
Jefferson City, MO 65109
573-556-0400
ilrcjcmo@earthlink.nc
http://www.ilrcjcmo.org
Disability Served: various

Life Skills Foundation
10176 Corporate Square Drive, Suite 100
St. Louis, MO 63132-2924
314-567-7705, 314-802-5299 (TDD)
http://www.lifeskills-stl.org
Disability Served: various

Midland Empire Resources for Independent Living
4420 South 40th Street
St. Joseph, MO 64503
816-279-8558, 816-279-4943 (TTY)
meril@meril.org
http://www.meril.org
Disability Served: various

NorthEast Independent Living Services
109 Virginia, Suite 560
Hannibal, MO 63401
573-221-8282 (Voice/TTY)
neils@nemonet.com
http://www.neilscenter.org
Disability Served: various

Ozark Independent Living
109 Aid Avenue
West Plains, MO 65775
417-257-0038, 888-440-7500 (TTY)
ozark@townsqr.com
http://users.townsqr.com/ozark
Disability Served: various

Paraquad Inc.
311 North Lindbergh Boulevard
St. Louis, MO 63141
314-567-1558, 314-567-5552 (TTY)
paraquad@paraquad.org
http://www.paraquad.org
Disability Served: various

Places for People Inc.
4130 Lindell Boulevard
St. Louis, MO 63108
314-535-5600
contact@placesforpeople.org
http://placesforpeople.org
Disability Served: mental health

Rehabilitation Institute of Kansas City
3011 Baltimore
Kansas City, MO 64108
816-751-7700
http://www.rehabkc.org
Disability Served: various

Rural Advocates for Independent Living
715 South Baltimore
Kirksville, MO 63501
660-627-7245, 800-681-7245
ritt@kvmo.net
http://www.nemr.net/~ritt
Disability Served: various

SEMO Alliance for Disability Independence Inc.
121 South Broadview, Suite 12
Cape Girardeau, MO 63703
573-651-6464 (Voice/TTY)
miki@mail.sadi.org
http://www.sadi.org
Disability Served: various

Services for Independent Living
1401 Hathman Place
Columbia, MO 65201

573-874-1646, 573-874-412l (TTY)
sil@silcolumbia.org
http://www.silcolumbia.org
Disability Served: various

Southwest Center for Independent Living
2864 South Nettleton Avenue
Springfield, MO 65807-5970
417-886-1188 (Voice/TTY)
scil@swcil.org
http://www.swcil.org
Disability Served: various

Tri-County Center for Independent Living
1420 Highway 72 East
Rolla, MO 65401
573-368-5933
tricil3@rollanet.org
http://www.tricountycenter.com
Disability Served: various

West-Central Independent Living Solutions
123 East Gay, Suite A1
Warrensburg, MO 64093
660-422-7883, 660-422-7894 (TTY)
wils@iland.net
http://www.w-ils.org
Disability Served: various

Whole Person Inc.-Kansas City Office
301 East Armour Boulevard, Suite 430
Kansas City, MO 64111
816-561-0304, 816-931-2202 (TTY)
Info@TheWholePerson.Org
http://www.thewholeperson.org
Disability Served: various

MONTANA
Living Independently for Today and Tomorrow Inc.
914 Wyoming Avenue
Billings, MT 59101
406-259-5181, 800-669-6319
daves@liftt.org
http://www.liftt.org
Disability Served: various

Montana Independent Living Project
PO Box 5415
Helena, MT 59604

406-442-5755
Disability Served: various

North Central Independent Living Services
1120 25th Avenue NE
Black Eagle, MT 59414
406-452-9834
Disability Served: various

Summit Independent Living Center
700 Southwest Higgins, Suite 101
Missoula, MT 59803
406-728-1630, 800-398-9002
sbushell@summitilc.org
http://www.summitilc.org
Disability Served: various

NEBRASKA
Center for Independent Living of Central Nebraska Inc.-Grand Island Office
3204 College Street
Grand Island, NE 68803-1730
308-382-9255, 308-382-9255 (TTY)
scook@cilne.org
http://www.cilne.org
Disability Served: various

Center for Independent Living of Central Nebraska Inc.-North Platte Office
1905 West A Street
North Platte, NE 69103
308-535-9930 (Voice/TTY)
ibritt@kdsi.net
http://www.cilne.org
Disability Served: various

League of Human Dignity-Lincoln Office
1701 P Street
Lincoln, NE 68508-1741
402-441-7871, 888-508-4758
info@leagueofhumandignity.com
http://www.leagueofhumandignity.com
Disability Served: various

League of Human Dignity-Norfolk Office
400 Elm Avenue
Norfolk, NE 68701
402-371-4475
Ninfo@leagueofhumandignity.com

http://www.leagueofhumandignity.com
Disability Served: various

League of Human Dignity-Omaha Office
5513 Center Street
Omaha, NE 68106
402-595-1256
Oinfo@leagueofhumandignity.com
http://www.leagueofhumandignity.com
Disability Served: various

NEVADA
Nevada Association for the Handicapped
6200 West Oakey
Las Vegas, NV 89102
702-870-7050
http://www.tyro.com/nah
Disability Served: various

Northern Nevada Center For Independent Living-Elko Office
350 West Silver Drive
Elko, NV 89801
775-753-4300
elkonncil@citlink.net
Disability Served: various

Northern Nevada Center For Independent Living-Fallon Office
1919 Grimes Street, Suite B
Fallon, NV 89406
775-423-4900
nncilf@cccomm.net
Disability Served: various

Northern Nevada Center For Independent Living-Sparks Office
999 Pyramid Way
Sparks, NV 89431
702-353-3599
Disability Served: various

Southern Nevada Center For Independent Living
6039 Eldora Avenue, Suite H-8
Las Vegas, NV 89146
702-889-4574
sncilnv@aol.com
http://www.sncil.org
Disability Served: various

NEW HAMPSHIRE
Granite State Independent Living Foundation
21 Chenell Drive
Concord, NH 03301
603-228-9680, 800-826-3700
http://www.gsil.org
Disability Served: various

NEW JERSEY
Camden Independent Living Center
2600 Mt. Ephraim Avenue, Suite 415
Camden, NJ 08104
856-966-0800, 856-966-0830 (TTY)
Disability Served: various

Center for Independent Living of South Jersey
1200 Delsea Drive, Suite 6
Westville, NJ 08093
609-853-6490, 973-532-2521 (TTY)
Disability Served: various

DAWN Inc.
400 South Main Street, Suite 3
Wharton, NJ 07885
973-361-5666, 888-383-DAWN
info@dawninc.org
http://www.dawninc.org
Disability Served: various

DIAL Inc.
66 Mt Prospect Avenue, Building C-1
Clifton, NJ 07013-1918
973-470-8090, 973-470-2521
info@dial-cil.org
http://www.dial-cil.org
Disability Served: various

**Heightened Independence and Progress-
    Bergen County Office**
131 Main Street, Suite 120
Hackensack, NJ 07601
201-996-9100, 201-996-9424 (TDD)
ber@hipcil.org
http://www.hipcil.org
Disability Served: various

**Heightened Independence and Progress-
    Hudson County Office**
26 Journal Square, Suite 602
Jersey City, NJ 07306

201-533-4407, 201-533-4409 (TDD)
hud@hipcil.org
http://www.hipcil.org
Disability Served: various

MOCEANS Center for Independent Living Inc.
279 Broadway, 2nd Floor
Long Branch, NJ 07740
732-571-4884, 732-571-4878 (TTY)
moceans@moceans.org
http://www.moceans.org
Disability Served: various

Resources for Independent Living in New Jersey
351 High Street, Suite 103
Burlington, NJ 08016
609-747-7745, 609-747-1875 (TTY)
info@rilnj.org
http://www.rilnj.org
Disability Served: various

Total Living Center Inc.
402A Whitehorsepike
Egg Harbor City, NJ 08215
609-965-3734, 609-965-5390 (TDD)
Disability Served: various

NEW MEXICO
Independent Living Resource Center
4401 B Lomas, NE
Albuquerque, NM 87110
505-266-5022
MoriartyILRC@aol.com
Disability Served: various

New Vistas Adult Services
1205 Parkway Drive, Suite A
Santa Fe, NM 87504
505-471-1001, 800-737-0330
http://www.newvistas.org
Disability Served: various

San Juan Center for Independence
3535 East 30th
Farmington, NM 87402
505-566-5827, 505-566-5827 (TDD)
http://www.sjci.org
Disability Served: various

Southern New Mexico Center for Independent Living
118 South Downtown Mall, Suite C
Las Cruces, NM 88001-1218
505-526-5016
Disability Served: various

NEW YORK

Access to Independence and Mobility
271 East First Street
Corning, NY 14830
607-962-8225 (Voice/TTY)
corning@aimcil.com
http://www.aimcil.com
Disability Served: various

Action Toward Independence Inc.
2927 Route 6
Slate Hill, NY 10973
914-355-2030 (Voice/TTY)
ati@warwick.net
http://www.angelfire.com/ny/ADVOCATE
Disability Served: various

ARISE Center for Independent Living
635 James Street
Syracuse, NY 13203
315-472-3171, 315-479-6363 (TTY)
advocate@ariseinc.org
http://www.ariseinc.org
Disability Served: various

Barrier Free Living
270 East Second Street
New York, NY 10009
212-677-6668 (Voice/TTY)
angelc@bflnyc.org
http://www.charityadvantage.com/barrierfreeliving/
    Home.asp
Disability Served: various

Bronx Independent Living Services
3525 Decatur Avenue
Bronx, NY 10467
718-515-2800
info@bils.org
http://www.bils.org
Disability Served: various

Brooklyn Center for Independence
2044 Ocean Avenue, Suite B3
Brooklyn, NY 11230
718-998-3000, 718-998-7406 (TTY)
zjama@bcid.org
http://www.bcid.org
Disability Served: various

Capital District Center for Independence
855 Central Avenue, Suite 110
Albany, NY 12206
518-459-6422 (Voice/TDD)
cdci@nobleharbor.com
http://www.cdciweb.com
Disability Served: various

Catskills Center for Independence
6104 State Highway 23
Oneonta, NY 13820
607-432-8000 (Voice/TTY)
ccfi@ccfi.us
http://www.ccfi.us
Disability Served: various

Center for Independence of the Disabled in New York
841 Broadway, Room 205
New York, NY 10003
212-674-2300
http://www.cidny.org
Disability Served: various

Directions in Independent Living
512 West State Street
Olean, NY 14760
716-373-4602
oleanilc@yahoo.com
Disability Served: various

Finger Lakes Independence Center
215 Fifth Street
Ithaca, NY 14850
607-272-2433 (Voice/TTY)
flic@clarityconnect.com
http://www.fliconline.org
Disability Served: various

Genesee Region Independent Living Center
61 Swan Street
Batavia, NY 14020

585-343-4524 (Voice/TTY)
grilc@freenet.buffalo.edu
http://bfn.org/~grilc
Disability Served: various

Glens Falls Independent Living Center
71 Glenwood Avenue
Queensbury, NY 12804
518-792-3537, 518-792-0505 (TDD)
gfilc@adelphia.net
http://www.gfilc.com
Disability Served: various

Harlem Independent Living Center
5-15 West 125th Street
New York, NY 10027
212-369-2371, 212 369-6475 (TTY)
HarlemILC@aol.com
http://www.retrofit.net/HILC/index.shtml
Disability Served: various

Independent Living Inc.
5 Washington Terrace
Newburgh, NY 12550-5338
914-565-1162 (Voice/TTY)
Disability Served: various

Independent Living of the Hudson Valley
49 Fourth Street
Troy, NY 12180
518-274-0701
admin@ilchv.org
http://www.ilchv.org
Disability Served: various

Long Island Center for Independent Living Inc.
3601 Hempstead Turnpike, Suite 312
Levittown, NY 11756
516-796-0144, 516-796-0135 (TTY)
licil@aol.com
http://www.licil.net
Disability Served: various

Massena Independent Living Center
156 Center Street
Massena, NY 13662
315-764-9442
milc@northnet.org
Disability Served: various

Nassau County Office for the Physically Challenged
1550 Franklin Avenue
Mineola, NY 11501
516-535-3147
Disability Served: physically disabled

Native American Independent Living Services
3108 Main Street
Buffalo, NY 14214
716-836-0822
info@wnyilp.org
http://www.wnyilp.org/NAILS/NAILS.html
Disability Served: various

Niagara Frontier Center for Independent Living
1522 Main Street
Niagara Falls, NY 14305-2522
716-284-2452
nfcil@iname.com
Disability Served: various

North Country Center for Independent Living
102 Sharron Avenue
Plattsburgh, NY 12901-1837
518-563-9058 (Voice/TTY)
andrew@ncci-online.com
http://www.ncci-online.com
Disability Served: various

Northern Regional Center for Independent Living
165 Mechanic Street
Watertown, NY 13601-2711
315-785-8703, 315-785-8704 (TTY)
aileeng@nrcil.net
http://www.nrcil.net
Disability Served: various

Options for Independence Inc.
75 Genesee Street
Auburn, NY 13021
315-255-3447 (Voice/TTY), 800-496-9148
options@optionsforindependence.org
http://www.optionsforindependence.org
Disability Served: various

Putnam Independent Living Services
1961 Route 6, 2nd Floor
Carmel, NY 10512
845-228-7457, 845-228-7459 (TTY)

http://www.putnamils.org
Disability Served: various

Queens Independent Living Center
140-40 Queens Boulevard
Jamaica, NY 11435
718-658-2526, 718-658-4720 (TTY)
aliberti@qilc.org
http://qilc.org
Disability Served: various

Regional Center for Independent Living
1641 East Avenue
Rochester, NY 14610
585-442-6470 (Voice/TTY)
http://www.rcil.org
Disability Served: various

Resource Center for Accessible Living Inc.
592 Ulster Avenue
Kingston, NY 12401
845-331-0541
RCAL@hvc.rr.com
http://www.rcal.org
Disability Served: various

Resource Center for Independent Living-Amsterdam
2540 Riverfront Center
Amsterdam, NY 12010
518-842-3561, 518-842-3593 (TTY)
Rodriguez@RCIL.com
http://www.RCIL.com
Disability Served: various

Rockland Independent Living Center
230 North Main Street
Spring Valley, NY 10977-4001
845-426-0707, 845-426-1180 (TTY)
mail@rilc.org
http://www.rilc.org
Disability Served: various

Southern Tier Independence Center
24 Prospect Avenue, 5th Floor
Binghamton, NY 13901
607-724-2111 (Voice/TTY)
mdibble@stic-cil.org
http://www.stic-cil.org
Disability Served: various

Southwestern Independent Living Center Inc.
843 North Main Street
Jamestown, NY 14701
716-661-3010, 716-661-3012 (TDD)
info@ilc-jamestown-ny.org
http://www.ilc-jamestown-ny.org
Disability Served: various

Staten Island Center for Independent Living Inc.
470 Castleton Avenue
Staten Island, NY 10301
718-720-9016, 718-720-9870 (TTY)
dorothy.doran@verizon.net
http://www.geocities.com/siciliving
Disability Served: various

Taconic Resources for Independence
82 Washington Street, Suite 214
Poughkeepsie, NY 12601
845-452-3913, 845-485-8110 (TTY)
trionline@taconicresources.net
http://www.taconicresources.net
Disability Served: various

Visions/Services for the Blind and Visually Impaired
500 Greenwich Street, 3rd Floor
New York, NY 10013
212-625-1616
Info@visionsvcb.org
http://www.visionsvcb.org
Disability Served: vision

Westchester Disabled on the Move
984 North Broadway, Suite L-1
Yonkers, NY 10701
914-968-4717 (Voice/TDD)
info@wdom.org
http://wdom.org
Disability Served: various

Westchester Independent Living Center Inc.
200 Hamilton Avenue, 2nd Floor
White Plains, NY 10607
914-682-3926, 914-682-0926 (TDD)
http://www.wilc.org
Disability Served: various

Western New York Independent Living Project Inc.
3108 Main Street
Buffalo, NY 14214

716-836-0822 (Voice/TDD)
info@wnyilp.org
http://www.wnyilp.org
Disability Served: various

NORTH CAROLINA
Joy A. Shabazz Center for Independent Living
235 North Greene Street
Greensboro, NC 27401
336-272-0501 (Voice/TDD)
Disability Served: various

Live Independently Networking Center
PO Box 1135
Newton, NC 28658
704-464-0331
Disability Served: various

Pathways for the Future
525 Mineral Springs Drive
Sylva, NC 28779
828-631-1167 (Voice/TTY)
bdaivis@pathwayscil.org
http://www.pathwayscil.org
Disability Served: various

Programs for Accessible Living
Doctor's Building, 1012 South King Drive, G-2
Charlotte, NC 28283
704-375-3977
Disability Served: various

NORTH DAKOTA
**Dakota Center for Independent Living-
  Bismarck Branch Office**
3111 East Broadway Avenue
Bismarck, ND 58501
701-222-3636 (Voice/TTY), 800-489-5013
bobg@dakotacil.org
http://www.dakotacil.org
Disability Served: various

**Dakota Center For Independent Living-
  Dickinson Branch Office**
40 First Avenue West, Park Square Mall
Dickinson, ND 58601
701-483-4363
kimdcil@ndsupernet.com

http://www.dakotacil.org
Disability Served: various

Fraser Ltd.
2902 South University Drive
Fargo, ND 58103
701-223-3301
fraser@fraserltd.org
http://www.fraserltd.org
Disability Served: various

Freedom Resource Center For Independent Living
2701 Ninth Avenue, SW
Fargo, ND 58103
701-478-0459 (Voice/TTY)
freedom@freedomrc.org
http://www.freedomrc.org
Disability Served: various

OHIO
**Ability Center of Greater Toledo-
  Defiance Branch Office**
1935 East Second Street
Defiance, OH 43512
419-782-5441 (Voice/TTY), 877-209-8336
knoe@abilitycenter.org
http://www.abilitycenter.org
Disability Served: various

Ability Center of Greater Toledo-Main Office
5605 Monroe Street
Sylvania, OH 43560
419-885-5733, 419-885-5733 (TTY)
sitemail@abilitycenter.org
http://www.abilitycenter.org
Disability Served: various

**Ability Center of Greater Toledo-
  Ottawa County Office**
400 West Third Street
Port Clinton, OH 43452
419-734-0330
mvanhoose@abilitycenter.org
http://www.abilitycenter.org
Disability Served: various

Access Center for Independent Living Inc.
35 South Jefferson Street
Dayton, OH 45402

937-341-5202
ryan@acils.com
http://www.acils.com
Disability Served: various

HELP Foundation
3622 Prospect Avenue
East Cleveland, OH 44115
216-432-4810
dwillis@helpfoundationinc.org
http://www.helpfoundationinc.org
Disability Served: various

Independent Living Center of North Central Ohio
1 Marion Avenue, Suite 115C
Mansfield, OH 44903
419-526-6770
Disability Served: various

Independent Living Options
632 Vine Street, Suite 601
Cincinnati, OH 45202
513-241-2600, 513-241-7170 (TTY)
cilo@cilo.com
http://www.cilo.net
Disability Served: various

MOBILE Inc. (Mid-Ohio Board for an Independent Living Environment Inc.
690 South High Street
Columbus, OH 43206
614-443-5936, 614-443-5957 (TTY)
bev@mobileonline.org
http://www.mobileonline.org
Disability Served: various

Services for Independent Living
25100 Euclid Avenue, Suite 105
Cleveland, OH 44117-2650
216-731-1529
Disability Served: various

Society for Equal Access Independent Living Center Inc.
821 Anola Avenue, Suite B
Dover, OH 44622
330-343-3668, 888-213-4452
http://web.tusco.net/seailc
Disability Served: various

Southeastern Ohio Center for Independent Living
418 South Broad Street
Lancaster, OH 43130
740-689-1494 (Voice/TTY), 888-957-6245
socil@sbcglobal.net
http://www.socil.org
Disability Served: various

Tri-County Independent Living Center Inc.
680 East Market Street, Suite 205
Akron, OH 44304
330-762-0007
http://www.tcilc.org
Disability Served: various

United Cerebral Palsy of Central Ohio
440 Industrial Mile Road
Columbus, OH 43228-2411
614-279-0109
tfitch@ucpofcentralohio.org
http://www.ucpofcentralohio.org
Disability Served: various

OKLAHOMA

Ability Resources
823 South Detroit Avenue, Suite 110
Tulsa, OK 74120
918-592-1235, 800-722-0886
clawson@ability-resources.org
http://www.ability-resources.org
Disability Served: various

Green County Independent Living Resource Center
4100 Southeast Adams Road, Suite C-106
Bartlesville, OK 74006
918-335-1314, 800-559-0567
vilesja@bartnet.net
Disability Served: various

Oklahomans for Independent Living
321 South Third, Suite 2
McAlester, OK 74501
918-426-6220 (Voice/TDD)
http://www.oil.cwis.net
Disability Served: various

Progressive Independence Inc.
121 North Porter Avenue
Norman, OK 73071

405-321-3203 (Voice/TDD)
jhughcs@progind.org
http://www.progind.org
Disability Served: various

Sandra Beasley Independent Living Center
705 South Oakwood Road, Suite B-1
Enid, OK 73703
580-237-8508, 800-375-4358
sbilcenter@coxinet.net
http://members.tripod.com/%7ELew_3/index.html
Disability Served: various

OREGON
Central Oregon Resources for Independent Living
20436 Clay Pigeon Court
Bend, OR 97702
541-388-8103
coril@coril.org
http://www.coril.org
Disability Served: various

Columbia Gorge Center
2940 Thomsen Road
Hood River, OR 97031
541-386-3520
cgc@gorge.net
http://www.cgc-direct.com
Disability Served: various

Eastern Oregon Center for Independent Living-Ontario Office
1021 Southwest Fifth Avenue
Ontario, OR 97914
541-889-3119 (Voice/TTY), 866-248-8369
eocil@eocil.org
http://www.eocil.org
Disability Served: various

Eastern Oregon Center for Independent Living-Pendleton Office
17 Southwest Frazer, Suite 325
Pendelton, OR 97801
541-235-2224, 866-248-8369
eocil@eocil.org
http://www.eocil.org
Disability Served: various

HASL Independent Abilities Center
1252 Redwood Avenue
Grants Pass, OR 97527

541-479-4275
hasl1@qwest.net
Disability Served: various

Independent Living Resources Inc.
2410 Southeast 11th Avenue
Portland, OR 97215
503-232-7411, 503-232-8408 (TTY)
ilrpdx@qwest.net
http://www.ilr.org
Disability Served: various

SPOKES Unlimited
415 Main Street
Klamath Falls, OR 97601
541-883-7547 (Voice/TTY)
info@spokesunlimited.org
http://www.spokesunlimited.org
Disability Served: various

PENNSYLVANIA
Abilities in Motion
416 Blair Avenue
Reading, PA 19601
610-376-0010, 888-376-0120, 610-288-2301 (TTY)
staff@abilitiesinmotion.org
http://www.abilitiesinmotion.org
Disability Served: various

Allied Services for the Handicapped
100 Abington Executive Park
Clarks Summit, PA 18411
570-348-1300, 570-348-1240 (TDD)
ngonde@allied-services.org
http://www.allied-services.org
Disability Served: various

Anthracite Region Center for Independent Living
44 West Broad Street
Hazelton, PA 18201
570-455-9800 (Voice/TTY), 800-777-9906
arcil@intergrafix.net
http://www.anthracitecil.org
Disability Served: various

Brian's House Inc.
1300 South Concord
West Chester, PA 19382
610-399-1175

http://www.brianshouse.org
Disability Served: various

Center for Independent Living of Central Pennsylvania

207 House Avenue, Suite 107
Camp Hill, PA 17011-4906
717-731-1900, 800-323-6060, 717-737-1335 (TTY)
http://www.cilcp.org
Disability Served: various

Center for Independent Living of North Central Pennsylvania

210 Market Street, Suite A
Williamsport, PA 17701-6633
570-327-9070, 800-984-7492
office@cilncp.org
http://www.cilncp.org
Disability Served: various

Center for Independent Living of Southcentral Pennsylvania

1603 Ninth Avenue
Altoona, PA 16602
814-949-1905, 800-237-9009
cilscpa@cilscpa.org
http://www.cilscpa.org
Disability Served: various

Center for Independent Living Opportunities

3450 Industrial Drive
York, PA 17402-9050
717-840-9653, 717-840-9653 (TTY)
cvicki@verizon.net
Disability Served: various

Community Resources for Independence- Main Office

2222 Filmore Avenue
Erie, PA 16506
814-838-7222, 814-838-8115 (TTY)
http://www.crinet.org
Disability Served: various

Community Resources for Independence- Oil City Office

255 Elm Street, Suite 1
Oil City, PA 16301
814-678-5052
http://www.crinet.org
Disability Served: various

Community Resources for Independence- Warren Office

Stone Building, 300 Hospital Drive, Rooms 113 & 114
Warren, PA 16365
814-723-5427
http://www.crinet.org
Disability Served: various

Freedom Valley Disability Center

3607 Chapel Road
Newton Square, PA 19073
610-353-6640, 800-427-4754, 610-353-8900 (TDD)
lynnfvdc@msn.com
http://www.fvdc.info
Disability Served: various

Lehigh Valley Center for Independent Living

435 Allentown Drive
Allentown, PA 18103
610-770-9781, 800-495-8245
info@lvcil.org
http://www.lvcil.org
Disability Served: various

Liberty Resources Inc.-Allentown Office

845 Wyoming Street
Allentown, PA 18103
610-432-3880, 888-879-1444, 610-432-3880 (TDD)
LRi@aln.libertyresources.org
http://www.libertyresources.org
Disability Served: various

Liberty Resources Inc.-Philadelphia Office

1341 North Delaware Avenue, Suite 105
Philadelphia, PA 19125
215-634-2000, 888-634-2155
LRInc@libertyresources.org
http://www.libertyresources.org
Disability Served: various

Life and Independence for Today

503 East Arch Street
St. Marys, PA 15857-1779
814-781-3050, 800-341-5438
lift@liftcil.org
http://www.liftcil.org
Disability Served: various

Northeastern Pennsylvania Center for Independent Living

431 Wyoming Avenue, Lower Level
Scranton, PA 18503-1228

570-344-7211, 570-344-5275 (TTY)
nepacilinfo@nepacil.org
http://www.nepacil.org
Disability Served: various

Three Rivers Center for Independent Living-Erie Office
3800 West 12th Street
Erie, PA 16505
814-833-8997, 877-833-8997
erieoffice@trcil.org
http://www.trcil.org
Disability Served: various

**Three Rivers Center for Independent Living-
    Main Office**
900 Rebecca Avenue
Pittsburgh, PA 15208-2434
412-371-7700, 412-371-9230 (TTY)
info@crinet.org
http://www.crinet.org
Disability Served: various

**Three Rivers Center for Independent Living-
    Washington Office**
150 West Beau Street, Suite 217
Washington, PA 15301
724-222-2910, 866-401-2910
washoffice@trcil.org
http://www.trcil.org
Disability Served: various

Tri-County Patriots for Independent Living
69 East Beau Street
Washington, PA 15301
412-223-5115, 724-228-4028 (TDD)
http://www.tripil.com
Disability Served: various

Voices for Independence
3711 West 12th Street
Erie, PA 16505
814-838-3702 (Voice/TTY)
vfi@voicesforindependence.org
http://www.voicesforindependence.org
Disability Served: various

RHODE ISLAND
Ocean State Center for Independent Living
1944 Warwick Avenue
Warwick, RI 02889

401-738-1013, 866-857-1161
oscil@oscil.org
http://www.oscil.org
Disability Served: various

PARI Independent Living Center
500 Prospect Street
Pawtucket, RI 02860
401-725-1966 (Voice/TTY)
info@pari-ilc.org
http://www.pari-ilc.org
Disability Served: various

SOUTH CAROLINA
Disability Action Center-Midlands Office
1115 Belleview Street
Columbia, SC 29201
803-779-5121, 803-779-0949 (TTY)
http://www.dacsc.org
Disability Served: various

Disability Action Center-Upstate Office
712 Laurens Road
Greenville, SC 29607
864-235-1421, 803-235-8798 (TTY)
http://www.dacsc.org
Disability Served: various

Walton Options for Independent Living-Aiken Office
Hitchcock Office Park, 33B Varden Drive
Aiken, SC 29803
803-648-2858 (Voice/TTY)
http://www.waltonoptions.org
Disability Served: various

**Walton Options for Independent Living-
    Gloverville Office**
Highway 421
Gloverville, SC 29828
803-593-8545 (Voice/TTY)
http://www.waltonoptions.org
Disability Served: various

SOUTH DAKOTA
Adjustment Training Center Inc.
607 North 4th Street
Aberdeen, SD 57401
605-229-0263
Disability Served: various

Opportunities for Independent Living
1200 South Main Street, Suite A
Aberdeen, SD 57401
605-626-2976, 800-406-2649
gary.oil@midconetwork.com
http://www.oil.org
Disability Served: various

**Prairie Freedom Center for Independent Living
of Sioux Falls**
301 South Garfield Avenue, Suite 8
Sioux Falls, SD 57104
605-339-6558
ccrisp@pfcil.org
Disability Served: various

**Prairie Freedom Center for Independent Living
of Yankton**
413 West 15th, Suite 107
Yankton, SD 57078
605-668-2940 (Voice/TTY)
ccrisp@pfcil.org
Disability Served: various

Western Resources for dis-ABLED Independence
405 East Omaha Street, Suite A
Rapid City, SD 57701
605-718-1930, 888-434-4943
Ann@wrdi.org
http://www.wrdi.org
Disability Served: various

TENNESSEE
Center for Independent Living of Middle Tennessee
480 Craighead Street, Suite 200
Nashville, TN 37204
615-292-5803, 615-292-7790 (TTY/TDD)
http://www.cil-mt.org
Disability Served: various

Jackson Center for Independent Living
1981 Hollywood Drive
Jackson, TN 38305
jcil05-info@yahoo.com
http://www.j-cil.com
Disability Served: various

Memphis Center for Independent Living
1633 Madison Avenue
Memphis, TN 38104

901-726-6404 (Voice/TTY)
mcil@mcil.org
http://www.mcil.org
Disability Served: various

Tri-State Resource and Advocacy Corporation Inc.
Building 5800, 5708 Uptain Road, Suite 350
Chattanooga, TN 37411
423-892-4774
ilctrac@bellsouth.net
http://www.4trac.org
Disability Served: various

TEXAS
ABLE Center for Independent Living
3641 North Dixie Boulevard
Odessa, TX 79762
432-580-3439
ablecil@ableCenter.org
http://ablecenter.org/AbleCenter
Disability Served: various

Austin Resource Center for Independent Living
618 South Guadalupe, #103
San Marcos, TX 78666
512-396-5790, 800-572-2973
sanmarcos@arcil.com
http://www.arcil.com
Disability Served: various

Crockett Resource Center for Independent Living
1020 Loop 304 East
Crockett, TX 75835
409-544-2811, 800-784-8710
crcil@txucom.net
Disability Served: various

Houston Center for Independent Living
7000 Regency Square Boulevard, #160
Houston, TX 77036-3209
713-974-4621
hcil@neosoft.com
http://www.coalitionforbarrierfreeliving.com
Disability Served: various

Independent Living Research Utilization
2323 South Shepherd, Suite 1000
Houston, TX 77019
713-520-0232 (Voice/TTY)
ilru@ilru.org

http://www.ilru.org
Disability Served: various

LIFE/RUN Centers for Independent Living
4902 34th Street, Suite 5
Lubbock, TX 79410
806-795-5433
wilmacrain@yahoo.com
http://www.liferun.org
Disability Served: various

**Panhandle Action Center for Independent Living
Skills**
3608 South Washington Street
Amarillo, TX 79110
806-352-1500
Disability Served: various

**REACH Resource Centers on Independent Living-
Dallas Office**
8625 King George, Suite 210
Dallas, TX 75235-2286
214-630-4796
reachdallas@reachcils.org
http://www.reachcils.org
Disability Served: various

**REACH Resource Centers on Independent Living-
Denton Office**
405 South Elm, Suite 202
Denton, TX 76201-6068
940-383-1062 (Voice/TTY)
reachden@reachcils.org
http://www.reachcils.org
Disability Served: various

**REACH Resource Centers on Independent Living-
Ft. Worth Office**
1205 Lake Street
Ft Worth, TX 76102-4501
817-870-9082
reachftw@reachcils.org
http://www.reachcils.org
Disability Served: various

San Antonio Independent Living Services
1028 South Alamo
San Antonio, TX 78210
210-281-1878
SAILS@swbell.net

http://www.sailstx.org
Disability Served: various

UTAH
OPTIONS for Independence
1095 North Main
Logan, UT 84341
435-753-5353
jbiggs@optionsind.org
http://www.optionsind.org
Disability Served: various

Redrock Center for Independence
515 West 300 North, #A
St. George, UT 84770
435-673-7501
rrci@rrci.org
http://www.rrci.org
Disability Served: various

Tri-County Independent Living Center of Utah
2726 Washington Boulevard
Ogden, UT 84401
801-612-3215, 801-612-3215 (TTY)
vickie@tri-county-ilc.co
http://www.tri-county-ilc.com
Disability Served: various

Utah Independent Living Center
3445 South Main Street
Salt Lake City, UT 84115-4453
801-466-5565, 800-355-2195
uilc@xmission.com
http://www.xmission.com/~uilc/main.php3
Disability Served: various

VERMONT
**Vermont Center for Independent Living-
Bennington Office**
532 Main Street
Bennington, VT 05201
802-447-0574 (Voice/TTY)
http://www.vcil.org
Disability Served: various

**Vermont Center for Independent Living-
Brattleboro Office**
167 Main Street, Suite 202
Brattleboro, VT 05301

802-254-6851(Voice/TTY)
http://www.vcil.org
Disability Served: various

Vermont Center for Independent Living-Burlington Office
59-63 Pearl Street
Burlington, VT 05401
802-862-0234 (Voice/TTY)
http://www.vcil.org
Disability Served: various

Vermont Center for Independent Living-Montpelier Office
11 East State Street
Montpelier, VT 05602
802-229-0501, 800-639-1522
http://www.vcil.org
Disability Served: various

VIRGINIA

Access Independence Inc.
403B South Loudoun Street
Winchester, VA 22601
540-662-4452, 540-722-9693 (TTY)
AskAI@accessindependence.org
http://www.accessindependence.org
Disability Served: various

Appalachian Independence Center-Bristol Office
PO Box 16744
Bristol, VA 24209
276-466-0567 (Voice/TTY)
aicadmin@ntelos.net
http://www.aicadvocates.org
Disability Served: various

Appalachian Independence Center-Galax Office
104 Rex Lane
Galax, VA 24333
276-236- 6055 (Voice/TTY)
aicadmin@ntelos.net
http://www.aicadvocates.org
Disability Served: various

Appalachian Independence Center-Main Office
230 Charwood Drive
Abingdon, VA 24210

276-628-2979, 276-676-0920 (TTY)
aicadmin@ntelos.net
http://www.aicadvocates.org
Disability Served: various

Appalachian Independence Center-Wytheville Office
680 West Main Street, PO Box 1073
Wytheville, VA 24382
276-228-8765 (Voice/TTY)
aicadmin@ntelos.net
http://www.aicadvocates.org
Disability Served: various

Blue Ridge Independent Living Center
1502-B Williamson Road, NE, Suite B
Roanoke, VA 24012
540-342-1231
brilc@brilc.org
http://www.brilc.org
Disability Served: various

Endependence Center Inc.
6320 North Center Drive, 15 Koger Center, Suite 100
Norfolk, VA 23502
757-461-8007, 757-461-7527 (TDD)
ecimain@whro.net
http://sites.communitylink.org/eci
Disability Served: various

Independence Resource Center
815 Cherry Avenue
Charlottesville, VA 22903
804-971-9629 (Voice/TTY)
tvandever@ntelos.net
Disability Served: various

Peninsula Center for Independent Living
2021-A Cunningham Drive, Suite 2
Hampton, VA 23666
757-827-0275, 757-827- 8800 (TDD)
youremail@yourdomain.com
http://www.iepcil.org
Disability Served: various

Resources for Independent Living Inc.
4009 Fitzhugh Avenue
Richmond, VA 23230
804-353-6503, 804-353-6583 (TTY)
Woodsonf@cavtel.net
Disability Served: various

Woodrow Wilson Center for Independent Living
PO Box 1500
Fishersville, VA 22939
540-332-7390, 800-345-9972
colemawl@wwrc.state.va.us
http://wwrc.virginia.gov
Disability Served: various

WASHINGTON

Center for Independence
325 East Pioneer Avenue
Puyallup, WA 98372
253-435-8490, 253-845-3174 (TTY)
cfi@goodsamhealth.org
Disability Served: various

Community Services Center for the Deaf and Hard of Hearing
1609 19th Avenue
Seattle, WA 98122
206-322-4996 (Voice/TTY)
sbernick@cscdhh.org
http://cscdhh.org
Disability Served: hearing

Designs for Independent Living
819 South Hatch
Spokane, WA 99202
509-535-9696
Disability Served: various

Epilepsy Association Northwest
3800 Aurora Avenue North, Suite 370
Seattle, WA 98103
206-547-4551
mail@epilepsyfoundationnw.org
Disability Served: epilepsy

Greater Lakes Mental Health Care Access Center
9330 59th Avenue, SW
Lakewood, WA 98499-6600
253-581-7020
http://www.glmhc.org
Disability Served: various

Independent Lifestyle Services
109 East 3rd, Suite 2
Ellensburg, WA 98926

509-962-9620
Disability Served: various

Independent Living Service Center
607 Southeast Everett Mall, Suite E
Everett, WA 98208
425-347-5768, 800-315-3583
ilsc@richpoor.net
Disability Served: various

Lilac Blind Foundation
1212 North Howard Street
Spokane, WA 99201
509-328-9116, 800-422-7893
info@lilacblindfoundation.org
http://www.lilacblindfoundation.org
Disability Served: vision

Tacoma Area Coalition of Individuals with Disabilities
6315 South 19th Street
Tacoma, WA 98466
253-565-9000, 253-565-5445 (TTY)
tacid@tacid.org
http://www.tacid.org
Disability Served: various

Washington Coalition of Citizens with Disabilities
4649 Sunnyside North, Suite 100
Seattle, WA 98103
206-545-7055, 866-545-7055
info@wccd.org
http://www.wccd.org
Disability Served: various

WEST VIRGINIA
Appalachian Center for Independent Living
Elk Office Center, 4710 Chimney Drive, Suite C
Charleston, WV 25302
304-965-0376, 800-642-3003 (TDD)
acil@yahoo.com
Disability Served: various

Mountain State Centers for Independent Living-Beckley Office
329 Prince Street
Beckley, WV 25801
304-255-0122, 304-255-0122 (TDD)

kmaynus@mtstcil.org
http://www.mtstcil.org
Disability Served: various

Mountain State Centers for Independent Living-Huntington Office
821 Fourth Avenue
Huntington, WV 25701
304-525-3324, 866-MTSTCIL
mtstcil@mtstcil.org
http://www.mtstcil.org
Disability Served: various

Mountain State Centers for Independent Living-Sistersville Office
PO Box 31
Sistersville, WV 26175
304-652-2116, 866-MTSTCIL
bgoodfellow@mtstcil.org
http://www.mtstcil.org
Disability Served: various

Northern West Virginia Center for Independent Living
601-3 East Brockway Avenue, Suites A&B
Morgantown, WV 26501
304-296-6091, 800-834-6408
nwvcil@westco.net
http://www.nwvcil.org
Disability Served: various

WISCONSIN
Access to Independence Inc.
2345 Atwood Avenue
Madison, WI 53704
608-242-8484, 608-242-8485 (TTY)
http://www.accesstoind.org
Disability Served: various

Center for Independent Living for Western Wisconsin Inc.-Main Office
2920 Schneider Avenue East
Menomonie, WI 54751
715-233-1070 (Voice/TTY)
info@cilww.com
http://www.cilww.com
Disability Served: various

Center for Independent Living for Western Wisconsin Inc.-Rice Lake Office
113 North Main Street
Rice Lake, WI 54868
715-736-1800 (Voice/TTY)
info@cilww.com
http://www.cilww.com
Disability Served: various

IndependenceFirst
600 West Virginia Street
Milwaukee, WI 53204
414-291-7520 (Voice/TTY)
dlangham@independencefirst.org
http://www.independencefirst.org
Disability Served: various

Independent Living Program
820 West College Avenue, Suite 5
Appleton, WI 54915
920-997-9999 (Voice/TTY)
Disability Served: various

Independent Living Resources
4439 Mormon Coulee Road
La Crosse, WI 54601
888-474-5745, 888-378-2198 (TTY)
advocacy@ilresources.org
http://www.ilresources.org
Disability Served: various

Inspiration Ministries
Corner State Road 67 and County F, PO Box 948
Walworth, WI 53184-0848
262-275-6131
info@inspirationministries.org
http://inspirationministries.org
Disability Served: various

North Country Independent Living
2231 Catlin Avenue, Suite 16
Superior, WI 54880
715-392-9118 (Voice/TTY), 800-924-1220
nciljeri@superior-nfp.org
http://www.northcountryil.com
Disability Served: various

Options for Independent Living Inc.
555 Country Club Road, PO Box 11967
Green Bay, WI 54308-9517

920-490-0500, 888-465-1515
info@optionsil.com
http://www.optionsil.com
Disability Served: various

WYOMING

**Rehabilitation Enterprises of North Eastern
   Wyoming Inc.-Gillette Office**
623 North Commercial
Gillette, WY 82716
307-686-2125
http://www.renew-wyo.com
Disability Served: various

**Rehabilitation Enterprises of North Eastern
   Wyoming Inc.-Newcastle Office**
35 Fairgrounds Road
Newcastle, WY 82701
307-746-4733
http://www.renew-wyo.com
Disability Served: various

**Rehabilitation Enterprises of North Eastern
   Wyoming Inc.-Sheridan Office**
1969 South Sheridan Avenue
Sheridan, WY 82801
307-672-7481, 888-309-2020
http://www.renew-wyo.com
Disability Served: various

Western Wyoming Center for Independent Living
190 Custer Street
Lander, WY 82520
307-332-4889 (Voice/TTY)
wwcfil@rmisp.com
Disability Served: various

Wyoming Independent Living Rehabilitation Center
305 West First Street
Casper, WY 82601
307-266-6956 (Voice/TTY)
khof@trib.com
http://www.wilr.org
Disability Served: various

CANADA

Breaking Down Barriers
275 First Street, Unit 9
Collingwood, ON L9Y 1A8
Canada

705-445-1543, 705-445-1658 (TDD)
bdb@georgian.net
http://www.breakingdownbarriers.org
Disability Served: various

Centre for Independent Living in Toronto
205 Richmond Street West, Suite 605
Toronto, ON M5V 1V3
Canada
416-599-2458, 416-599-5077 (TTY)
cilt@cilt.ca
http://www.cilt.ca
Disability Served: various

Disability Resource Centre for Independent Living
29 Byng Avenue, Suite 5
Kapuskasing, ON P5N 1W6
Canada
705-335-8778, 800-236-7417
krricl@nt.net
http://www.disabilityresourcecentre.netfirms.com
Disability Served: various

Independent Living Centre
433 King Street, Suite 101
London, ON N6B 3P3
Canada
519-660-4667
http://ilcla.tripod.com
Disability Served: various

Independent Living Centre Kingston
298 Concession Street
Kingston, ON K7K 2C1
Canada
613-542-8353, 613-542-8371 (TTY)
http://www.ilckingston.com
Disability Served: various

Independent Living Centre of Waterloo Region
127 Victoria Street South, Suite 2
Kitchener, ON N2G 2B4
Canada
519-571-6788, 519-571-7590 (TTY)
http://www.ilcwr.org
Disability Served: various

Independent Living Resource Centre
2786 Agricola Street, Suite 212
Halifax, NS B3K 4E1
Canada

902-453-0004 (Voice/TDD)
info@ilrc-halifax.ns.ca
http://www.ilrc-halifax.ns.ca/main.htm
Disability Served: various

Independent Living Resource Centre
4 Escasoni Place
St. John's, NF A1A 3R6
Canada
709-722-4031, 709-722-7998 (TTY)
http://www.ilrc.nf.ca
Disability Served: various

Independent Living Resource Centre
66 Elm Street, Suite 105
Sudbury, ON P3C 1R8
Canada
705-675-2121, 705-675-2121 (TTY)
http://www.ilrcsudbury.ca
Disability Served: various

Independent Living Resource Centre
125 South Syndicate Avenue, Victoriaville Mall, Suite 11
Thunder Bay, ON P7E 6H8
Canada
807-577-6166 (Voice/TTY)
http://www.ilrctbay.com/article/1.asp
Disability Served: various

Independent Living Resource Centre
311A-393 Portage Avenue
Winnipeg, MB R3B 3H6
Canada
204-947-0194 (Voice/TTY), 800-663-3043 (Voice/TTY)
http://www.ilrc.mb.ca
Disability Served: various

Independent Living Resource Centre of Calgary
7 -11 Street, NE
Calgary, AB T2E 4Z2
Canada
403-263 6880
http://www.ilrcc.ab.ca
Disability Served: various

Niagara Center for Independent Living
111 Church Street
St. Catharines, ON L2R 3C9
Canada
905-684-7111, 905-684-0420 (TTY)
http://www.ilcniagara.org
Disability Served: various

North Saskatchewan Independent Living Centre
237 Fifth Avenue, North
Saskatoon, SK S7K 2P2
Canada
306-665-5508
http://www.nsilc.com
Disability Served: various

Ottawa-Carleton Independent Living Center
B010 - 75 Albert Street
Ottawa, ON K1P 5E7
Canada
613-236-2558
http://www.magma.ca/%7Eocilc
Disability Served: various

South Saskatchewan Independent Living Centre
2240 Albert Street
Regina, SK S4P 2V2
Canada
306-757-7452 (Voice/TTY)
info@ssilc.ca
Disability Served: various

LEGAL ASSISTANCE ORGANIZATIONS

These organizations provide legal assistance and advocacy services for persons with disabilities. Some of the agencies are governmental entities that provide protection and advocacy services.

ALABAMA

Alabama Client Assistance Program
2125 East South Boulevard
Montgomery, AL 36116
800-228-3231 (Voice/TDD)
http://www.sacap.org
Disability Served: various

Alabama Disabilities Advocacy Program
PO Box 870395
Tuscaloosa, AL 35487-0395
205-348-4928, 800-826-1675 (Voice/TDD)
adap@adap.ua.edu
http://www.adap.net
Disability Served: various

ALASKA

Alaska Client Assistance Program-Anchorage Office
2900 Boniface Parkway, Suite 100
Anchorage, AK 99504
907-333-2211 (Voice/TTY)
akcap@alaska.com
http://home.gci.net/~alaskacap
Disability Served: various

Alaska Client Assistance Program-Bethel Office
PO Box 1321
Bethel, AK 99559
907-543-3806, 888-393-3805
akcap@alaska.com
http://home.gci.net/~alaskacap
Disability Served: various

Alaska Client Assistance Program-Fairbanks Office
PO Box 70223
Fairbanks, AK 99707
907-457-4576, 800-498-2960
akcap@alaska.com
http://home.gci.net/~alaskacap
Disability Served: various

Alaska Client Assistance Program-Juneau Office
PO Box 32526
Juneau, AK 99803-2526
907-790-3616, 800-966-0047
akcap@alaska.com

http://home.gci.net/~alaskacap
Disability Served: various

Disability Law Center of Alaska-Anchorage Office
3330 Arctic Boulevard, Suite 103
Anchorage, AK 99503
907-565-1002 (Voice/TTY), 800-478-1234 (Voice/TTY)
akpa@dlcak.org
http://www.dlcak.org
Disability Served: various

Disability Law Center of Alaska-Bethel Office
PO Box 2303
Bethel, AK 99559
907-543-3357, 888-557-3357
http://www.dlcak.org
Disability Served: various

Disability Law Center of Alaska-Fairbanks Office
250 Cushman, Suite 3H
Fairbanks, AK 99701
907-456-1070
http://www.dlcak.org
Disability Served: various

Disability Law Center of Alaska-Juneau Office
230 South Franklin, Suite 2
Juneau, AK 99801
907-586-1627
http://www.dlcak.org
Disability Served: various

ARIZONA

Arizona Center for Disability Law-Phoenix Office
3839 North Third Street, Suite 209
Phoenix, AZ 85012
602-274-6287 (Voice/TTY), 800-927-2260 (Voice/TTY)
center@acdl.com
http://www.acdl.com
Disability Served: various

Arizona Center for Disability Law-Tucson Office
100 North Stone Avenue, Suite 305
Tucson, AZ 85701
520-327-9547 (Voice/TTY), 800-922-1447 (Voice/TTY)
center@acdl.com

http://www.acdl.com
Disability Served: various

DNA-People's Legal Services, Inc.
PO Box 306
Window Rock, AZ 86515
928-871-4151
http://www.nativelegalnet.org/Home/PublicWeb/About/
    WhoWeAre
Disability Served: various

ARKANSAS

Disability Rights Center
1100 North University, Suite 201
Little Rock, AR 72207
501-296-1775 (Voice/TTY), 800-482-1174 (Voice/TTY)
panda@arkdisabilityrights.org
http://www.arkdisabilityrights.org
Disability Served: various

CALIFORNIA

California Client Assistance Program
California Department of Rehabilitation
2000 Evergreen Street
Sacramento, CA 95815
800-952-5544 (Voice), 866-712-1085 (TTY)
capinfo@dor.ca.gov
http://www.rehab.cahwnet.gov/cap
Disability Served: various

Disability Rights Advocates
449 15th Street, Suite 303
Oakland, CA 94612-2821
510-451-8644, 510-451-8716 (TTY)
general@dralegal.org
http://www.dralegal.org
Disability Served: various

Disability Rights Education and Defense Fund
2212 Sixth Street
Berkeley, CA 94710
510-644-2555 (Voice/TTY)
dredf@dredf.org
http://www.dredf.org
Disability Served: various

National Center for Youth Law
405 14th Street, 15th Floor
San Francisco, CA 94612-2701

510-835-8098
info@youthlaw.org
http://www.youthlaw.org
Disability Served: various

National Senior Citizens Law Center-
    Los Angeles Office
3435 Wilshire Boulevard, Suite 2860
Los Angeles, CA 90010-1938
213-639-0930
nsclc@nsclc.org
http://www.nsclc.org
Disability Served: elderly

National Senior Citizens Law Center-Oakland Office
405 14th Street, Suite 1400
Oakland, CA 94612
510-663-1055
nsclc@nsclc.org
http://www.nsclc.org
Disability Served: elderly

Protection and Advocacy Inc.-Developmental
    Disability Peer/Self Advocacy
100 Howe Avenue, Suite 200-N
Sacramento, CA 95825
916-488-7787, 916-488-7715 (TTY)
http://www.pai-ca.org
Disability Served: developmentally disabled

Protection and Advocacy Inc.-Los Angeles
    Legal Office
3580 Wilshire Boulevard, Suite 902
Los Angeles, CA 90010
213-427-8747, 800-781-4546 (TTY)
http://www.pai-ca.org
Disability Served: various

Protection and Advocacy Inc.-Oakland Legal Office
433 Hegenberger Road, Suite 220
Oakland, CA 94621
510-430-8033, 800-649-0154 (TTY)
http://www.pai-ca.org
Disability Served: various

Protection and Advocacy Inc.-Office of Clients' Rights
    Advocacy Los Angeles
3580 Wilshire Boulevard, Suite 925
Los Angeles, CA 90010
213-427-8761, 866-833-6712

http://www.pai-ca.org
Disability Served: various

Protection and Advocacy Inc.-Office of Clients' Rights Advocacy Sacramento
100 Howe Avenue, Suite 240-N
Sacramento, CA 95825
916-575-1615, 877-669-6023 (TTY)
http://www.pai-ca.org
Disability Served: various

Protection and Advocacy Inc.-Sacramento Legal Office
100 Howe Avenue, Suite 185-N
Sacramento, CA 95825
916-488-9950, 800-719-5798 (TTY)
http://www.pai-ca.org
Disability Served: various

Protection and Advocacy Inc.-San Diego Legal Office
1111 Sixth Avenue, Suite 200
San Diego, CA 92101
619-239-7861, 800-576-9269 (TTY)
http://www.pai-ca.org
Disability Served: various

COLORADO
Legal Center for People with Disabilities and Older People-Denver Office
455 Sherman Street, Suite 130
Denver, CO 80203-4403
303-722-0300 (Voice/TTY)
tlcmail@thelegalcenter.org
http://www.thelegalcenter.org
Disability Served: various

Legal Center for People with Disabilities and Older People-Grand Junction Office
322 North 8th Street
Grand Junction, CO 81501-3406
970-241-6371 (Voice/TTY)
tlcmail@thelegalcenter.org
http://www.thelegalcenter.org
Disability Served: various

CONNECTICUT
AIDS Legal Network for Connecticut
999 Asylum Avenue
Hartford, CT 06105-2465

860-541-5000, 860-541-5069 (TTY)
http://www.ghla.org/aln
Disability Served: AIDS

Protection and Advocacy for Persons with Disabilities
60B Weston Street
Hartford, CT 06120-1551
860-297-4300, 800-842-7303 (Voice/TTY)
http://www.ct.gov/opapd/site/default.asp
Disability Served: various

DELAWARE
Community Legal Aid Society, Inc.
100 West 10th Street, Suite 801
Wilmington, DE 19801
302-575-0660
http://www.declasi.org/dis.html
Disability Served: various

Delaware Client Assistance Program
254 East Camden-Wyoming Avenue
Camden, DE 19934
800-640-9336
capa2@magpage.com
Disability Served: various

DISTRICT OF COLUMBIA
Equal Employment Opportunity Commission
1801 L Street, NW, Suite 100
Washington, DC 20507
202-419-0700, 202-419-0702 (TTY)
http://www.eeoc.gov
Disability Served: various

Legal Action Center-Washington, DC Office
236 Massachusetts Avenue, NE, Suite 505
Washington, DC 20002-4980
202-544-5478
lacdc@lac.org
http://www.lac.org
Disability Served: AIDS, chemical dependency

National Disability Rights Network
900 Second Street, NE, Suite 211
Washington, DC 20002
202-408-9514
http://napas.org
Disability Served: various

National Senior Citizens Law Center-
Washington Office
1101 14th Street, NW, Suite 400
Washington, DC 20005
202-289-6976
nsclc@nsclc.org
http://www.nsclc.org
Disability Served: elderly

United States Department of Health and Human
Services Office for Civil Rights
HHH Building, 200 Independence Avenue, SW,
Room 509F
Washington, DC 20201
800-368-1019, 800-537-7697 (TDD)
OCRMail@hhs.gov
http://www.hhs.gov/ocr/hipaa
Disability Served: various

United States Department of Justice Civil Rights
Division
950 Pennsylvania Avenue, NW
Washington, DC 20530
800-514-0301, 800-514-0383 (TTY)
http://www.usdoj.gov/crt/ada/adahom1.htm
Disability Served: various

United States Department of Labor
200 Constitution Avenue, NW
Washington, DC 20210
4-USA-DOL, 877-889-5627 (TTY)
http://www.dol.gov
Disability Served: various

FLORIDA

Advocacy Center for Persons with Disabilities Inc.-
South Florida Office
441 Sheridan Street
Hollywood, FL 33021
954-967-1493, 866-478-0640 (TDD)
http://www.advocacycenter.org
Disability Served: various

Advocacy Center for Persons with Disabilities Inc.-
Tallahassee Office
2671 Executive Center Circle West, Suite 100
Tallahassee, FL 32301-5092
850-488-9071, 800-346-4127 (TDD)

http://www.advocacycenter.org
Disability Served: various

Advocacy Center for Persons with Disabilities Inc.-
Tampa Office
1000 North Ashley Drive, Suite 513
Tampa, FL 33602
813-233-2920, 866-875-1837 (TDD)
http://www.advocacycenter.org
Disability Served: various

GEORGIA

Georgia Advocacy Office Inc.
150 East Ponce de Leon Avenue, Suite 430
Decatur, GA 30030
404-885-1234, 800-537-2329
info@thegao.org
http://www.thegao.org
Disability Served: various

Georgia Client Assistance Program
123 North McDonough Street
Decatur, GA 30030
404-373-3116 (Voice/TTY), 800-822-9727 (Voice/TTY)
Disability Served: various

HAWAII

Hawaii Disability Rights Center
900 Fort Street Mall, Suite 1040
Honolulu, HI 96813
800-882-1057
info@hawaiidisabilityrights.org
http://www.hawaiidisabilityrights.org
Disability Served: various

Hawaii Protection and Advocacy Agency
1580 Makaloa Street, Suite 1060
Honolulu, HI 96814
808-949-2922 (Voice/TDD)
pahi@pixi.com
Disability Served: various

IDAHO

Comprehensive Advocacy Inc.-Boise Main Office
4477 Emerald, Suite B-100
Boise, ID 83706
208-336-5353 (Voice/TDD)

coadinc@cableone.net
http://users.moscow.com/co%2Dad
Disability Served: various

Comprehensive Advocacy Inc.-Moscow Field Office
428 West 3rd Street
Moscow, ID 83843
208-882-0962 (Voice/TDD)
co-ad@moscow.com
http://users.moscow.com/co%2Dad
Disability Served: various

Comprehensive Advocacy Inc.-Pocatello Field Office
845 West Center, C107
Pocatello, ID 83204
208-232-0922 (Voice/TDD)
coinc-tdd@qwest.net
http://users.moscow.com/co%2Dad
Disability Served: various

ILLINOIS
AIDS Legal Council of Chicago
188 West Randolph Street, Suite 2400
Chicago, IL 60601
312-427-8990
info@aidslegal.com
http://www.aidslegal.com
Disability Served: AIDS

Council for Disability Rights
30 East Adams, Suite 1130
Chicago, IL 60603
312-444-9484, 312-444-1967 (TDD)
http://www.disabilityrights.org
Disability Served: various

Equip for Equality-Central/Southern Illinois Office
235 South Fifth Street
Springfield, IL 62705
217-544-0464, 800-758-0464, 800-610-2779 (TTY)
http://www.equipforequality.org
Disability Served: various

Equip for Equality-Main/Chicago Office
20 North Michigan Avenue, Suite 300
Chicago, IL 60602
800-537-2632, 800-610-2779 (TTY)
http://www.equipforequality.org
Disability Served: various

Equip for Equality-Northwestern Illinois Office
1617 Second Avenue
Rock Island, IL 61204
309-786-6868, 800-758-6869, 800-610-2779 (TTY)
http://www.equipforequality.org
Disability Served: various

Illinois Client Assistance Program
100 North First Street, First Floor West
Springfield, IL 62702
800-641-3929 (Voice/TTY)
dhscap@dhs.state.il.us
http://www.dhs.state.il.us/ors/cap
Disability Served: various

INDIANA
Indiana Client Assistance Program
4701 North Keystone Avenue, Suite 222
Indianapolis, IN 46205
317-722-5555, 317-722-5563 (TTY)
sbeecher@ipas.state.in.us
http://www.in.gov/ipas/cap.html
Disability Served: various

Indiana Protection and Advocacy Services
4701 North Keystone Avenue, Suite 222
Indianapolis, IN 46205
317-722-5555, 317-722-5563 (TTY)
http://www.state.in.us/ipas
Disability Served: various

IOWA
Iowa Client Assistance Program
Division of Persons with Disabilities, Lucas State
    Office Building
Des Moines, IA 50310
800-652-4298
harlietta.helland@iowa.gov
http://www.state.ia.us/government/dhr/pd/client_assis_
    program
Disability Served: various

Iowa Protection and Advocacy Services Inc.
950 Office Park Road, Suite 221
West Des Moines, IA 50265
515-278-2502, 866-483-3342, 515-278-0571 (TTY)
info@ipna.org

http://www.ipna.org
Disability Served: various

KANSAS
Disability Rights Center of Kansas
3745 Southwest Wanamaker
Topeka, KS 66610
785-273-9661 (Voice/TDD), 877-776-1541 (Voice/TDD)
http://drckansas.org
Disability Served: various

KENTUCKY
Kentucky Client Assistance Program
209 St. Clair Street, 5th Floor
Frankfort, KY 40601
502-564-8035
VickiL.Staggs@.ky.gov
http://kycap.ky.gov
Disability Served: various

Kentucky Protection and Advocacy
100 Fair Oaks Lane, 3rd Floor
Frankfort, KY 40601
502-564-2967 (Voice/TTY), 800-372-2988 (Voice/TTY)
Info@kypa.net
http://www.kypa.net
Disability Served: various

LOUISIANA
The Advocacy Center-Baton Rouge Office
2704 Wooddale Boulevard, Suite B
Baton Rouge, LA 70805
225-925-8884
http://www.advocacyla.org
Disability Served: various

The Advocacy Center-Lafayette Office
600 Jefferson Street, Suite 812
Lafayette, LA 70501
337-237-7380
http://www.advocacyla.org
Disability Served: various

The Advocacy Center-Monroe Office
PO Drawer 310
Simsboro, LA 71275
318-247-0622

http://www.advocacyla.org
Disability Served: various

The Advocacy Center-New Orleans Office
225 Baronne Street, Suite 2112
New Orleans, LA 70112-1724
504-522-2337, 800-960-7705
http://www.advocacyla.org
Disability Served: various

The Advocacy Center-Shreveport Office
2620 Centenary Boulevard, Building 2, Suite 248
Shreveport, LA 71104
318-227-6186
http://www.advocacyla.org
Disability Served: various

MAINE
Disability Rights Center
PO Box 2007
Augusta, ME 04338-2007
800-452-1948 (Voice/TTY)
Advocate@drcme.org
http://www.drcme.org
Disability Served: various

Maine Client Assistance Program
47 Water Street
Hallowell, ME 04347
207-622-7055, 800-773-7055
capsite@aol.com
http://www.caresinc.org
Disability Served: various

MARYLAND
Maryland Client Assistance Program
2301 Argonne Drive
Baltimore, MD 21218
410-554-9361, 410-554-9360 (TTY/TDD)
cap@dors.state.md.us
http://www.dors.state.md.us/DORS/ProgramServices/
cap
Disability Served: various

Maryland Disability Law Center
1800 North Charles Street, 4th Floor
Baltimore, MD 21201
410-727-6352, 800-233-7201, 410-727-6387 (TDD)

http://www.mdlcbalto.org
Disability Served: various

Office of Federal Contract Compliance Programs
c/o United States Department of Labor,
103 South Gay Street
Baltimore, MD 21203
http://www.dol.gov/esa/contacts/ofccp/ofnation2.
  htm
Disability Served: various

MASSACHUSETTS
Center for Public Representation-Newton Office
246 Walnut Street
Newton, MA 02160
617-965-0776
http://www.centerforpublicrep.org
Disability Served: mental health

**Center for Public Representation-
  Northampton Office**
22 Green Street
Northampton, MA 01060
413-586-6024 (Voice/TTY)
info@cpr-ma.org
http://www.centerforpublicrep.org
Disability Served: mental health

Disability Law Center-Boston (Main) Office
11 Beacon Street, Suite 925
Boston, MA 02108
617-723-8455, 800-872-9992, 617-227-9464 (TTY)
mail@dlc-ma.org
http://www.dlc-ma.org
Disability Served: various

**Disability Law Center-Western Massachusetts
  Office**
32 Industrial Drive East
Northampton, MA 01060
413-584-6337, 800-222-5619, 413-582-6919 (TTY)
mail@dlc-ma.org
http://www.dlc-ma.org
Disability Served: various

Massachusetts Client Assistance Program
One Ashburton Place, Room 1305
Boston, MA 02108

800-322-2020
http://www.mass.gov/mod/ClientAssistance.html
Disability Served: various

MICHIGAN
Michigan Client Assistance Program
4095 Legacy Parkway, Suite 500
Lansing, MI 48911-4263
517-487-1755, 800-292-5896
http://www.mpas.org/AdvocacyServices.
  asp?TOPIC=10116
Disability Served: various

Michigan Protection and Advocacy Service Inc.
4095 Legacy Parkway, Suite 500
Lansing, MI 48911-4263
517-487-1755, 800-288-5923 (Voice/TTY)
molson@mpas.org
http://www.mpas.org
Disability Served: various

MINNESOTA
Legal Services of Northwest Minnesota
1015 7th Avenue North, PO Box 838
Moorhead, MN 56560
218-233-8585, 800-450-8585
legalaid@lsnmlaw.org
http://www.lsnmlaw.org
Disability Served: elderly

Minnesota Legal Services Coalition
2324 University Avenue West, Suite #101B
St. Paul, MN 55114
651-228-9105
statesuppport@mnlegalservices.org
http://www.mnlegalservices.org
Disability Served: various

MISSISSIPPI
Mississippi Client Assistance Program
3226 North State Street, PO Box 4958
Jackson, MS 39296-4958
601-362-2585 (Voice/TDD), 800-962-2400 (Voice/TDD)
http://www.mississippicap.com
Disability Served: various

Mississippi Protection and Advocacy System Inc.
5305 Executive Place
Jackson, MS 39206
601-981-8207 (Voice/TTY), 800-772-4057
info@mspas.com
http://www.mspas.com
Disability Served: various

MISSOURI

**Missouri Protection and Advocacy-
Cape Girardeau Office**
PO Box 69
Patton, MO 63662
573-866-3600, 888-398-3600
http://www.moadvocacy.org
Disability Served: various

**Missouri Protection and Advocacy-
Farmington Office**
614 Wal-Mart Drive, #111
Farmington, MO 63640
573-747-0500
http://www.moadvocacy.org
Disability Served: various

Missouri Protection and Advocacy-Fulton Office
PO Box 6187
Fulton, MO 65251
573-592-3320
http://www.moadvocacy.org
Disability Served: various

**Missouri Protection and Advocacy-
Jefferson City Main Office**
925 South Country Club Drive
Jefferson City, MO 65109
573-893-3333, 800-392-8667
mopasjc@earthlink.net
http://www.moadvocacy.org
Disability Served: various

**Missouri Protection and Advocacy-
Kansas City Office**
3100 Main Street, Suite 305
Kansas City, MO 64111
816-756-1001, 800-233-3959
http://www.moadvocacy.org
Disability Served: various

**Missouri Protection and Advocacy-
Poplar Bluff Office**
PO Box 186
Dexter, MO 63841
573-686-2300
http://www.moadvocacy.org
Disability Served: various

**Missouri Protection and Advocacy-
Springfield Office**
PO Box 3305
Springfield, MO 65808
417-833-2925, 888-632-9551
http://www.moadvocacy.org
Disability Served: various

**Missouri Protection and Advocacy-
St. Louis Office**
2941 South Brentwood Boulevard
Brentwood, MO 63144
314-961-0679, 800-233-3958
http://www.moadvocacy.org
Disability Served: various

MONTANA

Montana Advocacy Program
400 North Park, 2nd Floor, PO Box 1681
Helena, MT 59624
406-449-2344 (Voice/TDD), 800-245-4743 (Voice/TDD)
advocate@mtadv.org
http://www.mtadv.org
Disability Served: various

NEBRASKA

Nebraska Advocacy Services Inc.
134 South 13th Street, Suite 600
Lincoln, NE 68508
402-474-3183 (Voice/TDD), 800-422-6691
Disability Served: various

Nebraska Client Assistance Program
301 Centennial Mall South, Box 94987
Lincoln, NE 68509
800-742-7594 (Voice/TTY)
victoria@cap.state.ne.us
http://www.cap.state.ne.us
Disability Served: various

NEVADA

Nevada Client Assistance Program
1820 East Sahara Avenue, Suite 109
Las Vegas, NV 89104
800-633-9879
detrcap@nvdetr.org
http://detr.state.nv.us/rehab/reh_cap.htm#Client_
    Assistance_Program
Disability Served: various

Nevada Disability Advocacy and Law Center-
    Main Office
6039 Eldora Avenue, Suite C, Box 3
Las Vegas, NV 89146
702-257-8150, 888-349-3843, 702-257-8160 (TTY)
ndalc@ndalclv.org
http://www.ndalc.org
Disability Served: various

Nevada Disability Advocacy and Law Center-
    Northern Office
1311 North McCarran, #106
Sparks, NV 89431
775-333-7878, 800-992-5715, 775-788-7824 (TTY)
reno@ndalc.org
http://www.ndalc.org
Disability Served: various

NEW HAMPSHIRE

Disabilities Rights Center
18 Low Avenue
Concord, NH 03301-4971
603-228-0432 (Voice/TTY), 800-834-1721 (Voice/TTY)
advocacy@drcnh.org
http://www.drcnh.org
Disability Served: various

New Hampshire Client Assistance Program
57 Regional Drive
Concord, NH 03301
603-271-4175, 603-271-2774 (TTY)
http://www.state.nh.us/disability/caphomepage.html
Disability Served: various

NEW JERSEY

New Jersey Client Assistance Program
210 South Broad Street, 3rd Floor
Trenton, NJ 08608
800-922-7233, 609-633-7106 (TTY)

http://www.njpanda.org/capprogram.htm
Disability Served: various

New Jersey Protection and Advocacy, Inc.
210 South Broad Street, 3rd Floor
Trenton, NJ 08608
USA609-292-9742, 609-633-7106 (TTY)
advocate@njpanda.org
http://www.njpanda.org
Disability Served: various

NEW MEXICO

Native American Protection and Advocacy Project
PO Box 392
Shiprock, NM 87420
505-368-3216, 800-862-7271
http://www.navajoway.org/NAPAP.html
Disability Served: various

New Mexico Protection and Advocacy
1720 Louisiana Boulevard, NE, Suite 204
Albuquerque, NM 87110
505-256-3100, 800-432-4682
info@nmpanda.org
http://www.nmpanda.org
Disability Served: various

NEW YORK

American Civil Liberties Union
125 Broad Street, 18th Floor
New York, NY 10004
http://www.aclu.org/DisabilityRights/
    DisabilityRightsMain.cfm
Disability Served: various

Commission on Quality of Care and Advocacy
    for Persons with Disabilities
401 State Street, Schenectady
New York, NY 12305-2397
800-624-4143 (Voice/TDD)
http://www.cqc.state.ny.us
Disability Served: various

Legal Action Center-New York Office
153 Waverly Place
New York, NY 10014
212-243-1313, 800-223-4044
lacinfo@lac.org
http://www.lac.org
Disability Served: AIDS, chemical dependency

NORTH CAROLINA

North Carolina Client Assistance Program
2806 Mail Service Center
Raleigh, NC 27699-2806
919-855-3600 (Voice/TTY), 800-215-7227
Disability Served: various

NORTH DAKOTA

North Dakota Client Assistance Program
1237 West Divide Avenue, Suite 3
Bismarck, ND 58501-1208
701-328-8947, 701-328-8968 (TDD)
cap@state.nd.us
http://www.state.nd.us/cap
Disability Served: various

North Dakota Protection and Advocacy Project-Belcourt Office
St. Ann's Road & Highway 5, Office #1
Belcourt, ND 58316
701-477-5066
panda@state.nd.us
http://www.ndpanda.org
Disability Served: various

North Dakota Protection and Advocacy Project-Devils Lake Office
1401 College Drive
Devils Lake, ND 58301
701-662-9026
panda@state.nd.us
http://www.ndpanda.org
Disability Served: various

North Dakota Protection and Advocacy Project-Dickinson Office
135 Sims, Suite 206
Dickinson, ND 58601-5141
701-227-7444
panda@state.nd.us
http://www.ndpanda.org
Disability Served: various

North Dakota Protection and Advocacy Project-Fargo Office
1351 Page Drive, Suite 303
Fargo, ND 58103-3551
701-239-7222
panda@state.nd.us
http://www.ndpanda.org
Disability Served: various

North Dakota Protection and Advocacy Project-Grand Forks Office
311 South Fourth Street, Suite 112
Grand Forks, ND 58201-4792
701-795-3800
panda@state.nd.us
http://www.ndpanda.org
Disability Served: various

North Dakota Protection and Advocacy Project-Jamestown Office
311 First Avenue South
Jamestown, ND 58401-3373
701-253-3295
panda@state.nd.us
http://www.ndpanda.org
Disability Served: various

North Dakota Protection and Advocacy Project-Main Office
400 East Broadway, Suite 409
Bismarck, ND 58501-4071
701-328-2950
http://www.ndpanda.org
Disability Served: various

North Dakota Protection and Advocacy Project-Minot Office
900 North Broadway, Suite 210
Minot, ND 58703-2379
701-857-7686
panda@state.nd.us
http://www.ndpanda.org
Disability Served: various

North Dakota Protection and Advocacy Project-Williston Office
512 Fourth Avenue East, Room 220, PO Box 247
Williston, ND 58802-2472
701-774-4345
panda@state.nd.us
http://www.ndpanda.org
Disability Served: various

OHIO

Ohio Legal Rights Service
8 East Long Street
Columbus, OH 43215-2999
614-466-7264, 800-282-9181, 614-728-2553 (TTY)
http://olrs.ohio.gov/ASP/HomePage.asp
Disability Served: various

OKLAHOMA

Oklahoma Client Assistance Program
2712 Villa Prom
Oklahoma City, OK 73107-2423
405-521-3756, 800-522-8224, 405-522-6706 (TDD)
http://www.workworld.org/wwwebhelp/oklahoma_
    client_assistance_program.htm
Disability Served: various

Oklahoma Disability Law Center-Oklahoma City Office
300 Cameron Building, 2915 Classen Boulevard
Oklahoma City, OK 73106
405-525-7755 (Voice/TDD), 800-880-7755 (Voice/TDD)
http://home.flash.net/~odlcokc
Disability Served: various

Oklahoma Disability Law Center-Tulsa Office
2828 East 51 Street, Suite 302
Tulsa, OK 74105
918-743-6220 (Voice/TDD), 800-226-5883 (Voice/TDD)
http://www.workworld.org/wwwebhelp/oklahoma_
    disability_law_center.htm
Disability Served: various

OREGON

Oregon Advocacy Center
620 Southwest Fifth Avenue, 5th Floor
Portland, OR 97204-1428
503-243-2081, 503-323-9161 (TTY)
http://www.oradvocacy.org
Disability Served: various

PENNSYLVANIA

Legal Clinic for the Disabled Inc.
1513 Race Street
Philadelphia, PA 19102
215-587-3350, 215-587-3352 (TTY)
http://www.legalclinicforthedisabled.org
Disability Served: various

Pennsylvania Client Assistance Program-Harrisburg Office
2 North Second Street, Suite 100
Harrisburg, PA 17101
717-364-1733 (Voice/TDD)
info@equalemployment.org
http://www.equalemployment.org
Disability Served: various

Pennsylvania Client Assistance Program-Philadelphia Office
1617 JFK Boulevard, Suite 800
Philadelphia, PA 19103
215-557-7112 (Voice/TDD), 888-745-CDLP
info@equalemployment.org
http://www.equalemployment.org
Disability Served: various

Pennsylvania Client Assistance Program-Pittsburgh Office
Two Gateway Center, Suite 6
Pittsburgh, PA 15222-1450
412-255-4016, 888-745-2357 (TTD)
info@equalemployment.org
http://www.equalemployment.org
Disability Served: various

Pennsylvania Protection and Advocacy Inc.
1414 North Cameron Street, Suite C
Harrisburg, PA 17103
717-236-8110, 800-692-7443, 717-346-0293 (TTY)
http://www.ppainc.org
Disability Served: various

Public Interest Law Center of Philadelphia
125 South Ninth Street, Suite 700
Philadelphia, PA 19107
215-627-7100
http://www.pilcop.org
Disability Served: various

RHODE ISLAND

Rhode Island Disability Law Center Inc.
349 Eddy Street
Providence, RI 02903
401-831-3150, 401-831-5335 (TDD)
Disability Served: various

SOUTH CAROLINA

Protection and Advocacy for People with Disabilities Inc.-Central Office
3710 Landmark Drive, Suite 208
Columbia, SC 29204

803-782-0639, 866-232-4525 (TTY)
info@protectionandadvocacy-sc.org
http://www.protectionandadvocacy-sc.org
Disability Served: various

Protection and Advocacy for People with Disabilities Inc.-Low Country Office

1569 Sam Rittenberg Boulevard
Charleston, SC 29407
843-763-8571, 866-232-4525 (TTY)
info@protectionandadvocacy-sc.org
http://www.protectionandadvocacy-sc.org
Disability Served: various

Protection and Advocacy for People with Disabilities Inc.-Pee Dee Office

2137 B Hoffmeyer Road
Florence, SC 29501
866-275-7273, 866-232-4525 (TTY)
info@protectionandadvocacy-sc.org
http://www.protectionandadvocacy-sc.org
Disability Served: various

Protection and Advocacy for People with Disabilities, Inc.-Piedmont Office

1 Chick Springs Road, Suite 101-A
Greenville, SC 29069
866-275-7273, 866-232-4525 (TTY)
info@protectionandadvocacy-sc.org
http://www.protectionandadvocacy-sc.org
Disability Served: various

South Carolina Client Assistance Program

1205 Pendleton Street
Columbia, SC 29205
803-734-0285, 803-734-1147 (TDD)
http://www.govoepp.state.sc.us/cap
Disability Served: various

SOUTH DAKOTA

South Dakota Advocacy Services

221 South Central Avenue
Pierre, SD 57501
605-224-8294 (Voice/TTY), 800-658-4782 (Voice/TTY)
sdas@sdadvocacy.com
http://www.sdadvocacy.com
Disability Served: various

TENNESSEE

Disability Law and Advocacy Center of Tennessee Inc.

2416 21st Avenue South
Nashville, TN 37212
615-298-1080, 800-342-1660, 888-852-2852 (TTY)
GetHelp@TPAinc.org
http://www.tpainc.org
Disability Served: various

Tennessee Client Assistance Program

PO Box 121257
Nashville, TN 37212
800-342-1660
Disability Served: various

TEXAS

Advocacy Inc.-Beaumont Satellite Office

3420 Fannin Street, Suite 201
Beaumont, TX 77701
409-832-4872 (Voice/TDD)
http://www.advocacyinc.org
Disability Served: various

Advocacy Inc.-Central Texas Regional Office

7800 Shoal Creek Boulevard, Suite 142-S
Austin, TX 78757
512-454-4816 (Voice/TDD)
http://www.advocacyinc.org
Disability Served: various

Advocacy Inc.-Corpus Christi Satellite Office

c/o Coastal Bend Legal Services
Pueblo Law Center, 3825 Agnes Street
Corpus Christi, TX 78405-3002
361-883-3623 (Voice/TDD)
http://www.advocacyinc.org
Disability Served: various

Advocacy Inc.-East Texas Regional Office

1500 McGowen Street, Suite 100
Houston, TX 77004
713-974-7691 (Voice/TDD)
http://www.advocacyinc.org
Disability Served: various

Advocacy Inc.-El Paso Regional Office

300 East Main, Suite 205
El Paso, TX 79901

915-542-0585 (Voice/TDD)
http://www.advocacyinc.org
Disability Served: various

Advocacy Inc.-Ft. Worth Satellite Office
1300 West Lancaster, Suite 110
Ft. Worth, TX 76102
817-336-0075
http://www.advocacyinc.org
Disability Served: various

Advocacy Inc.-Laredo Satellite Office
c/o Coastal Bend Legal Services, 1702 Convent
Laredo, TX 78040-1413
956-722-7581 (Voice/TDD)
http://www.advocacyinc.org
Disability Served: various

Advocacy Inc.-Longview Satellite Office
211 West Tyler Street, Suite A
Longview, TX 75601
903-758-8888
http://www.advocacyinc.org
Disability Served: various

Advocacy Inc.-Main Office
7800 Shoal Creek Boulevard, #171-E
Austin, TX 78757-1024
512-454-4816 (Voice/TDD), 800-252-9108 (Voice/TDD)
infoai@advocacyinc.org
http://www.advocacyinc.org
Disability Served: various

Advocacy Inc.-McAllen Satellite Office
1418 Beech, Suite 113
McAllen, TX 78501
956-630-3013 (Voice/TDD)
http://www.advocacyinc.org
Disability Served: various

Advocacy Inc.-Nacogdoches Satellite Office
c/o East Texas Legal Services
414 East Pillar
Nacogdoches, TX 75963-1308
936-560-1455 (Voice/TDD)
http://www.advocacyinc.org
Disability Served: various

Advocacy Inc.-North Texas Regional Office
1420 West Mockingbird Lane, Suite 450
Dallas, TX 75247-4932

214-630-0916 (Voice/TDD)
http://www.advocacyinc.org
Disability Served: various

Advocacy Inc.-South Texas Regional Office
6800 Park Ten Boulevard, Suite 208-N
San Antonio, TX 78213
210-737-0499 (Voice/TDD)
http://www.advocacyinc.org
Disability Served: various

Advocacy Inc.-West Texas Regional Office
1001 Main Street, Suite 3
Lubbock, TX 79401-3200
806-765-7794 (Voice/TDD)
http://www.advocacyinc.org
Disability Served: various

Advocacy Inc.-Wichita Falls Satellite Office
801 Burnett Street, Suite 116
Wichita Falls, TX 76301-3290
940-761-1199 (Voice/TDD)
http://www.advocacyinc.org
Disability Served: various

UTAH
Disability Law Center
205 North 400 West
Salt Lake City, UT 84103
800-662-9080, 800-550-4182 (TTY)
info@disabilitylawcenter.org
http://www.disabilitylawcenter.org
Disability Served: various

VERMONT
Vermont Client Assistance Program
57 North Main Street
Rutland, VT 05701
802-775-0021, 800-769-7459
http://www.dad.state.vt.us/DVR/cap.htm
Disability Served: various

Vermont Protection and Advocacy Inc.
141 Main Street, Suite 7
Montpelier, VT 05602
802-229-1355, 800-834-7890, 802-229-2603 (TTY)
info@vtpa.org
http://www.vtpa.org
Disability Served: various

VIRGINIA

Council of Parent Attorneys and Advocates
296 Dover Road
Warrenton, VA 20186
http://www.copaa.org/find (searchable database of disability attorneys for children)
Disability Served: various

National Center for State Courts
300 Newport Avenue
Williamsburg, VA 23185-4147
800-616-6164
http://www.ncsconline.org
Disability Served: various

Virginia Office for Protection and Advocacy-Central Office
1910 Byrd Avenue, Suite 5
Richmond, VA 23230
804-225-2042 (Voice/TTY), 800-552-3962 (Voice/TTY)
general.vopa@vopa.virginia.gov
http://www.vopa.state.va.us
Disability Served: various

Virginia Office for Protection and Advocacy-Virginia Beach Field Office
287 Independence Boulevard, Suite 120
Virginia Beach, VA 23462
757-552-1148, 800-552-3962
general.vopa@vopa.virginia.gov
http://www.vopa.state.va.us
Disability Served: various

WASHINGTON

Washington Protection and Advocacy System
315 Fifth Avenue South, Suite 850
Seattle, WA 98104
206-324-1521, 800-562-2702, 206-957-0728 (TTY)
wpas@wpas-rights.org
http://www.wpas-rights.org
Disability Served: various

Washington State Client Assistance Program
2531 Rainier Avenue South
Seattle, WA 98144
888-721-6072 (Voice/TDD)
capseattle@att.net
http://www.capseattle.org
Disability Served: various

WEST VIRGINIA

West Virginia Advocates Inc.
Litton Building, 1207 Quarrier Street, Fourth Floor
Charleston, WV 25301
304-346-0847 (Voice/TDD), 800-950-5250 (Voice/TDD)
WVAinfo@wvadvocates.org
http://www.wvadvocates.org
Disability Served: various

WISCONSIN

Wisconsin Client Assistance Program
2811 Agriculture Drive, PO Box 8911
Madison, WI 53708-8911
800-362-1290
Disability Served: various

Wisconsin Coalition for Advocacy-Madison Office
16 North Carroll Street, Suite 400
Madison, WI 53703
608-267-0214 (Voice/TTY), 800-928-8778 (Voice/TTY)
http://www.w-c-a.org
Disability Served: various

Wisconsin Coalition for Advocacy-Milwaukee Office
6737 West Washington Street, #3230
Milwaukee, WI 53214
414-773-4646 (Voice/TTY), 800-708-3034 (Voice/TTY)
http://www.w-c-a.org
Disability Served: various

Wisconsin Coalition for Advocacy-Northern Wisconsin Office
801 Hammond Avenue
Rice Lake, WI 54868
715-736-1232 (Voice/TTY), 877-338-3724 (Voice/TTY)
http://www.w-c-a.org
Disability Served: various

WYOMING

Protection and Advocacy System Inc.-Evanston Field Office
350 City View Drive, #207A
Evanston, WY 82930
307-789-3035
wypande@vcn.com
http://www.wypanda.vcn.com
Disability Served: various

Protection and Advocacy System Inc.-Lander Field Office
PO Box 58
Lander, WY 82520

307-335-6908
wypandl@onewest.net
http://www.wypanda.vcn.com
Disability Served: various

Protection and Advocacy System Inc.-Main Office
320 West 25th Street, 2nd Floor
Cheyenne, WY 82001
307-632-3496
wypanda@vcn.com
http://www.wypanda.vcn.com
Disability Served: various

AMERICAN SAMOA
**Client Assistance Program and Protection
and Advocacy**
PO Box 3937
Pago Pago, AS 96799
marie@samoatelco.com
Disability Served: various

GUAM
Guam Legal Services
113 Bradley Place
Hagatna, Guam 96910
671-477-9811
glsc@netpci.com
Disability Served: various

NORTHERN MARIANA ISLANDS
**Northern Marianas Protection and Advocacy
Systems Inc.**
PO Box 503529
Saipan, MP 96950
670-235-7278 (TTY)
Disability Served: various

PUERTO RICO

Puerto Rico Client Assistance Program
PO Box 41309
San Juan, PR 00940-1309
mrosa@oppi.govierno.pr
Disability Served: various

CANADA
Canadian Law List
http://www.canadianlawlist.com (searchable database
of Canadian attorneys who specialize in disability
law)
Disability Served: various

Department of Justice Canada
284 Wellington Street
Ottawa, ON K1A 0H8
Canada
613-957-4222, 800-267-7777
http://canada.justice.gc.ca/en
Disability Served: various

PROFESSIONAL ORGANIZATIONS

Professional organizations comprise members who share a profession or are involved in the same industry. They provide assistance and information to people with disabilities.

Academy of Dispensing Audiologists
401 North Michigan Avenue, Suite 2200
Chicago, IL 60611
866-493-5544
http://www.audiologist.org
Disability Served: hearing
This organization supports the dispensing of hearing aids by qualified audiologists.

Academy of Rehabilitative Audiology
PO Box 952
DeSoto, TX 75123
ara@audrehab.org
http://www.audrehab.org
Disability Served: hearing
This organization promotes excellence in hearing care through the provision of comprehensive rehabilitative and habilitative services. It provides a forum for the exchange of ideas; fosters and encourages education and research; expands and improves on the delivery of services; receives, holds, and uses gifts and endowments for the organization to achieve its purposes; and serves as a public policy advocate for audiologic services.

Alliance of Cardiovascular Professionals
Building 2, 4356 Bonney Road, Thalia Landing Office, #103
Virginia Beach, VA 23452-1200
757-497-1225
peggymcelgunn@comcast.net
http://www.acp-online.org
Disability Served: various
This organization connects more than 3,000 professionals involved in all levels of cardiovascular service (administration, management, nursing, and technology) and all of its specialties (invasive, noninvasive, echo, and cardiopulmonary).

American Academy of Allergy, Asthma, and Immunology
555 East Wells Street, Suite 1100
Milwaukee, WI 53202-3823
414-272-6071
info@aaai.org
http://www.aaaai.org
Disability Served: asthma
This professional medical specialty organization represents allergists, asthma specialists, clinical immunologists, allied health professionals, and others with a special interest in the research and treatment of allergic disease. The organization publishes a professional journal and a number of newsletters, pamphlets, and booklets for both medical professionals and lay people to keep them informed of the latest news about allergies, asthma, and immunology.

American Academy of Child and Adolescent Psychiatry
3615 Wisconsin Avenue, NW
Washington, DC 20016-3007
202-966-7300
http://www.aacap.org
Disability Served: emotionally disabled adolescents, mental health
The academy is a professional medical organization of child and adolescent psychiatrists trained to promote healthy development and to evaluate, diagnose, and treat children and adolescents and their families who are affected by disorders of feeling, thinking, and behavior.

American Academy of Family Physicians
PO Box 11210
Shawnee Mission, KS 66207-1210
913-906-6095, 800-274-2237
fp@aafp.org
http://www.aafp.org
Disability Served: various
This organization aims to preserve and promote the science and art of family medicine and to ensure high-quality, cost-effective health care for patients of all ages.

American Academy of Nurse Practitioners
PO Box 12846
Austin, TX 78711
512-442-4262
admin@aanp.org
http://www.aanp.org
Disability Served: various

This organization for nurse practitioners promotes excellence in practice, education, and research; provides legislative leadership; strives to advance health policy; and advocates for access to quality, cost effective health care.

American Academy of Orthopaedic Surgeons

6300 North River Road
Rosemont, IL 60018-4262
847-823-7186, 800-346-AAOS
custserv@aaos.org
http://www.aaos.org
Disability Served: various
This organization's members champion the interests of patients suffering from spine and limb deformities and advance the highest quality of musculoskeletal health.

American Academy of Orthotists and Prosthetists

526 King Street, Suite 201
Alexandria, VA 22314
703-836-0788
academy@oandp.org
http://www.oandp.org
Disability Served: physically disabled
This organization is dedicated to promoting professionalism and advancing the standards of patient care through education, literature, research, advocacy, and collaboration.

American Academy of Pediatrics

141 Northwest Point Boulevard
Elk Grove Village, IL 60007-1098
847-434-4000
commun@aap.org
http://www.aap.org
Disability Served: various
This association of pediatricians focuses on the physical, mental, and social health of infants, children, adolescents, and young adults

American Academy of Physical Medicine and Rehabilitation

303 North Wabash Avenue, Suite 2500
Chicago, IL 60611
312-464-9700
info@aapmr.org
http://www.aapmr.org
Disability Served: various
This professional organization represents physical medicine and rehabilitation physicians who treat individuals with physical disabilities, chronic illnesses, and more.

American Academy of Physician Assistants

950 North Washington Street
Alexandria, VA 22314-1552
703-836-2272
aapa@aapa.org
http://www.aapa.org
Disability Served: various
This organization promotes quality, cost-effective, accessible health care, along with the professional and personal development of physician assistants.

American Association for Geriatric Psychiatry

7910 Woodmont Avenue, Suite 1050
Bethesda, MD 20814-3004
301-654-7850
cdevries@gmhfonline.org
http://www.aagpgpa.org
Disability Served: elderly, mental health
This association is dedicated to promoting the mental health and well being of older people and improving the care of those with late-life mental disorders. The association's foundation raises awareness of psychiatric and mental health disorders affecting the elderly, eliminates the stigma of mental illness and treatment, promotes healthy aging strategies, and increases access to quality mental health care for the elderly.

American Association for Homecare

625 Slaters Lane, Suite 200
Alexandria, VA 22314-1171
703-836-6263
info@aahomecare.org
http://www.aahomecare.org
Disability Served: various
This is the national association that represents every type of service in the homecare community, including home health and home medical equipment, respiratory and infusion therapy, telemedicine, telehealth, rehabilitation and assistive technology, and hospice.

American Association for Respiratory Care

9425 North MacArthur Boulevard, Suite 100
Irving, TX 75063-4706
972-243-2272
info@aarc.org

http://www.aarc.org
Disability Served: various
This national and international professional organization for respiratory care encourages and promotes professional excellence, advances the science and practice of respiratory care, and serves as an advocate for patients, their families, the public, the profession and the respiratory therapist.

American Association for the Advancement of Science
Project on Science, Technology and Disability
1200 New York Avenue, NW
Washington, DC 20005
202-326-6400
membership@aaas.org
http://www.aaas.org
Disability Served: various
This international nonprofit organization is dedicated to advancing science around the world by serving as an educator, leader, spokesperson, and professional association. In addition to organizing membership activities, the association publishes the journal *Science,* and many scientific newsletters, books, and reports, as well as spearheads programs that raise the bar of understanding for science worldwide.

American Association of Critical-Care Nurses
101 Columbia
Aliso Viejo, CA 92656-4109
949-362-2000, 800-899-2226
info@aacn.org
http://www.aacn.org
Disability Served: various
This association of critical care nurses is committed to providing the highest quality resources to maximize nurses' contribution to caring and improving the health care of critically ill patients and their families.

American Association of Homes and Services for the Aging
2519 Connecticut Avenue, NW
Washington, DC 20008-1520
202-783-2242
info@aahsa.org
http://www.aahsa.org
Disability Served: elderly
The members of this association serve two million people every day through mission-driven, not-for-profit organizations. Services provided by members include adult day services, home health, community services, senior housing, assisted living residences, continuing care retirement communities, and nursing homes.

American Association of Medical Assistants
20 North Wacker Drive, Suite 1575
Chicago, IL 60606
312-899-1500
http://www.aama-ntl.org
Disability Served: various
This association strives to enable medical assisting professionals to enhance and demonstrate the knowledge, skills, and professionalism required by employers and patients; protect medical assistants' right to practice; and promote effective, efficient health care delivery through optimal use of multiskilled certified medical assistants.

American Association of Neurological Surgeons
5550 Meadowbrook Drive
Rolling Meadows, IL 60008
847-378-0500, 888-566-2267
info@aans.org
http://www.neurosurgery.org/aans
Disability Served: various
This association of neurological surgeons is a scientific and educational association with over 6,500 members worldwide that is dedicated to advancing the specialty of neurological surgery in order to provide the highest quality of neurosurgical care to the public.

American Association of Neuroscience Nurses
4700 West Lake Avenue
Glenview, IL 60025
847-375-4733, 888-557-2266
info@aann.org
http://www.aann.org
Disability Served: various
This association serves as the leading authority in neuroscience nursing with a strong commitment to the advancement of neuroscience nursing as a specialty.

American Association of Occupational Health Nurses
2920 Brandywine Road, Suite 100
Atlanta, GA 30341
770-455-7757
http://www.aaohn.org
Disability Served: various

This association, representing the largest group of health care professionals serving the workplace, is driven by a mission to ensure that occupational and environmental nurses are the authority on health, safety, productivity, and disability management for worker populations.

American Association of Spinal Cord Injury Psychologists and Social Workers

75-20 Astoria Boulevard
Jackson Heights, NY 11370-1177
718-803-0414
aascipsw@unitedspinal.org
http://www.aascipsw.org
Disability Served: mental health, spinal-cord injury
The association establishes standards of care for those working in the field of spinal-cord injury, publishes educational materials, sponsors a research grant program, and holds an annual conference.

American Auditory Society

352 Sundial Ridge Circle
Dammeron Valley, UT 84783
435-574-0062
amaudsoc@aol.com
http://www.amauditorysoc.org
Disability Served: hearing
This society increase knowledge and understanding of the ear, hearing, and balance; disorders of the ear, hearing, and balance and preventions of these disorders; and habilitation and rehabilitation of individuals with hearing and balance dysfunction. The society coordinates and disseminates information, particularly through the holding of regular meetings, and through publication of professional, scientific, educational, and informational media.

American Back Society

2647 International Boulevard, Suite 401
Oakland, CA 94601
510-536-9929
info@americanbacksoc.org
http://www.americanbacksoc.org
Disability Served: back injury, spinal-cord injury
This membership organization is dedicated to finding cures and remedies for spinal injuries.

American Board for Certification in Orthotics and Prosthetics Inc.

330 John Carlyle Street, Suite 210
Alexandria, VA 22314
703-836-7114
info@abcob.org
http://www.abcop.org
Disability Served: physically disabled
The board is responsible for the credentialing of providers and organizations engaged in the delivery of orthotic and prosthetic services.

American Board of Transplant Coordinators

PO Box 15384
Lenexa, KS 66285-5384
913-599-0198
abtc-info@goamp.com
http://www.abtc.net
Disability Served: various
This board's purpose is to award a voluntary, non-governmental certification credential—certified clinical transplant coordinator or certified procurement transplant coordinator—to qualified transplant professionals who have successfully passed the certification examination.

American Chemical Society

Committee on Disabled Chemists
1155 16th Street, NW
Washington, DC 20036
202-872-4600, 800-227-5558
cwd@acs.org
http://www.acs.org
Disability Served: various
The committee's mission is to promote opportunities, both educational and professional, for persons with disabilities who are interested in pursuing careers in chemistry. The committee strives to demonstrate the capabilities of those persons to educators, employers, and peers.

American Counseling Association

5999 Stevenson Avenue
Alexandria, VA 22304
800-347-6647
http://www.counseling.org
Disability Served: chemical dependency, mental health
This not-for-profit association is dedicated to the growth and enhancement of the counseling profession. By providing leadership training, publications, continuing education opportunities, and advocacy services to its members, the association helps counseling professionals develop their skills and expand their knowledge base.

American Group Psychotherapy Association
25 East 21st Street, 6th Floor
New York, NY 10010
212-477-2677
info@agpa.org
http://www.agpa.org
Disability Served: mental health
This association is an interdisciplinary community that
    has been enhancing the practice, theory,
    and research of group therapy since 1942.

American Holistic Health Association
PO Box 17400
Anaheim, CA 92817-7400
714-779-6152
mail@ahha.org
http://ahha.org
Disability Served: various
This association is dedicated to promoting holistic
    principles: honoring the whole person (mind, body,
    and spirit) and encouraging people to actively
    participate in their own health and health care.

American Hospital Association
One North Franklin
Chicago, IL 60606-3421
312-422-3000
http://www.aha.org
Disability Served: various
This national organization represents and serves all
    types of hospitals, health care networks, and their
    patients and communities. Through representation
    and advocacy activities, the association ensures that
    members' perspectives and needs are heard and
    addressed in national health policy development,
    legislative and regulatory debates, and judicial
    matters.

American Hotel and Lodging Association
1201 New York Avenue, NW, Suite 600
Washington, DC 20005-3931
202-289-3100
regaffairs@ahla.com
http://www.ahla.com
Disability Served: various
This professional trade association provides members
    with national legislative advocacy; public relations
    and image management; education, research and
    information; ADA compliance; and other services to
    ensure a positive business climate for the U.S. lodging
    industry.

American Medical Association
515 North State Street
Chicago, IL 60610
800-621-8335
http://www.ama-assn.org
Disability Served: various
This association, the nation's largest physicians group,
    aims to be an essential part of the professional life
    of every physician and an essential force for progress
    in improving the nation's health.

American Medical Technologists
710 Higgins Road
Park Ridge, IL 60068
847-823-5169, 800-275-1268
http://www.amt1.com
Disability Served: various
This nonprofit association provides allied health
    professionals with professional certification
    services and membership programs to enhance
    their professional and personal growth.

American Nephrology Nurses' Association
East Holly Avenue, PO Box 56
Pitman, NJ 08071-0056
856-256-2320, 888-600-2662
anna@ajj.com
http://anna.inurse.com
Disability Served: kidney disease
This nonprofit association influences outcomes for
    patients with kidney or other disease processes
    requiring replacement therapies by advancing the
    practice of nephrology nursing through advocacy
    and scholarship.

**American Network of Community Options
    and Resources**
1101 King Street, Suite 380
Alexandria, VA 22314
730-535-7850
ancor@ancor.org
http://www.ancor.org
Disability Served: various
This nonprofit trade association represents private
    providers who offer support and services to
    people with disabilities. The network's efforts
    in the area of public policy, federal legislative
    and regulatory initiatives, judicial results, state-
    level initiatives, and of leading practices have
    positioned it as the national presence for private
    providers.

American Nurses Association
8515 Georgia Avenue, Suite 400
Silver Spring, MD 20910
301-628-5000, 800-274-4262
memberinfo@ana.org
http://www.nursingworld.org
Disability Served: various
This association is the only full-service professional organization representing the nation's entire registered nurse population. It advances the nursing profession by fostering high standards of nursing practice, promoting the economic and general welfare of nurses in the workplace, projecting a positive and realistic view of nursing, and by lobbying the Congress and regulatory agencies on health care issues affecting nurses and the general public.

American Occupational Therapy Association
4720 Montgomery Lane, PO Box 31220
Bethesda, MD 20814-1220
301-652-2682
http://www.aota.org
Disability Served: various
This professional association of occupational therapists, occupational therapy assistants, and students of occupational therapy supports those in the field of occupational therapy, including those who work with people experiencing health problems such as stroke, spinal-cord injuries, cancer, congenital conditions, developmental problems, and mental illness.

American Orthotic and Prosthetic Association
330 John Carlyle Street, Suite 200
Alexandria, VA 22314
571-431-0876
info@aopanet.org
http://www.aopanet.org
Disability Served: physically disabled
This national trade association committed to providing high quality, unprecedented business services and products to orthotic and prosthetic professionals raises awareness of the profession and impacts policies that affect the future of the orthotic and prosthetics industry.

American Osteopathic Association
142 East Ontario Street
Chicago, IL 60611
312-202-8000, 800-621-1773

info@osteotech.org
http://www.osteopathic.org
Disability Served: various
This member association representing osteopathic physicians serves as the primary certifying body for D.O.s and is the accrediting agency for all osteopathic medical colleges and health care facilities. It strives to advance the philosophy and practice of osteopathic medicine by promoting excellence in education, research, and the delivery of quality, cost-effective health care.

American Psychiatric Association
1000 Wilson Boulevard, Suite 1825
Arlington, VA 22209
703-907-7300, 888-35-PSYCH
apa@psych.org
http://www.psych.org
Disability Served: chemical dependency, mental health, mental retardation
The American Psychiatric Association is an organization of psychiatrists working together to ensure humane care and effective treatment for all persons with mental disorders, including mental retardation and substance-related disorders.

American Psychiatric Nurses Association
1555 Wilson Boulevard, Suite 602
Arlington, VA 22209
703-243-2443
inform@apna.org
http://www.apna.org
Disability Served: mental health
This membership organization promotes psychiatric-mental health nursing to improve mental health care for culturally diverse individuals, families, groups, and communities.

American Society of Clinical Oncology
1900 Duke Street, Suite 200
Alexandria, VA 22314
703-299-0150
asco@asco.org
http://www.asco.org
Disability Served: cancer patients and survivors
This professional organization, representing physicians who treat people with cancer, sets the standard for patient care worldwide and leads the way in carrying out clinical research aimed at improving the prevention, diagnosis, and treatment of cancer.

American Speech-Language-Hearing Association
10801 Rockville Pike
Rockville, MD 20852
301-897-5700, 800-638-8255
actioncenter@asha.org
http://www.asha.org
Disability Served: communication, hearing
This organization is a national professional, scientific, and credentialing organization for audiologists, speech-language pathologists, and speech, language, and hearing scientists. The association provides brochures and information about hearing, speech, and language problems.

American Spinal Injury Association
2020 Peachtree Road, NW
Atlanta, GA 30309-1402
404-355-9772
pat_duncan@shepherd.org
http://www.asia-spinalinjury.org
Disability Served: spinal-cord injury
This association educates members, other health care professionals, patients and their families, and the general public on all aspects of spinal-cord injury. It aims to prevent injury, improve care, increase availability of services, and maximize the injured individual's potential for full participation in community life. The association also fosters research, which aims at both prevention of spinal-cord injury and finding a cure.

Association for Advancement of Behavior Therapy
305 Seventh Avenue, 16th Floor
New York, NY 10001-6008
212-647-1890
http://www.aabt.org
Disability Served: mental health
This professional association serves as a resource and information center for matters related to behavior therapy. It also encourages the development of the scientific basis of the behavioral therapies and facilitates the growth of behavior therapy as a professional activity.

Association of University Centers on Disabilities
1010 Wayne Avenue, Suite 920
Silver Spring, MD 20910
301-588-8252
http://www.aucd.org
Disability Served: developmentally disabled

This nonprofit organization promotes and supports the national network of university centers on disabilities, which includes University Centers for Excellence in Developmental Disabilities Education, Research, and Service; Leadership Education in Neurodevelopmental and Related Disabilities Programs; and Developmental Disabilities Research Centers.

Association of Women's Health, Obstetric and Neonatal Nurses
2000 L Street, NW, Suite 740
Washington, DC 20036
202-261-2400, 800-673-8499
http://www.awhonn.org
Disability Served: various
This organization advances the nursing profession by providing nurses with critical information and support to help them deliver the highest quality care for women and newborns.

Association on Higher Education and Disability
PO Box 540666
Waltham, MA 02454
781-788-0003
ahead@ahead.org
http://www.ahead.org
Disability Served: various
This professional association addresses current and emerging issues with respect to disability, education, and accessibility in order to achieve universal access. It offers training to higher education personnel through conferences, workshops, publications, and consultation.

Canadian Medical Association
1867 Alta Vista Drive
Ottawa, ON K1G 3Y6
Canada
800-267-9703
cmamsc.cma.ca
http://www.cma.ca
Disability Served: various
This association strives to ensure a healthy population and a vibrant medical profession in Canada by serving as the national advocate, in partnership with the people of Canada, for the highest standards of health and health care.

Center for Applied Special Technology
40 Harvard Mills Square, Suite 3
Wakefield, MA 01880-3233

781-245-2212
cast@cast.org
http://www.cast.org
Disability Served: various
This nonprofit research and development organization
uses technology to make education more accessible
and flexible for students with disabilities.

Centers for Disease Control and Prevention
1600 Clifton Road
Atlanta, GA 30333
404-639-3534, 800-311-3435
http://www.cdc.gov
Disability Served: various
The Centers for Disease Control and Prevention is one of
the 13 major operating components of the Department
of Health and Human Services, which is the principal
agency in the United States government for protecting
the health and safety of all Americans and for providing
essential human services, especially for those people
who are least able to help themselves. Its priorities lie
in two health protection goals: health promotion and
prevention of disease, injury, and disability.

Communication Aid Manufacturers Association
205 West Randolph, Suite 1830
Chicago, IL 60606
800-441-2262
cama@northshore.net
http://www.aacproducts.org
Disability Served: communication
This is a professional association of augmentative and
alternative communication software and hardware
manufacturers. It provides continuing education
activities in speech-language pathology and audiology.

**Conference of Educational Administrators Serving
the Deaf**
PO Box 1778
St. Augustine, FL 32085-1778
nationaloffice@ceasd.org
http://www.ceasd.org
Disability Served: hearing
This organization works to improve educational
outcomes of persons with hearing impairments
through training, advocacy, and research.

Convention of American Instructors of the Deaf
PO Box 377
Bedford, TX 76095-0377

817-354-8414 (Voice/TTY)
caid@swbell.net
http://www.caid.org
Disability Served: hearing
This organization of teachers, and other education-
related personnel of deaf and hard of hearing
children, promotes student learning and
development by bringing together local, state,
regional, and national interest organizations.

Council for Learning Disabilities
PO Box 4014
Leesburg, VA 20177
571-258-1010
http://www.cldinternational.org
Disability Served: learning disabled
This organization, composed of professionals who
are committed to enhancing the education and
lifespan development of individuals with learning
disabilities, promotes effective teaching and research.
The council establishes standards of excellence
and promotes innovative strategies for research
and practice through interdisciplinary collegiality,
collaboration, and advocacy.

**Council of State Administrators of Vocational
Rehabilitation**
4733 Bethesda Avenue, Suite 330
Bethesda, MD 20814
301-654-8414
carlsuter@rehabnetwork.org
http://www.rehabnetwork.org
Disability Served: various
This organization's mission is to maintain and enhance
a strong, effective, and efficient national program
of public vocational rehabilitation services, which
empowers individuals with disabilities to achieve
employment, economic self-sufficiency, independence,
and inclusion and integration into our communities.

International Agency for the Prevention of Blindness
LV Prasad Eye Institute
Banjara Hills, Hyderabad 500 034
India
91-40-235-45-389
IAPB@lvpei.org
http://www.iapb.org
Disability Served: vision
This international organization of health care
professionals supports research on blindness.

International Association for Medical Assistance to Travelers

1623 Military Road, #279
Niagara Falls, NY 14304-1745
716-754-4883
info@iamat.org
http://www.iamat.org
Disability Served: various
This nonprofit organization makes competent medical care available to travelers by doctors who speak English.

International Hearing Society

16880 Middlebelt Road, Suite 4
Livonia, MI 48154
734-522-7200
chelms@ihsinfo.org
http://www.ihsinfo.org
Disability Served: hearing
The International Hearing Society is the nonprofit, professional association that represents hearing instrument specialists in the United States, Canada, Japan, and several other countries. Its members are engaged in the practice of testing human hearing and selecting, fitting, and dispensing hearing instruments.

International Transplant Nurses Society

1739 East Carson Street
PO Box 351
Pittsburgh, PA 15203-1700
412-343-ITNS
itns@msn.com
http://www.itns.org
Disability Served: various
This nonprofit organization promotes excellence in transplant clinical nursing through the provision of educational and professional growth opportunities, interdisciplinary networking and collaborative activities, and transplant nursing research.

National Adult Day Services Association

2519 Connecticut Avenue, NW
Washington, DC 20008
800-558-5301
info@nadsa.org
http://www.nadsa.org
Disability Served: various
This association is the leading voice of the rapidly growing adult day service industry in the United States. Adult day services are community-based group programs designed to meet the needs of functionally and/or cognitively impaired adults through an individual plan of care. The association provides its members with effective national advocacy, educational and networking opportunities, research, and communication.

National Alliance for Caregiving

4720 Montgomery Lane, 5th Floor
Bethesda, MD 20814
info@caregiving.org
http://www.caregiving.org
Disability Served: various
The alliance's members include grassroots organizations, professional associations, service organizations, disease-specific organizations, government, and corporations. Its purpose is to conduct research, do policy analysis, develop national programs, and increase public awareness of family caregiving issues though publications, reports and policy papers, and national conferences.

National Association for Home Care and Hospice

228 Seventh Street, SE
Washington, DC 20003
202-547-7424
http://www.nahc.org
Disability Served: various
This trade association represents the interests and concerns of home care agencies, hospices, home care aide organizations, and medical equipment suppliers. It advocates for senior citizens and other vulnerable groups to be able to live in independence through the assistance of home care services.

National Association of Area Agencies on Aging

1730 Rhode Island Avenue, NW, Suite 1200
Washington, DC 20036
202-872-0888
smarkwood@n4a.org
http://www.n4a.org
Disability Served: elderly
This association is the umbrella organization for the 655 area agencies on aging in the United States. It advocates on behalf of the local aging agencies to ensure that needed resources and support services are available to older Americans. These agencies coordinate and support a wide range of home- and community-based services, including information and referral, home-delivered and congregate meals, transportation,

employment services, senior centers, adult day care, and a long-term care ombudsman program.

National Association of Clinical Nurse Specialists
2090 Linglestown Road, Suite 107
Harrisburg, PA 17110
717-234-6799
http://www.nacns.org
Disability Served: various
This association enhances and promotes the contribution of the clinical nurse specialist to the health and well being of individuals, families, groups, and communities.

National Association of Geriatric Nursing Assistants
1201 L Street, NW
Washington, DC 20005
202-454-1288, 800-784-6049
http://www.nagna.org
Disability Served: elderly
This nonprofit association works to ensure that the highest quality of care is provided to the elderly living in nursing homes. It provides recognition for outstanding achievements, development training for certified nursing assistants (CNAs), mentoring programs to reduce CNA turnover, and advocacy for issues important to long term care and CNAs.

National Association of Home Builders
1201 15th Street, NW
Washington, DC 20005
800-368-8400
http://www.nahb.org
Disability Served: various
This association provides information and education on accessible housing.

National Association of Neonatal Nurses
4700 West Lake Avenue
Glenview, IL 60025-1485
847-375-3660, 800-451-3795
info@nann.org
http://www.nann.org
Disability Served: various
This organization strives to improve the lives of all newborns, infants, and their families through excellence in neonatal nursing practice, education, research, and professional development.

National Association of Nephrology Technicians/ Technologists
PO Box 2307
Dayton, OH 45401-2307
937-586-3705, 877-607-6268
nant@nant.meinet.com
http://www.dialysistech.org
Disability Served: kidney disease
This nonprofit professional organization strives to improve the quality of care in the dialysis industry while promoting education, recognition through certification and licensing, job security, and employment opportunities for nephrology professionals.

National Association of Pediatric Nurse Associates and Practitioners
20 Brace Road, Suite 200
Cherry Hill, NJ 08034-2634
856-857-9700
info@napnap.org
http://www.napnap.org
Disability Served: various
This professional association for pediatric nursing professionals, and other advanced practice nurses who care for children, advocates for children's health by providing funding, education, and research opportunities to pediatric nursing professionals; influencing legislation that affects maternal/child health care; and producing and distributing educational materials to parents and families.

National Association of RSVP Directors
PO Box 852
Athens, AL 35612
256-232-7207
bruth@al-rsvp.com
http://www.narsvpd.com
Disability Served: elderly
This association provides a network of communications among RSVP Directors and projects as well as serving as a vehicle for expression on behalf of older Americans to the Corporation for National and Community Service, Congress, and other appropriate government agencies.

National Association of School Psychologists
4340 East West Highway, Suite 402
Bethesda, MD 20814

301-657-0270
center@naspweb.org
http://www.nasponline.org
Disability Served: mental health
This professional organization represents and
supports school psychologists in order to
enhance the mental health and educational
competence of all children.

National Association of Social Workers (NASW)
750 First Street, NE
Washington, DC 20002-4241
202-408-8600
membership@naswdc.org
http://www.naswdc.org
Disability Served: various
The largest membership organization of professional
social workers in the world, the NASW works to
enhance the professional growth and development of its members, to create and maintain
professional standards, and to advance sound
social policies.

**National Association of State Directors
of Developmental Disabilities Services**
113 Oronoco Street
Alexandria, VA 22314
703-683-4202
http://www.nasddds.org
Disability Served: developmentally disabled
This nonprofit professional association focuses its efforts
on improving services for the developmentally
disabled. The association is active in disseminating
information and advocating for legislation.

National Association of the Deaf (NAD)
814 Thayer Avenue
Silver Spring, MD 20910-4500
301-587-1788, 301-587-1789 (TTY)
nadinfo@nad.org
http://www.nad.org
Disability Served: hearing
The association is the nation's largest organization
safeguarding the accessibility and civil rights of
28 million deaf and hard of hearing Americans
in education, employment, health care, and
telecommunications. The NAD publications
department produces many books and
web-based publications.

**National Conference of Gerontological Nurse
Practitioners**
4824 Edgemoor Lane
Bethesda, MD 20814-5306
301-654-3776
lmartin@ncgnp.org
http://www.ncgnp.org
Disability Served: elderly
This organization, which advocates for quality care for
older adults, provides continuing gerontological
education for advanced practice nurses. It promotes
the professional development of advanced practice
nursing, promotes communication and professional
collaboration among health care providers, and
supports research related to the care of older adults.

National Council on Spinal Cord Injury
151 Tremont Street
Boston, MA 02111
617-338-7777
Disability Served: spinal-cord injury
This membership organization promotes research and
provides informational services regarding spinal-cord
injury.

National Disability Rights Network
900 Second Street, NE, Suite 211
Washington, DC 20002
202-408-9514
info@napas.org
http://www.napas.org
Disability Served: various
The network is a national association of protection and
advocacy systems and client assistance programs.

National Education Association of the United States
1201 16th Street, NW
Washington, DC 20036-3290
202-833-4000
www-registration@list.nea.org
http://www.nea.org
Disability Served: various
This professional association provides information and
services to educators and other professionals, some
of whom serve students with disabilities.

National Federation of Licensed Practical Nurses
605 Poole Drive
Garner, NC 27529

919-779-0046
cbarbour@mgmt4u.com
http://www.nflpn.org
Disability Served: various
This professional organization for licensed practical
nurses, licensed vocational nurses, and practical/
vocational nursing students in the United States,
strives to foster high standards of nursing care and
promote continued competence through education,
certification, and lifelong learning.

National Gerontological Nursing Association

7794 Grow Drive
Pensacola, FL 32514
850-473-1174, 800-723-0560
ngna@puetzamc.com
http://www.ngna.org
Disability Served: elderly
This organization, whose members included clinicians,
educators, and researchers, is dedicated to the clinical
care of older adults in diverse care settings.

National Hospice and Palliative Care Organization

1700 Diagonal Road, Suite 625
Alexandria, VA 22314
703-837-1500, 800-658-8898
nhpco_info@nhpco.org
http://www.nhpco.org
Disability Served: various
This nonprofit membership organization represents
hospice and palliative care programs and
professionals in the United States. It is committed to
improving end of life care and expanding access to
hospice care with the goal of enhancing quality of
life for people who are dying. Hospice care involves a
team-oriented approach of expert medical care, pain
management, and emotional and spiritual support
expressly tailored to the patient's wishes, within a
home or home-like setting.

National League for Nursing

61 Broadway, 33rd Floor
New York, NY 10006
212-363-5555, 800-669-1656
http://www.nln.org
Disability Served: various
This organization, with the purpose of providing
leadership in nursing education, aims to prepare
the nursing workforce to meet the needs of diverse

populations in an ever-changing health care
environment.

National Mental Health Association (NMHA)

2001 North Beauregard Street, 12th Floor
Alexandria, VA 22311
703-684-7722, 800-969-6642
http://www.nmha.org
Disability Served: mental health
This nonprofit association addresses all aspects of
mental health and mental illness. With more than
340 affiliates nationwide. The NMHA works to
improve the mental health of all Americans through
advocacy, education, research, and service. The
association's programs educate the public, encourage
reform, and promote the use of effective local and
regional prevention and recovery programs.

National Mobility Equipment Dealers Association

3327 West Bearss Avenue
Tampa, FL 33618
800-833-0427
nmeda@aol.com
http://www.nmeda.org
Disability Served: various
This association is dedicated to providing safe and
quality adaptive transportation and mobility
equipment for consumers with disabilities.

National Network of Career Nursing Assistants

3577 Easton Road
Norton, OH 44203
330-825-9342
cnajeni@aol.com
http://www.cna-network.org
Disability Served: various
This nonprofit, educational organization promotes
recognition, education, research, advocacy and
peer support development for nursing assistants
in nursing homes and other long term care
settings.

National Spinal Cord Injury Association

6701 Democracy Boulevard, Suite 300-9
Bethesda, MD 20817
800-962-9629
info@spinalcord.org
http://www.spinalcord.org
Disability Served: spinal-cord injury

This association is dedicated to improving the quality of life for Americans living with the results of spinal-cord injury and disease, and their families.

North American Transplant Coordinators Organization

PO Box 15384
Lenexa, KS 66285-5384
913-492-3600
natco-info@goAMP.com
http://www.natco1.org
Disability Served: various
This organization supports, develops, and advances the knowledge and practice of its members in an effort to influence the effectiveness, quality, and integrity of organ donation and transplantation.

Oncology Nursing Society

125 Enterprise Drive
RIDC Park West
Pittsburgh, PA 15275-1214
412-859-6100, 866-257-4ONS
http://www.ons.org
Disability Served: cancer patients and survivors
This professional organization of more than 30,000 registered nurses and other health care providers is dedicated to excellence in patient care, education, research, and administration in oncology nursing.

Professionals Networking for Excellence in Service Delivery with Individuals Who Are Deaf or Hard of Hearing

c/o ADARA
PO Box 480
Myersville, MD 21773
ADARAorgn@aol.com
http://www.adara.org
Disability Served: hearing
This organization facilitates excellence in human service delivery for individuals who are deaf or hard of hearing. This mission is accomplished by enhancing the professional competencies of the membership, expanding opportunities for networking among colleagues, and supporting positive public policies for individuals who are deaf or hard of hearing.

Registry of Interpreters for the Deaf

333 Commerce Street
Alexandria, VA 22314

703-838-0030, 703-838-0459 TTY
info@rid.org
http://www.rid.org
Disability Served: hearing
This national membership organization consists of professionals who provide sign language interpreting/transliterating services for deaf and hard of hearing persons. The organization advocates for the increased quality, qualifications, and quantity of interpreters through professional certifications, and professional development through continuing education programs.

Society for Healthcare Consumer Advocacy

One North Franklin, Suite 31N
Chicago, IL 60606
312-422-3851
shca@aha.org
http://www.shca-aha.org
Disability Served: various
This organization advances health care consumer advocacy by supporting the role of professionals who represent and advocate for consumers across the health care continuum. It provides its members with education, information, and networking opportunities and serves as a resource for consumers, payers, the community, and health care professions regarding issues such as patient education, patients' rights, ethics, patient satisfaction/measurement, complaint management, and customer service.

United States Society for Augmentative and Alternative Communication

15 West 72nd Street, Suite 10B
New York, NY 10023
877-8USSAAC
info@ussaac.org
http://www.ussaac.org
Disability Served: communication
This society helps provide communication for individuals who are unable to verbalize. It is dedicated to providing information on the technology, tools, and therapies within the world of augmentative and alternative communication. Everyone from therapists to families to educators is served by the organization.

REHABILITATION CENTERS

Rehabilitation facilities provide a variety of services and programs for persons with all types of disabilities. Programs can range from short term to long term and from residential to nonresidential day programs. Services may include evaluation and training in assistive devices, employment counseling and support services, medical rehabilitation, adult day care, and developmental therapy.

ALABAMA

Alabama Department of Rehabilitation Services
2129 East South Boulevard
Montgomery, AL 36116-2455
334-281-8780, 800-543-3098
http://www.rehab.state.al.us
Disability Served: various

Alabama Goodwill Industries Inc.
2350 Green Springs Highway South
Birmingham, AL 35205
205-323-6331
algoodwill@aol.com
http://www.goodwill.org/states/al/index.htm
Disability Served: various

The Arc of Jefferson County
215 21st Avenue South
Birmingham, AL 35205
205-323-6383
hunter2549@aol.com
http://www.thearcofalabama.com
Disability Served: developmentally disabled

Briarcliff Nursing Center
850 Northwest 9th Street
Alabaster, AL 35007
205-620-3200
Disability Served: various

Cheaha Regional Mental Health/Caradale
1623 Old Birmingham Highway, PO Box 1248
Sylacauga, AL 35150
205-245-2201
Disability Served: mental health

**Easter Seals Rehabilitation Center
    of Central Alabama**
2125 East South Boulevard
Montgomery, AL 36116-2454
334-288-0240
ljohnson@eastersealsca.org
http://www.alabama.easter-seals.org
Disability Served: various

**Easter Seals Rehabilitation Center
    of Northwest Alabama**
1450 East Avalon Avenue
Muscle Shoals, AL 35661
205-381-1110
http://alabama.easterseals.com
Disability Served: various

**Easter Seals Rehabilitation Center-
    West Central Alabama**
2906 Citizens Parkway, PO Box 1347
Selma, AL 36702-0338
334-872-8421
Disability Served: various

Easter Seals West Alabama
1110 Sixth Avenue East
Tuscaloosa, AL 35401
203-759-1211
eswa@eastersealswestal.org
http://www.alabama.easter-seals.org
Disability Served: various

EL Darden Rehabilitation Center
1001 East Broad Street
Gadsden, AL 35999
205-547-5751
Disability Served: various

Fort Payne-Dekalb Rehab Center
311 North Gault Avenue
Ft. Payne, AL 35967
256-845-9367
Disability Served: various

Goodwill Easter Seals of the Gulf Coast
2448 Gordon Smith Drive
Mobile, AL 36617
251-471-1581
http://www.goodwill-easterseals.org
Disability Served: various

HealthSouth Lakeshore Outpatient
3800 Ridgeway Drive
Birmingham, AL 35209

205-868-2290
http://www.healthsouth.com
Disability Served: various

HealthSouth Rehabilitation Hospital
4465 Narrow Lane Road
Montgomery, AL 36116
334-284-7700
Disability Served: various

Huntsville Rehabilitation Foundation
2929 Johnson Road, SW
Huntsville, AL 35805-0671
256-880-0671
info@hsvrehab.org
http://www.hsvrehab.org
Disability Served: various

**Indian Rivers Mental Health and Mental
    Retardation Center**
1914 Seventh Street, PO Box 2190
Tuscaloosa, AL 35403
205-391-0107
Disability Served: mental health, mental retardation

Lighthouse Inc.
925 Convent Road, NE
Cullman, AL 35055
256-739-2777
http://www.geocities.com/lighthouse_cullman
Disability Served: chemical dependency

North Alabama Rehabilitation Hospital
107 Governors Drive, SW
Huntsville, AL 35801
205-535-2300
Disability Served: various

**North Central Alabama Mental Retardation
    Authority Inc.**
1621 Wolverine Drive, SE, Box 597
Decatur, AL 35603
205-355-7315
ncamra@hiwaay.net
Disability Served: developmentally disabled, mental
    retardation

Southeastern Blind Rehabilitation Center
700 South 19th Street (124)
Birmingham, AL 35233

205-558-4706, ext. 6997
George.Sands@med.va.gov
Disability Served: vision

UAB Model SCI System
619 Nineteenth Street South, SRC 529
Birmingham, AL 35249-7330
205-934-3283
sciweb@uab.edu
http://www.spinalcord.uab.edu
Disability Served: spinal-cord injury

Vaughn-Blumberg Center
2715 Flynn Road
Dothan, AL 36303
205-793-3102
Disability Served: various

Wiregrass Rehabilitation Center Inc.
795 Ross Clark Circle, NE, PO Box 338
Dothan, AL 36302-0338
334-792-0022
wrcadmin@ala.net
Disability Served: various

ALASKA
Alaska Center for the Blind and Visually Impaired
3903 Taft Drive
Anchorage, AK 99517
907-248-7770
info@alaskabvi.org
http://www.alaskabvi.org
Disability Served: vision

Alaska Division of Vocational Rehabilitation
801 West 10th Street, Suite A
Juneau, AK 99801-1894
907-465-2814, 800-478-2815
anne_knight@labor.state.ak.us
http://www.labor.state.ak.us/dvr/home.htm
Disability Served: various

Alaska Veterans Facility
4201 Tudor Centre Drive, Suite 115
Anchorage, AK 99508
907-563-6966
Disability Served: various

Center for Blind and Deaf Adults
731 Gambell, Suite 200
Anchorage, AK 99501
907-276-3456, 907-258-0510 (TTY)
Disability Served: hearing, vision

ARIZONA

Arizona Center for the Blind and Visually Impaired
3100 East Roosevelt Street
Phoenix, AZ 85008
602-273-7411
jlamay@acbvi.org
http://www.acbvi.org
Disability Served: vision

Arizona Industries for the Blind
3013 West Lincoln Street
Phoenix, AZ 85009
602-269-5131
tfarnsworth@azdes.gov
http://www.azdes.gov/aib
Disability Served: vision

Arizona Rehabilitation Services Administration
1789 West Jefferson
Phoenix, AZ 85007
602-542-3332, 602-542-6049 (TTY)
http://www.azdes.gov/rsa
Disability Served: various

Banner Good Samaritan Medical Center
1111 East McDowell Road
Phoenix, AZ 85006
602-239-2317
Disability Served: various

Barrow Neurological Institute Rehab Center
350 West Thomas Road
Phoenix, AZ 85013
602-406-3000
http://www.thebarrow.com
Disability Served: traumatic brain injury

Carondelet Brain Injury Programs and Services-St. Joseph's Hospital
350 North Wilmot Road
Tucson, AZ 85711
520-721-3856
http://www.carondelet.org
Disability Served: traumatic brain injury

Carondelet Rehabilitation Services of Arizona-St. Mary's Hospital
1601 West St. Mary's Road
Tucson, AZ 85703
520-622-5833
http://www.carondelet.org
Disability Served: various

Children's Clinics For Rehabilitative Services
2600 North Wyatt Drive
Tucson, AZ 85712
520-324-5437
contact@childrensclinics.org
http://www.childrensclinics.org
Disability Served: various

Desert Life Rehabilitation and Care Center
1919 West Medical Street
Tucson, AZ 85704
520-297-8311
http://www.desertlifercc.com
Disability Served: various

El Dorado Hospital and Medical Center
1400 North Wilmot Road
Tucson, AZ 85712
520-886-6361
http://www.eldoradoHospital.com
Disability Served: various

Freestone Rehabilitation Center
10617 East Oasis Drive
Mesa, AZ 85208
602-986-1531
Disability Served: various

HealthSouth Meridian Point Rehabilitation Hospital
11250 North 92nd Street
Scottsdale, AZ 85260
602-860-0671
http://www.healthsouth.com
Disability Served: various

HealthSouth Rehabilitation Institute of Tucson
2650 North Wyatt Drive
Tucson, AZ 85712
520-325-1300, 800-333-8628
http://www.healthsouth.com
Disability Served: various

HealthSouth Rehabilitation Center of Tucson
75 North Wilmot Road
Tucson, AZ 85711
520-790-0900
http://www.healthsouth.com
Disability Served: various

HealthSouth Valley of the Sun Rehabilitation Hospital
13460 North 67th Avenue
Glendale, AZ 85304-1042
623-878-8800
http://www.healthsouth.com
Disability Served: various

Institute for Human Development
PO Box 5630
Flagstaff, AZ 86011
520-523-4791
http://www.nau.edu/ihd
Disability Served: various

La Frontera Center Inc.
502 West 29th Street
Tucson, AZ 85713
520-770-7432
Disability Served: various

ManorCare Health Services-Tucson
3705 North Swan Road
Tucson, AZ 85718
520-299-7088
tucson@manorcare.com
http://www.hcr-manorcare.com
Disability Served: various

Progress Valley III
10505 North 69th Street, Suite 1100
Scottsdale, AZ 85253
480-315-1999
info@progressvalley.org
http://www.progressvalley.org
Disability Served: chemical dependency

Saint Joseph's Hospital and Medical Center
Home Care Services
350 West Thomas Road
Phoenix, AZ 85004
602-406-3000
http://www.ichosestjoes.com
Disability Served: various

Scottsdale Memorial Hospital Rehabilitation Services
7400 East Osborn Road
Scottsdale, AZ 85251
602-481-4000
Disability Served: various

Sterling Ranch Inc.
PO Box 36
Skull Valley, AZ 86338
928-442-3289
info@sterlingranch.info
http://www.sterlingranch.info
Disability Served: developmentally disabled

Toyei Industries Inc.
Building #6
Ganado, AZ 86505
928-755-6257
Disability Served: various

Tucson Association for the Blind and Visually Impaired
3767 East Grant Road
Tucson, AZ 85716
520-795-1331
Disability Served: vision

Yavapai Rehabilitation Center
436 North Washington Avenue
Prescott, AZ 86301
520-445-0991
Disability Served: various

ARKANSAS
Arkansas Division of Services for the Blind
700 Main Street, PO Box 3237
Little Rock, AR 72203
800-960-9270, 501-682-0093 (TDD)
http://www.arkansas.gov/dhs/dsb/NEWDSB
Disability Served: vision

Arkansas Easter Seal Society
3920 Woodland Heights Road
Little Rock, AR 72212
501-227-3600 (Voice/TTY)
adc@cei.net
http://ar.easterseals.org
Disability Served: various

Arkansas Lighthouse for the Blind
69th & Murray Streets, PO Box 192666
Little Rock, AR 72219
501-562-2222
Disability Served: vision

Arkansas Rehabilitation Services
1616 Brookwood Drive, PO Box 3781
Little Rock, AR 72203
501-296-1600, 501-296-1669 (TDD)
http://www.arsinfo.org
Disability Served: various

HealthSouth Rehabilitation Hospital of Fort Smith
1401 South J Street
Ft. Smith, AR 72901
479-785-3300
Disability Served: various

HealthSouth Rehabilitation Hospital of Jonesboro
1201 Fleming Avenue
Jonesboro, AR 72401-4311
870-932-0440
http://www.healthsouth.com
Disability Served: various

Hot Springs Rehabilitation Center
PO Box 1358
Hot Springs, AR 71902
501-624-4411
ktaylor@ars.state.ar.us
http://www.arsinfo.org/hsrehab.html
Disability Served: various

Lions World Services for the Blind
2811 Fair Park Boulevard, PO Box 4055
Little Rock, AR 72204
501-664-7100
trn72204@lwsb.org
http://www.lwsb.org
Disability Served: vision

Northwest Arkansas Rehabilitation Hospital
153 East Monte Painter Drive
Fayetteville, AR 72703
501-444-2200
Disability Served: various

Rebsamen Rehabilitation Center
1400 Braden Street
Jacksonville, AR 72076

501-985-7381
Disability Served: various

Saint Michael Hospital-Rehabilitation Unit
2400 St. Michael Drive
Texarkana, AR 75503
501-614-4000
Disability Served: various

Saint Vincent North Rehabilitation Hospital
2201 Wildwood Avenue
Sherwood, AR 72110
501-834-1800
Disability Served: various

CALIFORNIA

Adult Care Services
800 South Broadway, #309
Walnut Creek, CA 94596
510-944-5800
Disability Served: various

Alvarado Hospital Medical Center/San Diego Rehabilitation Hospital
6645 Alvarado Road
San Diego, CA 92120
619-287-3270
http://www.alvaradoHospital.com
Disability Served: various

Arc of San Diego Parent-Infant Program
2770 Glebe Road
Lemon Grove, CA 91945
619-697-8068
http://www.arc-sd.com
Disability Served: various

Arc of Southeast Los Angeles County
12049 Woodruff Avenue
Downey, CA 90242
562-803-4606
http://www.arcselac.org
Disability Served: developmentally disabled

Arc Ventura County
5103 Walker Street
Ventura, CA 93003
805-650-8611
jduran@arcvc.org
http://www.arcvc.org
Disability Served: developmentally disabled

Arrow Center
3035 G Street
San Diego, CA 92102-3245
619-233-8855
http://www.arc-sd.com/Locations.htm
Disability Served: developmentally disabled

Asian Rehabilitation Services Inc.
1701 East Washington Boulevard
Los Angeles, CA 90021
213-743-9242
admin@asianrehab.org
http://www.asianrehab.org
Disability Served: various

Assistance League of Los Altos
169 State Street
Los Altos, CA 94022
650-941-4625
http://www.assistanceleague.org/chaptersdetail.
   cfm?ID=100&state=5&path=1
Disability Served: various

Azure Acres Chemical Dependency Recovery Center
2264 Green Hill Road
Sebastopol, CA 95472
866-762-3766
cfiser@azureacres.com
http://www.azureacres.com/?source=4therapy
Disability Served: chemical dependency

Back in the Saddle
9775 Mockingbird Avenue
Apple Valley, CA 92308-8341
760-240-3217
Disability Served: elderly

Bakersfield Association for Retarded Citizens
2240 South Union Avenue
Bakersfield, CA 93307-4158
661-834-2272
http://www.barc-inc.org
*Disability Served: developmentally disabled,
   mental retardation*

Brotman Medical Center
3828 Delmas Terrace
Culver City, CA 90231
310-836-7000
http://www.brotmanmedicalCenter.com
Disability Served: various

Build Rehabilitation Industries
1323 Truman Street
San Fernando, CA 91340
818-898-0020
brosen@buildrehab.org
http://buildindustries.com
Disability Served: various

California Department of Rehabilitation
2000 Evergreen Street, PO Box 944222
Sacramento, CA 95815
916-263-8981, 916-263-7477 (TTY)
http://www.rehab.cahwnet.gov
Disability Served: various

California Elwyn
18325 Mount Baldy Circle
Fountain Valley, CA 92708
714-557-6313
info@caelwyn.org
http://www.caelwyn.org
Disability Served: various

Camp Campbell Outpatient Programs
256 East Hamilton, Suite J & K
Campbell, CA 95008
408-367-2190
http://www.camprecovery.com
Disability Served: chemical dependency

Camp Recovery Center
3192 Glen Canyon Road
Scotts Valley, CA 95066
800-924-2879
http://www.camprecovery.com
Disability Served: chemical dependency

Camp Santa Cruz Intensive Outpatient Program
215 River Street
Santa Cruz, CA 95060
831-425-1350
http://www.camprecovery.com
Disability Served: chemical dependency

Casa Colina Centers for Rehabilitation
255 East Bonita Avenue, PO Box 6001
Pomona, CA 91769-6001
909-596-7733, 800-926-5462
rehab@casacolina.org
http://www.casacolina.org
Disability Served: various

Cedars Development Foundation of Marin
PO Box 947
Ross, CA 94957
415-454-5310
Disability Served: various

Cedars-Sinai Medical Center
8700 Beverly Boulevard
Los Angeles, CA 90048
213-423-3277
http://www.csmc.edu
Disability Served: various

Center for Applied Rehabilitation Technology
Rancho Los Amigos Medical Center
7601 East Imperial Highway
Downey, CA 90242
562-401-6800
CARTinfo@gmail.com
http://www.rancho.org/cart/default.htm
Disability Served: physically disabled

Center for the Partially Sighted
12301 Wilshire Boulevard, Suite 600
Los Angeles, CA 90025
310-458-3501, 800-481-EYES
http://www.low-vision.org
Disability Served: vision

Centre for Neuro Skills
2658 Mt Vernon Avenue
Bakersfield, CA 93306
661-872-3408, 800-922-4994
bakersfield@neuroskills.com
http://www.neuroskills.com
Disability Served: traumatic brain injury

Centre for Neuro Skills
16542 Ventura Boulevard, #500
Encino, CA 91436
818-783-3800
losangeles@neuroskills.com
http://www.neuroskills.com
Disability Served: traumatic brain injury

Children's Hospital and Health Center
Speech-Language Pathology Department
3020 Children's Way
San Diego, CA 92123
858-576-1700

http://www.chsd.org
Disability Served: communication

Children's Hospital Los Angeles Rehabilitation Program
4650 Sunset Boulevard, Box 6
Los Angeles, CA 90027
323-669-2450
http://chla.usc.edu
Disability Served: various

Children's Therapy Center
770 Paseo Camarillo, Suite 120
Camarillo, CA 93010
805-383-1501
Disability Served: various

Clausen House
88 Vernon Street
Oakland, CA 94610
510-839-0050
nan@clausenhouse.org
http://www.clausenhouse.org
Disability Served: developmentally disabled

Community Center for the Blind and Visually Impaired
130 West Flora Street
Stockton, CA 95202-1636
209-466-3836
ccbviinfo@sbcglobal.net
http://www.communityblindCenter.org
Disability Served: vision

Community Gatepath
1764 Marco Polo Way
Burlingame, CA 94010
650-259-8544
info@gatepath.com
http://www.communitygatepath.com
Disability Served: various

Community Hospital of Los Gatos
815 Pollard Road
Los Gatos, CA 95030
408-866-4020
http://www.communityHospitallg.com
Disability Served: various

Community Rehabilitation Industries
1500 East Anaheim Street
Long Beach, CA 90813

562-591-0539
rose@cri-lb.org
Disability Served: various

Compobello Chemical Dependency Recovery Center
3400 Guerneville Road
Santa Rosa, CA 94501
707-579-4066
Disability Served: chemical dependency

Corona Regional Medical Center
800 South Main Street
Corona, CA 92882
951-737-4343
http://www.coronaregional.com
Disability Served: various

Crutcher's Serenity House
50 Hillcrest Drive, PO Box D
Deer Park, CA 94576
877-274-4968
crutcherssh@earthlink.net
http://www.crutcherssh.com/page3.html
Disability Served: chemical dependency

Daniel Freeman Hospitals Rehabilitation Centers
333 North Prairie Avenue
Inglewood, CA 90301
310-674-7050
http://www.netadvantage.com/dfreeman/rc_main.html
Disability Served: spinal-cord injury, traumatic brain injury

Delano Regional Medical Center
1401 Garces Highway
Delano, CA 93215
661-725-4800
drmc@drmc.com
http://www.drmc.com
Disability Served: various

Desert Area Resources and Training
201 East Ridgecrest Boulevard
Ridgecrest, CA 93555
706-375-9787
dart@dartontarget.org
http://www.dartontarget.org
Disability Served: various

Desert Hospital Acute Inpatient Rehabilitation
1150 North Indian Canyon Drive
Palm Springs, CA 92262
760-323-6511
http://www.desertmedctr.com
Disability Served: various

Devereux California
PO Box 6784
Santa Barbara, CA 93160
805-968-2525
http://www.devereux.org
Disability Served: autism, developmentally disabled

Easter Seals Bay Area
180 Grand Avenue, Suite 300
Oakland, CA 94612
510-835-2131
info@easterseals.com
http://bayarea.easterseals.com
Disability Served: various

Easter Seals Superior California
Sacramento Center & Regional Offices
3205 Hurley Way
Sacramento, CA 95864
916-485-6711
http://superiorca.easterseals.com
Disability Served: various

East Los Angeles Doctors Hospital
4060 Whittier Boulevard
Los Angeles, CA 90023
323-268-5514
http://www.health-plus.net/hosp_eastla.html
Disability Served: various

Enchanted Hills Camp
3410 Mount Veeder Road
Napa, CA 94558
707-224-4023
http://www.lighthouse-sf.org
Disability Served: vision

Eye Medical Clinic of Fresno Inc.
1122 South Street
Fresno, CA 93721
209-486-5000
Disability Served: vision

Feather River Industries
1811 Kusel Road
Oroville, CA 95966
530-534-1112
info@wtcinc.org
http://www.featherriverindustries.com
Disability Served: various

Fontana Rehabilitation Workshop Inc.
Industrial Support Systems
8333 Almeria Avenue
Fontana, CA 92334
909-428-3833
Disability Served: various

Foothill Workshop for the Handicapped Inc.
789 North Fair Oaks Avenue
Pasadena, CA 91103
626-449-0218
Disability Served: various

Fred Finch Youth Center
3800 Coolidge Avenue
Oakland, CA 94602
510-482-2244
swankeyes@fredfinch.org
http://www.fredfinch.org
Disability Served: developmentally disabled

Gabriel Valley Training Center
400 South Covina Boulevard
La Puente, CA 91746
626-968-8479
Disability Served: various

Garfield Medical Center
525 North Garfield Avenue
Monterey Park, CA 91754
626-573-2222
http://www.whittierHospital.com
Disability Served: various

Gateway Center of Monterey County Inc.
850 Congress Avenue
Pacific Grove, CA 93950
831-372-8002
info@gatewayCenter.org
http://www.gatewayCenter.org
Disability Served: various

Glendale Adventist Medical Center Rehabilitation Institute
1509 Wilson Terrace
Glendale, CA 91206
818-409-8000
http://www.glendaleadventist.com
Disability Served: various

Glendale Memorial Hospital and Health Center Rehabilitation Unit
1420 South Central Avenue
Glendale, CA 91204
818-502-1900
http://www.glendalememorial.com
Disability Served: various

Grossmont Hospital Rehabilitation Center
5555 Grossmont Center Drive
La Mesa, CA 91942
619-740-4100
http://www.sharp.com/Hospital/index.cfm?id=917
Disability Served: various

Hacienda La Puente Adult Education
15959 East Gale Avenue
City of Industry, CA 91716-0002
626-933-1915
Disability Served: various

HealthSouth Bakersfield Regional Rehabilitation Hospital
5001 Commerce Drive
Bakersfield, CA 93309
805-323-5500, 800-288-9829
http://www.bakersfield.org
Disability Served: various

Hi-Desert Continuing Care Center
6722 White Feather Road
Joshua Tree, CA 92252
760-366-1500
admindept@hdmc.org
http://serv1.hdmc.org
Disability Served: various

Hillhaven Alameda
516 Willow Street
Oakland, CA 94501-6132
510-521-5600
Disability Served: various

Hillhaven Extended Care
1115 Capitola Road
Santa Cruz, CA 95062-2844
408-475-4055
Disability Served: various

Home of the Guiding Hands
1825 Gillespie Way
El Cajon, CA 92020
619-938-2850
http://guidinghands.org
Disability Served: developmentally disabled

The Independent Way
575 Independent Road
Oakland, CA 94621
510-639-4680, 510-567-9705 (TTY)
http://www.arc-alameda.com
Disability Served: developmentally disabled

Janus Alcoholism Services Inc.
200 Seventh Avenue, Suite 150
Santa Cruz, CA 95062
831-462-1060
jtice@janussc.org
http://www.janussc.org
Disability Served: chemical dependency

Joe McGie Center
2812 Hegan Lane
Chico, CA 95928
530-343-3406
tam@ewtc.org
http://www.wtcinc.org/joemcgie.htm
Disability Served: various

John Muir Medical Center Rehabilitation Services
1601 Ygnacio Valley Road
Walnut Creek, CA 94598
925-939-3000
http://www.jmmdhs.com
Disability Served: various

Kentfield Rehabilitation Hospital
1125 Sir Francis Drake Boulevard
Kentfield, CA 94904
415-485-3527
Disability Served: various

LaPalma Intercommunity Hospital
7901 Walker Street
La Palma, CA 90623
714-670-7400
info@lpihoc.com
http://www.lapalmaintercommunityHospital.com
Disability Served: various

Laurel Grove Hospital-Rehab Care Unit
19933 Lake Chabot Road
Castro Valley, CA 94546
510-727-2755
nissims@sutterhealth.org
http://www.edenmedCenter.org
Disability Served: various

Learning Services-Escondido
2335 Bear Valley Parkway
Escondido, CA 92027
888-419-9955, ext. 12
http://www.learningservices.com/escondido.htm
Disability Served: traumatic brain injury

Learning Services-Gilroy
10855 DeBruin Way
Gilroy, CA 95020
888-419-9955, ext. 12
http://www.learningservices.com/gilroy.htm
Disability Served: traumatic brain injury

Leon S. Peters Rehabilitation Center
2823 Fresno Street
Fresno, CA 93721
209-442-3957
jlau@communitymedical.org
http://www.communitymedical.org
Disability Served: various

LightHouse for the Blind and Visually Impaired
214 Van Ness Avenue
San Francisco, CA 94102
415-441-1981, 415-431-4572 (TTY)
http://www.lighthouse-sf.org
Disability Served: vision

LightHouse of Marin
1137 4th Street
San Rafael, CA 94901
415-258-8496

http://www.lighthouse-sf.org
Disability Served: vision

LightHouse of the North Coast
2830 G Street, Suite B-1
Eureka, CA 95501
707-268-5646
http://www.lighthouse-sf.org
Disability Served: vision

Lions Blind Center of Diablo Valley
175 Alvarado Avenue
Pittsburg, CA 94565
925-432-3013, 800-750-3937
Disability Served: vision

Lion's Center for the Blind
3834 Opal Street
Oakland, CA 94609
510-450-1580
Kathyrine_Brown@lbCenter.org
Disability Served: vision

Living Skills Center for the Visually Impaired
2430 Road 20, #B112
San Pablo, CA 94086
510-234-4984
patty@livingskillsCenter.org
http://www.livingskillsCenter.org
Disability Served: vision

Loma Linda University Rehabilitation Institute
11406 Loma Linda Drive
Loma Linda, CA 92354
909-558-6144
http://www.llu.edu/lluhc/rehabilitation/rehab.htm
Disability Served: various

**Long Beach Memorial Medical Center Memorial
    Rehabilitation Hospital**
2801 Atlantic Avenue
Long Beach, CA 90806
562-933-9001
http://www.memorialcare.org
Disability Served: various

Lucile Packard Children's Hospital at Stanford
725 Welch Road
Palo Alto, CA 94304
650-497-8199, 650-497-8170

http://www.lpch.org
Disability Served: various

ManorCare Health Services-Hemet
1717 West Stetson Street
Hemet, CA 92343
714-925-9171
hemet@manorcare.com
http://www.hcr-manorcare.com
Disability Served: various

ManorCare Health Services-Rossmoor
1975 Tice Valley Boulevard
Walnut Creek, CA 94595
925-906-0200
rossmoor@manorcare.com
http://www.hcr-manorcare.com
Disability Served: various

ManorCare Nursing-Citrus Heights
7807 Uplands Way
Citrus Heights, CA 95610
916-967-2929
citrusheights@manorcare.com
http://www.hcr-manorcare.com
Disability Served: various

ManorCare Nursing-Fountain Valley
11680 Warner Avenue
Fountain Valley, CA 92708
714-241-9800
fountainvalley@manorcare.com
http://www.hcr-manorcare.com
Disability Served: various

ManorCare Nursing-Palm Desert
74-350 Country Club Drive
Palm Desert, CA 92260
619-341-0261
palmdesert@manorcare.com
http://www.hcr-manorcare.com
Disability Served: various

ManorCare Nursing-Sunnyvale
1150 Tilton Drive
Sunnyvale, CA 94087
408-735-7200
sunnyvale@manorcare.com
http://www.hcr-manorcare.com
Disability Served: various

Martin Luther King-Drew Medical Center
12021 South Wilmington Avenue
Los Angeles, CA 90059
310-668-4321
http://www.ladhs.org/mlk
Disability Served: various

Motherlode Rehabilitation Enterprises
399 Placerville Drive
Placerville, CA 95667
916-622-4848
Disability Served: various

Napa County Mental Health
2344 Old Sonoma Road, Building D
Napa, CA 94559
707-253-4711
Disability Served: mental health

Napa Valley Support Systems
650 Imperial Way, Suite 202
Napa, CA 94559
707-253-7490
Disability Served: various

North Bay Rehabilitation Services Inc.
649 Martin Avenue
Rohnert Park, CA 94928-2050
707-585-1991
regina@nbrs.org
http://www.nbrs.org
Disability Served: various

North Coast Rehabilitation Center
151 Sotoyome Street
Santa Rosa, CA 95405
707-542-2771
Disability Served: various

Northridge Hospital Medical Center
18300 Roscoe Boulevard
Northridge, CA 91328
818-885-5338
http://www.northridgeHospital.org
Disability Served: various

Old Adobe Developmental Services Inc.
235 Casa Grande Road
Petaluma, CA 94954

707-763-9807
http://www.oadsinc.org
Disability Served: developmentally disabled

Palomar Pomerado Rehabilitation Service
555 East Valley Parkway
Escondido, CA 92025
800-628-2880
tlc@pph.org
http://www.pphs.org/body.cfm?id=20&action=detail&
    ref=9
Disability Served: various

Peninsula Center for the Blind
2470 El Camino Real, Suite 107
Palo Alto, CA 94306-1701
650-858-0202
Center@pcbvi.org
http://www.pcbvi.org
Disability Served: vision

People Services Inc.
4195 Lakeshore Boulevard
Lakeport, CA 95453
707-263-3810
peopleservices@mindspring.com
http://www.peopleservices.org
Disability Served: various

Petaluma Recycling Center
315 Second Street
Petaluma, CA 94952
707-763-4761
http://www.oadsinc.org
Disability Served: developmentally disabled

Phoenix Programs Inc.
1875 Willow Pass Road
Concord, CA 94520
925-825-4700
http://www.phoenixprograms.org
Disability Served: various

Pride Industries
10030 Foothills Boulevard
Roseville, CA 95747-7102
916-788-2100, 800-550-6005
http://www.prideindustries.com
Disability Served: various

Pride Industries-Auburn
13080 Earhart Avenue
Auburn, CA 95603
530-888-0331
http://www.prideindustries.com
Disability Served: various

Pride Industries-Grass Valley
12451 Loma Rica Drive
Grass Valley, CA 95945
530-477-1832
http://www.prideindustries.com
Disability Served: various

**Providence Holy Cross Comprehensive Rehabilitation
    Center**
15031 Rinaldi Street North
Mission Hills, CA 91346
818-365-8051
http://www.providence.org/LosAngeles/Facilities/
    Providence_Holy_Cross
Disability Served: various

**Queen of Angels/Hollywood Presbyterian
    Medical Center**
1300 North Vermont Avenue
Los Angeles, CA 90027
213-413-3000
http://www.tenethealth.com
Disability Served: various

Ramona Adult Center
2138 San Vicente Road, # A
Ramona, CA 92065
760-789-1553
Disability Served: various

Rancho Los Amigos National Rehabilitation Center
7601 East Imperial Highway
Downey, CA 90242
562-401-7111
radsCenter@aol.com
http://www.rancho.org
Disability Served: various

Regional Center of Orange County
PO Box 22010
Santa Ana, CA 92702-2010
714-685-5555
http://www.rcocdd.com
Disability Served: various

Rehabilitation Institute of Southern California
1800 East LaVeta Avenue
Orange, CA 92666
714-633-7400
psingh@rio-rehab.com
http://www.rio-rehab.com
Disability Served: various

Robert H. Ballard Rehabilitation Hospital
1760 West 16th Street
San Bernardino, CA 92411-2411
909-473-1200
Disability Served: various

Rubicon Programs Inc.
2500 Bissell Avenue
Richmond, CA 94804
510-235-1516, 800-735-2929 (TTY)
http://www.rubiconprograms.org
Disability Served: various

Saint Joseph Hospital-General Hospital Campus
2200 Harrison Avenue
Eureka, CA 95501
707-445-5111
http://www.stjhs.org
Disability Served: various

Saint Jude Medical Center
101 East Valencia Mesa Drive
Fullerton, CA 92635
714-871-3280
https://www.stjudemedicalCenter.org
Disability Served: various

Saint Mary's Low Vision Center
Health Enhancement Center
1055 Linden Avenue
Long Beach, CA 90813
562-491-9275
http://www.sc.chw.edu/wwwroot/smmc/docs/index.
    htm
Disability Served: vision

Saint Mary's Medical Center
1050 Linden Avenue
Long Beach, CA 90813
562-491-9000
http://www.stmarymedicalCenter.com
Disability Served: various

Saint Mary's Medical Center Acute Rehab
450 Stanyan Street
San Francisco, CA 94117
415-668-1000
http://www.stmarysmedicalcenter.org
Disability Served: various

San Bernardino Valley Lighthouse for the Blind Inc.
762 North Sierra Way
San Bernardino, CA 92410
909-884-3121
Jeff@lighthouse4theblind.org
http://www.lighthouse4theblind.org
Disability Served: vision

San Francisco Vocational Services
814 Mission Street, Suite 600
San Francisco, CA 94103-3018
415-512-9500 (Voice/TTY)
sfvs@sfvocationalservices.org
http://www.sfvocationalservices.org
Disability Served: various

San Joaquin Valley Rehabilitation Hospital
7173 North Sharon Avenue
Fresno, CA 93720
559-436-3600
jpage@sjvrehab.com
http://www.sanjoaquinrehab.com
Disability Served: various

Santa Barbara Cottage Hospital
PO Box 689
Santa Barbara, CA 93102
805-682-7111
http://www.sbch.org
Disability Served: various

Santa Clara Valley Medical Center
751 South Bascom Avenue
San Jose, CA 95128
408-885-5000
http://www.scvmed.org
Disability Served: various

Scripps Memorial Hospital
354 Santa Fe Drive
Encinitas, CA 92024
760-633-6501
http://www.scrippshealth.org
Disability Served: various

Scripps Memorial Hospital at La Jolla
9888 Genesee Avenue
La Jolla, CA 92037
858-626-4123
http://www.scrippshealth.org
Disability Served: various

Sharp Coronado Hospital
250 Prospect Street
Coronado, CA 92118
619-522-3600
info@sharp.com
http://www.sharp.com
Disability Served: various

Sierra Gates Rehabilitation
7150 Sierra Ponds Lane
Granite Bay, CA 95650
916-791-7067
helpdesk@winwaysrehab.com
http://www.sierragates.com
Disability Served: traumatic brain injury

Sierra Vista Regional Medical Center
1010 Murray Avenue
San Luis Obispo, CA 93405
805-546-7600
http://www.sierravistaregional.com
Disability Served: various

Sober Living by the Sea Treatment Centers
2811 Villa Way
Newport Beach, CA 92663
800-647-0042
http://www.soberliving.com
Disability Served: chemical dependency

Society for the Blind
2750 24th Street
Sacramento, CA 95818
916-452-8271
programs@societyfortheblind.org
http://www.societyfortheblind.org
Disability Served: vision

Solutions at Santa Barbara-Transitional Living Center
1135 North Patterson Avenue
Santa Barbara, CA 93111
805-683-1995
sol1135@aol.com

http://www.jodihouse.org/solutions.htm
Disability Served: physically disabled

South Bay Rehabilitation Center at Paradise Valley Hospital
2400 East Fourth Street
National City, CA 91950
619-470-4227 (inpatient), 619-470-4300 (outpatient)
http://www.paradisevalleyHospital.org
Disability Served: various

Stepping Stones Growth Center
311 MacArthur Boulevard
San Leandro, CA 94577
510-568-3331
http://www.steppingstonesgrowth.org
Disability Served: various

Subacute Saratoga Hospital
13425 Sousa Lane
Saratoga, CA 95070
408-378-8875
http://www.subacutesaratoga.com
Disability Served: various

Sunnyside Rehabilitation and Nursing Center
22617 South Vermont Avenue
Torrance, CA 90502
310-320-4130
Disability Served: various

Temple Community Hospital
235 North Hoover Street
Los Angeles, CA 90004
213-382-7252
info@templecommunityHospital.com
http://www.templecommunityHospital.com
Disability Served: various

Tustin Rehabilitation Hospital
14851 Yorba Street
Tustin, CA 92780
714-832-9200
http://www.healthsouth.com
Disability Served: various

Ukiah Valley Association
564 South Dora Street, Suite D
Ukiah, CA 95482
707-468-8824

pamjensen@uvah.org
http://www.uvah.org
Disability Served: various

University of California-Los Angeles Intervention Program
23-10 Rehabilitation Center, 1000 Veteran Avenue
Los Angeles, CA 90024
310-825-4821
http://www.bol.ucla.edu/~kloo/IP/Home.htm
Disability Served: various

University of Southern California University Hospital
1500 San Pablo Street
Los Angeles, CA 90033
323-442-8500
http://www.uscuh.com
Disability Served: various

Valley Center for the Blind
4421 North Cedar Avenue, Suite #200
Fresno, CA 93721
559-222-4447
valleycntrblind@sbcglobal.net
Disability Served: vision

Valley Hospital Medical Center for Rehabilitative Medicine
14500 Sherman Circle
Van Nuys, CA 91405
818-908-8676
Disability Served: various

Veterans Affairs Rehabilitation Research and Development Center
3801 Miranda Avenue, Mail Stop 153
Palo Alto, CA 94304-1290
650-493-5000
http://www.palo-alto.med.va.gov
Disability Served: various

Village Square Nursing and Rehabilitation Center
1586 West San Marcos Boulevard
San Marcos, CA 92069
706-471-2986
http://www.kindredhealthcare.com
Disability Served: various

Westside Community Hospital
151 South Highway 33
Newman, CA 95360-9603

209-862-2951
Disability Served: various

White Memorial Medical Center
1720 Cesar E. Chavez Avenue
Los Angeles, CA 90033
323-268-5000
http://www.whitememorial.com
Disability Served: various

Winways
7732 Santiago Canyon Road
Orange, CA 92869
714-771-5276
helpdesk@winwaysrehab.com
http://www.winwaysrehab.com
Disability Served: various

Work Training Center
2255 Fair Street
Chico, CA 95928
530-343-7994
karen@ewtc.org
http://www.wtcinc.org
Disability Served: various

COLORADO
Boulder County Enterprises Inc.
900 Coffman
Longmont, CO 80501
303-772-6278
http://bcn.boulder.co.us/oscn/agencies/bce.html
Disability Served: various

Cherry Hills Health Care Center
3575 South Washington Street
Englewood, CO 80110
303-789-2265
http://www.cherryhillshc.com
Disability Served: various

Cheyenne Village Inc.
6275 Lehman Drive
Colorado Springs, CO 80918
719-592-0200, 719-592-0224 (TTY)
info@cheyennevillage.org
http://www.cheyennevillage.org
Disability Served: developmentally disabled

Children's Hospital Rehabilitation Center
1056 East 19th Avenue
Denver, CO 80218
303-861-6633
http://www.thechildrensHospital.org
Disability Served: various

Colorado Division of Vocational Rehabilitation
1575 Sherman Street, 4th Floor
Denver, CO 80023
303-866-4150 (Voice/TDD), 866-870-4595
debbie.powell@state.co.us
http://www.cdhs.state.co.us/ods/dvr
Disability Served: various

Community Hospital Back and Conditioning Clinic
2021 North 12th Street
Grand Junction, CO 81501
970-242-0920
http://www.gjhosp.org
Disability Served: back injury

Eastern Colorado Services for the Developmentally Disabled
617 South 10th Avenue, PO Box 1682
Sterling, CO 80751
970-522-7121
ramona@ecsdd.org
http://www.easterncoloradoservices.org
Disability Served: developmentally disabled

Las Animas County Rehabilitation Center
1205 Congress Drive
Trinidad, CO 81082
719-846-3388
Disability Served: various

Learning Services-Bear Creek
7201 West Hampden Avenue
Lakewood, CO 80227
888-419-9955, ext. 12
http://www.learningservices.com/lakewood.htm
Disability Served: traumatic brain injury

ManorCare Health Services-Denver
290 South Monaco Parkway
Denver, CO 80224
303-355-2525
denver@manorcare.com
http://www.hcr-manorcare.com
Disability Served: various

ManorCare Nursing and Rehabilitation Center-Boulder
2800 Palo Parkway
Boulder, CO 80301
303-440-9100
boulder@manorcare.com
http://www.hcr-manorcare.com
Disability Served: various

Mapleton Center for Rehabilitation
311 Mapleton Avenue
Boulder, CO 80301
303-440-2273
http://www.bch.org
Disability Served: various

Mosaic-Colorado Springs
1785 North Academy Boulevard, Suite 127
Colorado Springs, CO 80909-2733
719-380-0451
integrity@mosaicinfo.org
http://www.mosaicinfo.org
Disability Served: various

Mosaic-Ft. Collins
109 Cameron Drive, Suite A
Ft. Collins, CO 80525-3802
970-223-1751
integrity@mosaicinfo.org
http://www.mosaicinfo.org
Disability Served: various

Mosaic-Grand Junction
436 Independent Avenue
Grand Junction, CO 81505-6128
970-245-0519
integrity@mosaicinfo.org
http://www.mosaicinfo.org
Disability Served: various

Penrose/St. Francis Healthcare Services
Capron Rehabilitation Unit
2215 North Cascade Street
Colorado Springs, CO 80907
719-776-5200
psfrehab@centura.org
http://www.penrosestfrancis.org
Disability Served: various

Platte River Industries Inc.
490 Bryant Street
Denver, CO 80204
303-825-0041
Disability Served: various

Pueblo Diversified Industries Inc.
2828 Granada Boulevard
Pueblo, CO 81005-3104
800-466-8393
http://www.pdipueblo.net
Disability Served: various

Rehabilitation Hospital of Colorado Springs
325 Parkside Drive
Colorado Springs, CO 80910
719-630-8000
Disability Served: various

SHALOM Denver
2498 West 2nd Avenue
Denver, CO 80223
303-623-0251
sgehrke@jewishfamilyservice.org
http://www.shalomdenver.com
Disability Served: various

Spalding Rehabilitation Hospital
900 Potomac Street
Aurora, CO 80011
303-367-1166
http://www.spaldingrehab.com
Disability Served: various

United Cerebral Palsy of Colorado
2200 South Jasmine Street
Denver, CO 80222-5708
303-691-9339
jham@cpco.org
Disability Served: cerebral palsy

CONNECTICUT
Ahlbin Centers for Rehabilitation Medicine
Bridgeport Hospital
267 Grant Street
Bridgeport, CT 06610
203-366-7551
http://www.bridgeporthospital.org/ahlbin
Disability Served: various

Bristol Association for Retarded Citizens
621 Jerome Avenue, PO Box 726
Bristol, CT 06011

860-582-9102
Brstl.Assoc.Rtrdd@snet.net
http://www.geocities.com/BristolARC
Disability Served: developmentally disabled, mental
    retardation

Central Connecticut Association for Retarded Citizens
950 Slater Road
New Britain, CT 06051
860-229-6665
dseeger@ccarc.com
http://www.ccarc.com
Disability Served: developmentally disabled, mental
    retardation

Connecticut Board of Education and Services for the Blind
184 Windsor Avenue
Windsor, CT 06095
860-602-4000, 800-842-4510, 860-602-4221 (TDD)
besb@po.state.ct.us
http://www.besb.state.ct.us
Disability Served: vision

Connecticut Bureau of Rehabilitation Services
25 Sigourney Street
Hartford, CT 06106
800-537-2549, 860-424-4839 (TDD/TTY)
judith.moeckel@po.state.ct.us
http://www.brs.state.ct.us
Disability Served: various

DATAHR Rehabilitation Institute
135 Old State Road
Brookfield, CT 06804
203-775-4700
Disability Served: various

Eastern Blind Rehabilitation Center and Clinic
VA Connecticut Healthcare System, West Haven
    Campus
950 Campbell Avenue
West Haven, CT 06516
203-932-5711
http://www.visn1.med.va.gov/vact
Disability Served: vision

Employment Opportunities and Community Inclusion Program
333 State Street
North Haven, CT 06473

203-456-5995
Disability Served: various

Gaylord Hospital Inc.
PO Box 400
Wallingford, CT 06492
203-284-2800
http://www.gaylord.org
Disability Served: various

Hockanum Industries Inc.
40 Hale Street
Vernon, CT 06066
203-429-6724
thalstead@hockanumindustries.org
http://www.hockanumindustries.org
Disability Served: developmentally disabled

Kuhn Employment Opportunities Inc.
165 Pratt Street
Meriden, CT 06450
203-235-2583
info@kuhngroup.org
http://www.kuhngroup.org
Disability Served: various

Lake Grove at Durham
459R Wallingford Road
Durham, CT 06422
203-349-3467
Disability Served: various

Litchfield County Association for Retarded Citizens
84R Main Street
Torrington, CT 06790
860-482-9364
larc@litchfieldarc.org
http://www.litchfieldarc.org
Disability Served: developmentally disabled, mental
    retardation

Meriden-Wallingford Society
224-226 Cook Avenue
Meriden, CT 06451
203-237-9975
info@mwsinc.org
http://www.mwsinc.org
Disability Served: various

Norwalk Hospital
Physical Medicine and Rehabilitation
698 West Avenue

Norwalk, CT 06856
203-852-3400
http://www.norwalkhosp.org
Disability Served: various

Rehabilitation Associates Inc.
60 Katana Drive
Fairfield, CT 06824
203-384-8681
Disability Served: various

Reliance House Inc.
40 Broadway
Norwich, CT 06360
860-887-6536
JEdmo@reliancehouse.org
http://www.reliancehouse.org
Disability Served: mental health

SARAH Inc.
45 Boston Street
Guilford, CT 06437
203-458-8532
cshanley@sarah-inc.org
http://www.sarah-inc.org
Disability Served: various

DELAWARE
Alfred I. duPont Hospital for Children
Rehabilitation Program
1600 Rockland Road, PO Box 269
Wilmington, DE 19803
302-651-5605
http://www.nemours.org
Disability Served: various

Delaware Association for the Blind
800 West Street
Wilmington, DE 19801
302-655-2111
Disability Served: vision

Delaware Division of Vocational Rehabilitation
4425 North Market Street
Wilmington, DE 19802
302-761-8300
http://www.delawareworks.com/dvr
Disability Served: various

Delaware Elwyn Institute
321 East 11th Street
Wilmington, DE 19801
302-658-8860
http://www.elwyn.org/contact_de.html
Disability Served: various

Easter Seals
61 Corporate Circle, New Castle Common
New Castle, DE 19720
302-324-4444
http://de.easterseals.com
Disability Served: various

Edgemoor Day Program
500 Duncan Road, Suite A
Wilmington, DE 19809
302-762-9077
Disability Served: various

First State Senior Center
291A North Rehoboth Boulevard
Milford, DE 19963
302-422-1510
dhssinfo@state.de.us
http://www.dhss.delaware.gov/dhss/main/maps/
  other/dddssrctr.htm
Disability Served: elderly

Mosaic-Newark
260 Chapman Road, Suite 104A
Newark, DE 19720-5410
302-456-5995
integrity@mosaicinfo.org
http://www.mosaicinfo.org
Disability Served: various

**Salvation Army Delaware Developmental
  Disabilities Program**
559 East Dupont Highway
Georgetown, DE 19966
302-934-3730
Disability Served: various

DISTRICT OF COLUMBIA
Barbara Chambers Children's Center
1470 Irving Street, NW
Washington, DC 20010

202-387-6755
http://barbarachambers.org
Disability Served: various

Children's Hospital Spina Bifida Program
111 Michigan Avenue, NW
Washington, DC 20010
202-884-3094
http://www.dcchildrens.com/dcchildrens/about/
    ProgramDisplay.aspx?ProgramId=326
Disability Served: spina bifida

Columbia Lighthouse for the Blind
1120 20th Street, NW, Suite 750 South
Washington, DC 20036
202-454-6400
info@clb.org
http://www.clb.org
Disability Served: vision

**District of Columbia Rehabilitation Services
    Administration**
1350 Pennsylvania Avenue, NW
Washington, DC 20004
202-442-8400, 202-442-8600 (TTY/TDD)
http://dhs.dc.gov/dhs/cwp/view,a,3,q,492432.asp
Disability Served: various

Georgetown University Hospital
3800 Reservoir Road, NW
Washington, DC 20007
202-342-2400
Disability Served: various

George Washington University Medical Center
2300 Eye Street, NW
Washington, DC 20037
202-994-5179
sphhsinfo@gwumc.edu
http://www.gwumc.edu
Disability Served: various

Green Door Clubhouse
1623 16th Street, NW
Washington, DC 20009
202-462-4092
http://www.greendoor.org
Disability Served: mental health

Hospital for Sick Children
1731 Bunker Hill Road, NE
Washington, DC 20017
202-832-4400, 202-832-7848 (TTY)
http://www.hfscsite.org
Disability Served: various

Psychiatric Institute of Washington
4228 Wisconsin Avenue, NW
Washington, DC 20016
202-885-5600
http://www.psychinstitute.com
Disability Served: mental health, chemical dependency

FLORIDA
**Baptist Hospital of Miami Davis Center for
    Rehabilitation**
8900 North Kendall Drive
Miami, FL 33176
786-596-5188
http://www.baptisthealth.net/bhs/en/hospital/
    front/0,2250,3418,00.html
Disability Served: various

Bayfront Rehabilitation Center
Bayfront Medical Center
701 Sixth Street South
St. Petersburg, FL 33701-4814
http://www.bayfront.org
Disability Served: various

BIRC Day Treatment
9430 Turkey Lake Road
Orlando, FL 32819
407-363-0455
Disability Served: various

Central Florida Sheltered Workshop Inc.
1600 Aaron Avenue
Orlando, FL 32811
407-299-6050
Disability Served: various

Conklin Center for the Blind
405 White Street
Daytona Beach, FL 32114
386-258-3441

info@conklinCenter.org
http://www.conklincenter.org
Disability Served: vision

Easter Seals Broward County, Florida
6951 West Sunrise Boulevard
Plantation, FL 33313
954-792-8772
nvulgaris@esbc-fl.easter-seals.org
http://broward.easterseals.com
Disability Served: various

Easter Seals/MARC Southwest Florida
350 Braden Avenue
Sarasota, FL 34243
941-355-7637
http://swfl.easterseals.com
Disability Served: various

Easter Seal Society of Dade County Inc.
1475 Northwest 14th Avenue
Miami, FL 33125
305-325-0470
essdade@aol.com
http://miami.easterseals.com
Disability Served: various

Easter Seals Volusia and Flagler Counties Inc.
1219 Dunn Avenue, PO Box 9117
Daytona Beach, FL 32120
386-255-4568
http://fl-vf.easterseals.com
Disability Served: various

Florida Department of Health and Rehabilitative Services
1317 Winewood Boulevard
Tallahassee, FL 32399-0700
940-488-6811
http://www.cehn.org/cehn/resourceguide/fdhrs.html
Disability Served: various

Florida Division of Blind Services
1320 Executive Center Drive
Tallahassee, FL 32399
850-245-0300
Ana_Saint-Fort@dbs.doe.state.fl.us
http://dbs.myflorida.com/index.shtml
Disability Served: vision

Florida Division of Vocational Rehabilitation
Building A, 2002 Old Saint Augustine Road
Tallahassee, FL 32301
850-245-3399 (Voice/TDD)
http://www.rehabworks.org
Disability Served: various

Florida Hospital Rehabilitation Center
601 East Rollins Street
Orlando, FL 32803
407-303-1928
http://www.flhosp.org
Disability Served: various

Goodwill Industries-Suncoast Inc.
10596 Gandy Boulevard, PO Box 14456
St. Petersburg, FL 33702
727-523-1512
gw.marketing@goodwill-suncoast.com
http://www.goodwill-suncoast.org
Disability Served: various

Halifax Hospital Medical Center Eye Clinic Professional Center
303 North Clyde Morris Boulevard
Daytona Beach, FL 32114
904-255-7409
http://www.hfch.org
Disability Served: vision

HealthSouth Rehabilitation Center-Treasure Coast
3755 7th Terrace, Suite 201
Vero Beach, FL 32960
772-562-5888
http://www.healthsouth.com
Disability Served: various

HealthSouth Rehabilitation Hospital of Largo
901 Clearwater Largo Road North
Largo, FL 33770
727-586-2999
http://www.healthsouth.com
Disability Served: various

HealthSouth Rehabilitation Hospital of Miami
20601 Old Cutler Road
Miami, FL 33189
305-2551-3800
http://www.healthsouth.com
Disability Served: various

HealthSouth Rehabilitation Hospital of Sarasota
3251 Proctor Road
Sarasota, FL 34231
941-921-8600, 800-873-4222
http://www.healthsouth.com
Disability Served: various

HealthSouth Rehabilitation Hospital of Tallahassee
1675 Riggins Road
Tallahassee, FL 32308
850-656-4800
http://www.healthsouth.com
Disability Served: various

HealthSouth Sea Pines Rehabilitation Hospital
101 East Florida Avenue
Melbourne, FL 32901
321-984-4600
http://www.healthsouth.com
Disability Served: various

HealthSouth Sports Medicine and Rehabilitation Center
3280 Ponce de Leon Boulevard
Coral Gables, FL 33134
305-444-0909
http://www.healthsouth.com
Disability Served: various

HealthSouth Sports Medicine and Rehabilitation Center
2141 Alternate A1A South, Suite 300
Jupiter, FL 33477
561-743-8890
http://www.healthsouth.com
Disability Served: various

Holy Cross Hospital
4725 North Federal Highway
Ft. Lauderdale, FL 33308
954-771-8000
http://www.holy-cross.com
Disability Served: various

Independence for the Blind Inc.
1278 Paul Russell Road
Tallahassee, FL 32301
850-942-3658
Blind@noblestar.net
Disability Served: vision

Independence for the Blind of West Florida
1302 Dunmire Street
Pensacola, FL 32504
850-477-2663
http://www.ibwest.org
Disability Served: vision

Independent Living for Adult Blind
101 West State Street
Jacksonville, FL 32202
904-633-8307
bsimpson@fccj.edu
Disability Served: vision

Lee Memorial Hospital
2776 Cleveland Avenue
Ft. Myers, FL 33901
941-332-1111
http://www.leememorial.org
Disability Served: various

Lighthouse for the Blind of Palm Beach
7810 South Dixie Highway
West Palm Beach, FL 33405
561-586-5600
Disability Served: vision

Lighthouse for the Visually Impaired and Blind-Brooksville
6492 California Street
Brooksville, FL 34609
352-754-1132
cpaquin@lighthouse-pasco.org
http://www.lighthouse-hernando.org
Disability Served: vision

Lighthouse for the Visually Impaired and Blind-Port Richey
8610 Galen Wilson Boulevard
Port Richey, FL 34668
727-815-0303
cpaquin@lighthouse-pasco.org
http://www.lighthouse-hernando.org
Disability Served: vision

MacDonald Training Center Inc.-Plant City
2902 North Cork Road
Plant City, FL 33565
813-752-6508
http://www.macdonaldCenter.org
Disability Served: various

MacDonald Training Center Inc.-Tampa
5420 West Cypress Street
Tampa, FL 33607-1706
813-870-1300
http://www.macdonaldCenter.org
Disability Served: various

Mediplex Rehab-Bradenton
5627 Ninth Street East
Bradenton, FL 34203
813-753-8941
Disability Served: various

Miami Lighthouse for the Blind and Visually Impaired
601 Southwest 8th Avenue
Miami, FL 33130
305-856-2288
info@miamilighthouse.org
http://www.miamilighthouse.com
Disability Served: vision

Mount Sinai Medical Center Rehabilitation Unit
4300 Alton Road, Warner Building
Miami Beach, FL 33140
305-674-2064
http://www.msmc.com
Disability Served: various

**Naples Community Hospital Comprehensive
    Rehabilitation Center**
350 7th Street North
Naples, FL 34102
239-436-5000
http://www.nchmd.org
Disability Served: various

Pain Institute of Tampa
15267 Amberly Drive
Tampa, FL 33647
813-977-6688
http://www.newtampapain.com
Disability Served: chronic pain

Palm Beach Habilitation Center
4522 South Congress Avenue
Lake Worth, FL 33461-4797
561-965-8500
postman@pbhab.com
http://www.pbhab.com
Disability Served: various

Pine Castle Inc.
4911 Spring Park Road
Jacksonville, FL 32207
904-733-2650
info@pinecastle.org
http://www.pinecastle.org
Disability Served: developmentally disabled

Pinecrest Rehabilitation Hospital
5360 Linton Boulevard
Delray Beach, FL 33484
561-495-0400
http://www.pinecrestrehab.com
Disability Served: various

Polk County Association for Handicapped Citizens
1038 Sunshine Drive East
Lakeland, FL 33801
863-665-3846
http://www.pcahc.org
Disability Served: various

Rosomoff Comprehensive Pain Center
5200 Northeast 2nd Avenue
Miami Beach, FL 33137
305-532-7246
http://www.rosomoffpaincenter.com
Disability Served: chronic pain

Sand Lake Hospital Brain Injury Rehabilitation Center
9400 Turkey Lake Road
Orlando, FL 32819
407-351-8501
http://www.orhs.org/comm_hosp/sand_lake/brain.cfm
Disability Served: traumatic brain injury

**Sarasota Memorial Hospital/Comprehensive
    Rehabilitation Unit**
1700 South Tamiami Trail
Sarasota, FL 34239
941-917-9000
http://www.smh.com
Disability Served: various

SCARC Inc.
213 West McCollum Avenue
Bushnell, FL 33513
352-793-5156
http://www.sumtercounty.com/scarc
Disability Served: developmentally disabled

Seagull Industries for the Disabled
3879 West Industrial Way
Riviera Beach, FL 33404
561-842-5814
main@seagull.org
http://www.seagull.org
Disability Served: developmentally disabled

Shands Rehab Hospital
4101 Northwest 89th Boulevard
Gainesville, FL 32606
352-265-5491
http://www.shands.org
Disability Served: various

South Miami Hospital
6200 Southwest 73 Street
Miami, FL 33143
786-662-4000
 http://www.baptisthealth.net/bhs/en/hospital/
    front/0,2250,3644,00.html
Disability Served: various

Strive Physical Therapy Center
2620 Southeast Maricamp Road
Ocala, FL 34471
352-351-8883
http://www.striverehab.com
Disability Served: physically disabled

Tampa Bay Academy
12012 Boyette Road
Riverview, FL 33569
813-677-6700, 800-678-3838, 813-677-2502 (TTY)
info@tampa.yfcs.com
http://www.tampabay-academy.com
Disability Served: chemical dependency, mental health

Tampa General Hospital Rehabilitation Center
2 Columbia Drive
Tampa, FL 33606
813-844-7000
jstone@tgh.org
http://www.tgh.org
Disability Served: various

Tampa Lighthouse for the Blind
1106 West Platt Street
Tampa, FL 33606-2142
813-251-2407

tlh@tampalighthouse.org
http://www.tampalighthouse.org
Disability Served: vision

Tampa Shriners Hospital
12502 North Pine Drive
Tampa, FL 33612
813-972-2250
http://www.shrinershq.org/shc/tampa
Disability Served: physically disabled

Tri-County Rehabilitation Center Inc.
1650 South Kanner Highway
Stuart, FL 34994
772-221-4050
http://www.tricountytec.org
Disability Served: various

**University of Miami-Jackson Memorial
   Rehabilitation Center**
1611 Northwest 12th Avenue
Miami, FL 33136-1094
305-585-1111
http://www.um-jmh.org
Disability Served: various

Upper Pinellas Association for Retarded Citizens
1501 North Belcher Road, Suite 249
Clearwater, FL 33765
727-799-3330
Veronica@uparc.com
http://www.uparc.com
*Disability Served: developmentally disabled, mental
   retardation*

**Visually Impaired Persons of Southwest
   Florida Inc.**
35 West Mariana Avenue
North Ft. Myers, FL 33903
239-997-7797
http://www.vipCenter.org
Disability Served: vision

West Florida Rehabilitation Institute
8383 North Davis Highway
Pensacola, FL 32514
850-494-4000
http://www.westfloridaHospital.com
Disability Served: various

Willough at Naples
9001 Tamiami Trail East
Naples, FL 34113
800-722-0100
info@thewilloughatnaples.com
http://thewilloughatnaples.com
Disability Served: chemical dependency

GEORGIA

Annandale Village
3500 Annandale Lane
Suwanee, GA 30024-2150
770-945-8381
administration@annandale.org
http://www.annandale.org
Disability Served: developmentally disabled

Augusta Easter Seals Rehabilitation Center
1241 Reynolds Street, PO Box 2441
Augusta, GA 30903
706-667-9695
Disability Served: various

Bobby Dodd Center
2120 Marietta Boulevard, NW
Atlanta, GA 30318-2122
678-365-0071
http://www.bobbydodd.org
Disability Served: various

Candler General Hospital-Rehabilitation Unit
5353 Reynolds Street
Savannah, GA 31405
912-819-6000
http://www.sjchs.org
Disability Served: various

Cave Spring Rehabilitation Center
7 Georgia Avenue, PO Box 385
Cave Spring, GA 30124
706-777-2301
Disability Served: various

Children's Healthcare of Atlanta-Egleston
1405 Clifton Road
Atlanta, GA 30322-1062
404-785-5252
http://www.choa.org
Disability Served: various

Children's Healthcare of Atlanta-Office Park
1600 Tullie Circle
Atlanta, GA 30329
404-250-kids
http://www.choa.org
Disability Served: various

Children's Healthcare of Atlanta-Scottish Rite
1001 Johnson Ferry Road, NE
Atlanta, GA 30342-1600
404-256-8252
http://www.choa.org
Disability Served: various

Devereux Georgia Treatment Network
PO Box 1688
Kennesaw, GA 30156-8688
800-342-3357
http://www.devereux.org
Disability Served: developmentally disabled, learning
    disabled, mental health

Emory Crawford Long Hospital
550 Peachtree Street, NE
Atlanta, GA 30308
404-686-2387
http://www.emoryhealthcare.org/departments/rehab
Disability Served: various

**Emory University Center for Rehabilitation
    Medicine**
1441 Clifton Road, NE
Atlanta, GA 30322
404-712-5527
http://www.emoryhealthcare.org/departments/rehab
Disability Served: various

Georgia Industries for the Blind
700 Faceville Highway, PO Box 218
Bainbridge, GA 31718
912-248-2666
Disability Served: vision

**Georgia Institute of Technology Center for
    Rehabilitation Technology**
Atlanta, GA 30332-0156
404-894-4960, 800-726-9119
http://www.gatech.edu
Disability Served: various

Georgia Rehabilitation Services
148 Andrew Young International Boulevard, NE
Atlanta, GA 30303
404-232-3001, 877-709-8185
http://www.vocrehabga.org
Disability Served: various

HealthSouth Central Georgia Rehabilitation Hospital
3351 Northside Drive
Macon, GA 31210
478-471-3500
http://www.healthsouth.com
Disability Served: various

Learning Services-Peachtree
2400 Highway 29 South
Lawrenceville, GA 30245
888-419-9955, ext. 12
http://www.learningservices.com/atlanta.htm
Disability Served: traumatic brain injury

Pain Control and Rehabilitation Institute of Georgia
2786 North Decatur Road, Suite 220
Decatur, GA 30030
404-297-1400
Disability Served: various

Savannah Association for the Blind Inc.
214 Drayton Street, PO Box 81
Savannah, GA 31401
912-236-4473
Disability Served: vision

Shepherd Center
2020 Peachtree Road, NW
Atlanta, GA 30309-1402
404-352-2020
http://www.shepherd.org/shepherdhomepage.nsf/
    Home?OpenForm
Disability Served: physically disabled

Walton Rehabilitation Hospital
1355 Independence Drive
Augusta, GA 30901
706-724-7746, 800-366-6055
http://www.wrh.org
Disability Served: various

WellStar/Cobb Hospital
3950 Austell Road
Austell, GA 30106

770-732-4000
http://www.wellstar.org
Disability Served: various

Wesley Woods Center
1821 Clifton Road, NE
Atlanta, GA 30329
404-728-4900
http://www.emoryhealthcare.org/departments/rehab
Disability Served: various

HAWAII
**Hawaii Vocational Rehabilitation and Services
    for the Blind Division**
PO Box 339
Honolulu, HI 96809
808-586-5355
http://www.state.hi.us/dhs/vr.pdf
Disability Served: vision

Honolulu Shriners Hospital
1310 Punahou Street
Honolulu, HI 96826-1099
808-941-4466
http://www.shrinershq.org/shc/honolulu/index.html
Disability Served: physically disabled

Lanakila Rehabilitation Center
1809 Bachelot Street
Honolulu, HI 96817
808-531-0555
communityrelations@lanakilahawaii.org
http://www.lanakilahawaii.org
Disability Served: various

Rehabilitation Hospital of the Pacific
226 North Kuakini Street
Honolulu, HI 96817
808-531-3511
marketing@rehabHospital.org
http://www.rehabHospital.org
Disability Served: various

IDAHO
Eastern Idaho Regional Medical Center
3100 Channing Way
Idaho Falls, ID 83404
208-529-7660

http://www.eirmc.org
Disability Served: various

Easter Seals-Goodwill Center
1465 South Vinnell Way
Boise, ID
208-378-9924
http://esgw-nrm.easterseals.com
Disability Served: various

Idaho Division of Vocational Rehabilitation
PO Box 83720
Boise, ID 83720
208-287-6443
rthomas@idvr.state.id.us
http://www.vr.idaho.gov
Disability Served: various

Idaho Elks Rehabilitation Hospital
600 North Robbins Road
Boise, ID 83702
208-489-4003
http://www.idahoelksrehab.org
Disability Served: various

Pocatello Regional Medical Center
777 Hospital Way
Pocatello, ID 83201
208-234-0777
Disability Served: various

ILLINOIS

Accelerated Rehabilitation Centers LLC
205 West Wacker Drive, Suite 820
Chicago, IL 60606
877-977-3422
info@acceleratedrehab.com
http://www.acceleratedrehab.com
Disability Served: physically disabled

Albany Park Community Center Inc.
3403 West Lawrence Avenue, Suite 300
Chicago, IL 60625
773-583-5111
http://www.albanyparkcommunityCenter.org
Disability Served: mental health

Alexian Brothers Medical Center
800 Biesterfield Road, Niehoff Pavilion
Elk Grove Village, IL 60007

847-437-5500, 847-956-5116 (TDD)
http://www.alexian.org
Disability Served: various

Anixter Rehabilitation Center
6610 North Clark Street
Chicago, IL 60626-4062
773-973-7900, 773-973-2180 (TTY)
AskAnixter@anixter.org
http://www.anixter.org
Disability Served: various

The Arc of Illinois
18207-A-Dixie Highway
Homewood, IL 60430
708-206-1930
janet@thearcofil.org
http://www.thearcofil.org
Disability Served: various

Aspire of Illinois
9901 Derby Lane
Westchester, IL 60154-3709
708-547-3550, 708-547-9379 (TDD)
info@aspireofillinois.org
http://www.aspireofillinois.org
Disability Served: developmentally disabled

**Back in the Saddle Hippotherapy Program
  at Glen Grove Equestrian Center**
9453 Harms Road
Morton Grove, IL 60053
773-286-2266, 847-966-8032
http://www.infinitec.org/live/special%20animals/
  saddlehippotherapy.htm
Disability Served: cerebral palsy, developmentally disabled

**Beacon Therapeutic Diagnostic and Treatment
  Center-Calumet Park**
12440 South Ada
Calumet Park, IL 60827
708-388-3183
Beacon@Beacon-Therapeutic.org
http://www.beacon-therapeutic.org
Disability Served: various

**Beacon Therapeutic Diagnostic and Treatment
  Center-Chicago**
10650 South Longwood Drive
Chicago, IL 60643
773-881-1005, 708-388-3183 (TTY)

Beacon@Beacon-Therapeutic.org
http://www.beacon-therapeutic.org
Disability Served: *various*

Blind Service Association
22 West Monroe, 11th Floor
Chicago, IL 60603
312-236-0808
Disability Served: *vision*

Brain Injury Association of Illinois
PO Box 64420
Chicago, IL 60664-0420
312-726-5699, 800-699-6443
http://www.biail.org
Disability Served: *traumatic brain injury*

Caremark Healthcare Services
2211 Sanders Road
Northbrook, IL 60062
800-423-1411
https://www.caremark.com
Disability Served: *various*

Centegra Northern Illinois Medical Center
4201 Medical Center Drive
McHenry, IL 60050
815-344-5000
http://www.centegra.org
Disability Served: *various*

Center for Comprehensive Services
306 West Mill Street
Carbondale, IL 62902
800-203-5394
http://www.ccs-rehab.com
Disability Served: *traumatic brain injury*

Chicago Association for Retarded Citizens
8 South Michigan Avenue, Suite 1700
Chicago, IL 60603
312-346-6230
relations@chgoarc.org
http://www.chgoarc.org
Disability Served: *developmentally disabled,*
mental retardation

Children's Home and Aid Society of Illinois
125 South Wacker Drive, 14th Floor
Chicago, IL 60606
312-424-0200

http://www.chasi.org
Disability Served: *various*

Clearbrook
1835 West Central Road
Arlington Heights, IL 60008
847-870-7711
Disability Served: *developmentally disabled*

Clinton County Rehabilitation
1665 North 4th Street, PO Box 157
Breese, IL 62230
618-526-8800
Disability Served: *various*

Cornerstone Services Inc.
777B Joyce Road
Joliet, IL 60436
815-730-4580
http://www.cornerstoneservices.org
Disability Served: *developmentally disabled, mental health*

Developmental Services Center
1304 West Bradley Avenue
Champaign, IL 61821
217-356-9176
bparks@dsc-illinois.org
http://www.dsc-illinois.org
Disability Served: *developmentally disabled*

Disability Services at the University of Illinois
1207 South Oak Street
Champaign, IL 61820
217-333-1970 (Voice/TTY)
http://www.disability.uiuc.edu
Disability Served: *various*

Easter Seals Jayne Shover Center
799 South McLean Boulevard
Elgin, IL 60123
847-742-3264, 847-742-3203 (TDD)
http://www.jayneshover.org
Disability Served: *various*

Easter Seals Reaching for Adulthood Program
120 West Madison Avenue
Oak Park, IL 60302
708-524-8700
ddemus@eastersealschicago.org
http://www.eastersealschicago.org
Disability Served: *various*

Easter Seals Rehabilitation Center-Aurora
1230 North Highland Avenue
Aurora, IL 60506
630-896-1961
Disability Served: various

**Easter Seals Rehabilitation Center of Will Grundy
Counties Inc.**
22 Barney Avenue
Joliet, IL 60435
815-725-2194
Disability Served: various

Easter Seals Society-Brandecker Center
9455 South Hoyne Avenue
Chicago, IL 60620
773-239-1799
mcooney@eastersealschicago.org
http://chicago.easterseals.com
Disability Served: various

**Edward Hines Jr. Hospital Central Blind
Rehabilitation Center**
PO Box 5000 (124)
Hines, IL 60141
708-216-2343
sharon.foley@med.va.gov
http://www.va.gov/nfs/HinesVAInternship/default.htm
Disability Served: vision

El Valor Corporation
Early Intervention Program
1850 West 21st Street
Chicago, IL 60608
312-666-4511, 312-666-3361 (TTY)
info@elvalor.net
Disability Served: various

Franklin-Williamson Rehabilitation Center
902 West Main Street
West Frankfort, IL 62896
618-937-6483
ed.conner@fwhs.org
http://www.fwhs.org
Disability Served: various

Fulton County Rehabilitation Center
500 North Main Street
Canton, IL 61520
309-647-6510
Disability Served: various

Gilchrist-Marchman Rehabilitation Center
2345 West North Street
Chicago, IL 60647
773-276-4000
ahamilton@eastersealschicago.org
http://chicago.easterseals.com
Disability Served: various

Glenkirk
3504 Commercial Avenue
Northbrook, IL 60062-1821
847-272-5111
http://www.glenkirk.org
Disability Served: developmentally disabled

Illinois Center for Autism
548 South Ruby Lane
Fairview Heights, IL 62208-2614
618-398-7500
http://www.illinoisCenterforautism.org
Disability Served: autism

Illinois Center for Rehabilitation and Education
1151 South Wood Street
Chicago, IL 60612
773-633-3546
http://www.uic.edu/ahp/OT/AT/prov.html#wood
Disability Served: vision

Illinois Division of Rehabilitation Services
100 South Grand Avenue East
Springfield, IL 62762
800-843-6154, 800-447-6404 (TTY)
DRS@dhs.state.il.us
http://www.dhs.state.il.us/ors
Disability Served: various

Illinois Masonic Medical Center
836 West Wellington
Chicago, IL 60657
773-975-1600, 773-296-7684 (TTD)
http://www.advocatehealth.com/immc
Disability Served: various

Institute of Physical Medicine and Rehabilitation
6501 North Sheridan Road
Peoria, IL 61614
309-692-8110
quality@ipmr.org
http://www.ipmrrehab.org
Disability Served: various

Integrated Health Services-Burbank
5400 West 87th Street
Burbank, IL 60459
708-423-1200
Disability Served: various

Interpersonal Learning Center Enterprises
6415 Stanley Avenue
Berwyn, IL 60402
708-788-0511
Disability Served: mental health

Jesse Brown VA Medical Center
VA Chicago Healthcare System
820 South Damen
Chicago, IL 60612
312-569-8387
http://www.visn12.med.va.gov/chicago
Disability Served: various

Jewish Vocational Service
600 West Van Buren Street
Chicago, IL 60607
312-454-9002, 312-454-1048 (TTY)
Disability Served: various

Lake County Mental Health-Waukegan
3012 Grand Avenue
Waukegan, IL 60085-2321
847-746-0701
http://www.dpaillinois.com/mch/county/lake.html
Disability Served: mental health

Lambs Farm
14245 West Rockland Road
Libertyville, IL 60048
847-362-4636
info@lambsfarm.org
http://lambsfarm.org
Disability Served: developmentally disabled

Land of Lincoln Goodwill Industries
800 North 10th Street
Springfield, IL 62791
217-789-0400
http://locator.goodwill.org
Disability Served: various

LaRabida Children's Hospital and Research Center
East 65th and Lake Michigan
Chicago, IL 60649

773-363-6700
info@larabida.org
http://www.larabida.org
Disability Served: various

Little City Foundation-Chicago
700 North Sacramento, Suite 220
Chicago, IL 60612-1026
773-265-1539
ltaylor@littlecity.org
http://www.littlecity.org
Disability Served: developmentally disabled

Little City Foundation-Palatine
1760 West Algonquin Road
Palatine, IL 60067-4799
847-358-5510
ltaylor@littlecity.org
http://www.littlecity.org
Disability Served: developmentally disabled

Little Friends Community Living Program
140 North Wright Street
Naperville, IL 60540
630-355-9858
tniemeyer@lilfriends.com
http://www.littlefriendsinc.com
Disability Served: developmentally disabled

Macon Resources Inc.
2121 Hubbard Avenue, PO Box 2760
Decatur, IL 62524-2760
217-875-1910
http://www.maconresources.org
Disability Served: developmentally disabled

ManorCare Health Services-Oak Lawn East
9401 South Kostner Avenue
Oak Lawn, IL 60453
708-423-7882
oaklawneast@manorcare.com
http://www.hcr-manorcare.com
Disability Served: various

Marianjoy Rehabilitation Hospital and Clinics
26 West 171 Roosevelt Road
Wheaton, IL 60187
630-462-4000
dlebloch@marianjoy.org
http://www.marianjoy.org
Disability Served: various

Mary Bryant Home for the Blind
2960 Stanton
Springfield, IL 62703
217-529-1611
Disability Served: vision

Mosaic
725 West Madison Street
Pontiac, IL 61764-1621
815-842-4166
integrity@mosaicinfo.org
http://www.mosaicinfo.org
Disability Served: various

Nanon Wood Center for Children
Arc Community Support Systems
2502 South Veterans Drive
Effingham, IL 62401
217-347-5601
http://www.arc-css.org
Disability Served: various

Northern Illinois Special Recreation Association
820 East Terra Cotta Avenue, Suite 125
Crystal Lake, IL 60014
815-459-0737
info@nisra.org
http://www.nisra.org
Disability Served: various

Oak Forest Hospital of Cook County
15900 South Cicero Avenue
Oak Forest, IL 60452
708-687-7344
http://www.cchil.org/Cch/oak.htm
Disability Served: various

Parent Place
314 South Grand Avenue West
Springfield, IL 62704
217-546-5257
theparentplace@famvid.com
Disability Served: various

Peoria Association for Retarded Citizens
1913 Townline Road
Peoria, IL 61612
309-689-3718
phyllisjordan1@yahoo.com

Disability Served: developmentally disabled, mental retardation

Peoria Blind People's Center
2905 West Garden Street
Peoria, IL 61605
309-637-3693
Disability Served: vision

Pilsen-Little Village Community Mental Health Center
2319 South Damen Avenue
Chicago, IL 60608
773-579-0832
plvcmhc@pilsenmh.org
http://www.pilsenmh.org
Disability Served: various

Ray Graham Association for People with Disabilities
2801 Finley Road
Downers Grove, IL 60515
630-620-2222
http://www.ray-graham.org
Disability Served: various

Rehabilitation Institute of Chicago
345 East Superior Street
Chicago, IL 60611
800-354 REHAB
http://www.ric.org
Disability Served: various

REHAB Products and Services
3715 North Vermillion Street
Danville, IL 61832
217-446-1146
http://www.co.vermilion.il.us
Disability Served: various

Riverside Medical Center
800 Riverside Drive
Waupaca, IL 54981
800-924-4442
http://www.riversidemedical.org
Disability Served: various

Rush-Copley Medical Center
2000 Ogden Avenue
Aurora, IL 60504
630-978-6200

http://www.rushcopley.com
Disability Served: various

Rush University Center for Rehabilitation
1653 West Congress Parkway
Chicago, IL 60612
312-942-7161
http://www.rush.edu
Disability Served: various

Saint Elizabeth's Hospital Physical Rehabilitation Unit
211 South Third Street, 8th Floor
Belleville, IL 62220-1998
618-234-2120, ext. 1129
http://www.steliz.org
Disability Served: various

Shelby County Community Services Inc.
101 East North 12th Street
Shelbyville, IL 62565
217-774-1400
Disability Served: various

Shriners Hospitals for Children, Chicago
2211 North Oak Park Avenue
Chicago, IL 60707-3392
773-622-5400
http://www.shrinerschicago.org
Disability Served: physically disabled

Special Children Inc.
1306 Wabash Drive
Belleville, IL 62221
618-234-6876
http://www.specialchildren.net
Disability Served: developmentally disabled

Spine and Sports Rehabilitation Center
1030 North Clark Street
Chicago, IL 60610
312-354-7767
http://www.ric.org/about/cssor.php
Disability Served: various

Streator Unlimited Inc.
305 North Sterling Street
Streator, IL 61364
815-673-5574

mail@streatorunlimited.org
http://www.streatorunlimited.org
Disability Served: developmentally disabled

TCRC Sight Center
117 East Washington Street
East Peoria, IL 61611
309-698-4001
Disability Served: developmentally disabled, vision

Technology Center for Environment, Computer and Communication
Rehabilitation Institute of Chicago
345 East Superior Street, Room 980
Chicago, IL 60611
312-908-2556
http://www.ric.org
Disability Served: communication

Thresholds Bridge for the Deaf
4101 North Ravenswood Avenue
Chicago, IL 60613
888-99 REHAB
Thresholds@thresholds.org
http://www.thresholds.org
Disability Served: hearing, mental health

Thresholds Psychiatric Rehabilitation Centers
4101 North Ravenswood Avenue
Chicago, IL 60613
888-99 REHAB
Thresholds@thresholds.org
http://www.thresholds.org
Disability Served: mental health

Trinity Regional Health System
2701 17th Street
Rock Island, IL 61201
309-779-5000
http://www.trinityqc.com/body.cfm?id=88
Disability Served: various

United Cerebral Palsy of Greater Chicago-Julius and Betty Levinson Building
332 West Harrison Street
Oak Park, IL 60304-1557
708-383-8887
http://www.ucpnet.org/locations.html
Disability Served: various

University of Illinois Medical Center
1740 West Taylor Street
Chicago, IL 60612
888-842-1801
http://uillinoismedCenter.org/content.cfm/content.
  cfm/neuro_services
Disability Served: various

Van Matre HealthSouth Rehabilitation Hospital
950 South Mulford Road
Rockford, IL 61108
815-964-8500
http://www.rhsnet.org/Excellence/rehabilitation.aspx
Disability Served: various

Warren Achievement Center Inc.
1220 East 2nd Avenue
Monmouth, IL 61462
309-734-3131
info@warrenachievement.com
http://warrenachievement.com
Disability Served: developmentally disabled

West Suburban Medical Center
3 Erie Court
Oak Park, IL 60302
708-383-6200
http://www.reshealth.org
Disability Served: various

INDIANA
Ball Memorial Hospital Inc.
2401 West University Avenue
Muncie, IN 47303
765-747-3111
http://www.cardinalhealthsystem.org
Disability Served: various

Clark Memorial Hospital-Rehabilitation Unit
1220 Missouri Avenue
Jeffersonville, IN 47130
812-283-2210
www.information@clarkmemorial.org
http://www.clarkmemorial.org
Disability Served: various

Community Health Network
1500 North Ritter Avenue
Indianapolis, IN 46219

317-355-1411
http://www.ecommunity.com
Disability Served: various

Crossroads Industrial Services
8302 East 33rd Street
Indianapolis, IN 46228
317-897-7320
mgillum@crossroadsindustrialservices.com
http://www.crossroadsindustrialservices.com
Disability Served: various

Deaconess Hospital
600 Mary Street
Evansville, IN 47747
812-426-3642, 800-334-9224
http://www.deaconess.com
Disability Served: various

Evansville Association for the Blind
500 Second Avenue, PO Box 6445
Evansville, IN 47719-6445
812-422-1181
eabcdc@evansville.net
http://eab.evansville.edu
Disability Served: vision

**HealthSouth Tri-State Regional Rehabilitation
  Hospital**
4100 Covert Avenue
Evansville, IN 47714
812-476-9983, 800-677-3422
http://www.healthsouth.com
Disability Served: various

Healthwin Hospital
20531 Darden Road, PO Box 4136
South Bend, IN 46634
219-272-0100
Disability Served: various

Howard Regional Health System Specialty Hospital
829 North Dixon Road
Kokomo, IN 46901
317-452-6700
Disability Served: various

Indiana Bureau of Vocational Rehabilitation
402 West Washington Street, Room W-451, PO Box 7083
Indianapolis, IN 46207

317-232-1147
scook3@fssa.state.in.us
http://www.in.gov/fssa/servicedisabl/ddars
Disability Served: various

Indiana Easter Seals Crossroads Rehabilitation Center
4740 Kingsway Drive
Indianapolis, IN 46205-1521
Disability Served: various

Martin Luther Homes of Indiana Inc.
2740 South Seventh Street
Terre Haute, IN 47802
812-235-3399
abean@mlhs.com
Disability Served: various

Memorial Regional Rehabilitation Center
615 North Michigan
South Bend, IN 46601
574-647-7312
http://www.qualityoflife.org/services/Rehab
Disability Served: spinal-cord injury, stroke, traumatic
brain injury

Methodist Hospital Rehabilitation Institute
303 East 89th Avenue
Merrillville, IN 46410
219-738-3500
http://www.methodistHospitals.org
Disability Served: various

Methodist Hospital Rehabilitation Institute-Midlake
2269 West 25th Avenue
Gary, IN 46402
219-944-4160
http://www.methodistHospitals.org
Disability Served: various

Parkview Regional Rehabilitation Center
2200 Randallia Drive
Ft. Wayne, IN 46805
888-480-5151
http://www.parkview.com
Disability Served: various

Saint Anthony Memorial-Indiana Rehabilitation Unit
301 West Homer Street
Michigan City, IN 46360
219-879-8511

http://www.samhc.org
Disability Served: various

Saint Joseph Community Hospital-Mishawaka
215 West 4th Street
Mishawaka, IN 46544
574-259-2431
mcinteet@sjrmc.com
http://www.sjmed.com
Disability Served: various

Saint Joseph Medical Center-Plymouth Campus
1915 Lake Avenue
Plymouth, IN 46563
574-936-3181
mcinteet@sjrmc.com
http://www.sjmed.com
Disability Served: various

Saint Joseph's Medical Center-South Bend Campus
801 East LaSalle Avenue
South Bend, IN 46617
574-237-7111
mcinteet@sjrmc.com
http://www.sjmed.com/default.htm
Disability Served: various

Trade Winds Rehabilitation Center
5901 West Seventh Avenue
Gary, IN 46406
219-949-4000
http://www.tradewindservices.org
Disability Served: various

IOWA
Genesis Medical Center
Genesis Regional Rehabilitation Program
1227 East Rusholme Street
Davenport, IA 52803
563-421-1000
http://www.genesishealth.com
Disability Served: various

Genesis Medical Center-West Campus
1401 West Central Park
Davenport, IA 52804
563-421-1000
http://www.genesishealth.com/facilities/genesis/gmc_
index1.aspx
Disability Served: vision

Homelink
Van G. Miller & Associates
PO Box 1860
Waterloo, IA 50704
800-482-1993
http://www.vgmhomelink.com
Disability Served: various

Iowa Methodist Medical Center Younker Rehabilitation Center
1200 Pleasant Street
Des Moines, IA 50309-1459
515-241-4499
http://www.iowahealth.org
Disability Served: various

Iowa Vocational Rehabilitation Services
510 East 12th Street
Des Moines, IA 50319-0240
515-281-4211 (Voice/TTY)
http://www.dvrs.state.ia.us
Disability Served: various

Mercy Medical Center Physical Rehabilitation Unit
250 Mercy Drive
Dubuque, IA 52001
563-589-8000
http://www.mercydubuque.com
Disability Served: various

Mercy Pain Center
1111 Sixth Avenue
Des Moines, IA 50314
515-247-3121
http://www.mercydesmoines.org
Disability Served: chronic pain

Mid-Iowa Workshops Inc.
PO Box 966
Marshalltown, IA 50158
641-752-3697
miwi@marshallnet.com
http://www.unitedwaymarshalltown.org
Disability Served: various

Nishna Productions Inc.
902 Day Street
Shenandoah, IA 51601
712-623-4362
Disability Served: various

Tenco Industries Inc.
710 Gateway Drive, PO Box 1287
Ottumwa, IA 52501
641-682-8114
pamwilliams@lisco.com
http://www.tenco.org
Disability Served: various

Winifred Law Opportunity Center
106 East Second Avenue, PO Box 516
Indianola, IA 50125
515-961-5341
Disability Served: various

KANSAS

Arrowhead West Inc.
1100 East Wyatt Earp Boulevard
Dodge City, KS 67801
620-227-8803
http://www.arrowheadwest.org
Disability Served: developmentally disabled

Arrowhead West Inc.-Central Kansas Division
9505 West Central, Suite 110
Wichita, KS 67212
316-722-8314
http://www.arrowheadwest.org
Disability Served: developmentally disabled

Arrowhead West Inc.-Medicine Lodge Division
Junction of Highway 160 & 281
Medicine Lodge, KS 67104
620-886-3711
http://www.arrowheadwest.org
Disability Served: developmentally disabled

Bethany Rehabilitation Center
155 South 18th Street, # 185
Kansas City, KS 66102
913-281-8400
Disability Served: various

Big Lakes Developmental Center Inc.
1416 Hayes Drive
Manhattan, KS 66502
785-776-9201
sfunk@biglakes.org
http://www.biglakes.org
Disability Served: developmentally disabled

Heartspring
8700 East 29th Street North
Wichita, KS 67226
800-835-1043
http://heartspring.org
Disability Served: various

Hillsboro Community Medical Center
701 South Main
Hillsboro, KS 67063
620-947-3114
pt@hcmcks.org
http://www.hcmcks.org
Disability Served: various

Indian Creek Nursing Center
6515 West 103rd Street
Overland Park, KS 66212
913-642-5545
Disability Served: various

Johnson County Developmental Supports
10501 Lackman Road
Lenexa, KS 66219-1223
913-492-6161
jcdsinfo@jocoks.com
http://www.jcds.org
Disability Served: developmentally disabled

**Kansas Department of Social and Rehabilitation
Services**
915 Southwest Harrison Street
Topeka, KS 66606
785-296-3959, 785-296-1491 (TTY)
http://www.srskansas.org/rehab
Disability Served: various

Kansas Rehabilitation Hospital
1504 South West 8th Avenue
Topeka, KS 66606
785-235-6600
http://www.kansasrehab.com
Disability Served: various

KETCH
1006 East Waterman
Wichita, KS 67211
316-383-8700
http://www.ketch.org
Disability Served: various

Lakemary Center-Olathe
15145 South Keeler
Olathe, KS 66062
913-768-6831
http://www.lakemaryctr.org
Disability Served: developmentally disabled

Lakemary Center-Paola
100 Lakemary Drive
Paola, KS 66071
913-557-4000
http://www.lakemaryctr.org
Disability Served: developmentally disabled

Northview Developmental Services Inc.
700 East 14th
Newton, KS 67114
316-283-5170
Disability Served: various

Via Christi Regional Medical Center-St. Joseph's Campus
3600 East Harry Street
Wichita, KS 67218
316-685-1111
http://www.via-christi.org
Disability Served: various

KENTUCKY

Cardinal Hill of Northern Kentucky
31 Spiral Drive
Florence, KY 41042
859-525-1128
http://www.cardinalhill-northernky.org/northern
Disability Served: various

Cardinal Hill Rehabilitation Hospital
2050 Versailles Road
Lexington, KY 40504
606-254-5701, 800-843-1408
http://www.cardinalhill.org/rehabilitation
Disability Served: various

**Cardinal Hill Rehabilitation Hospital-Easter Seals
Center of Louisville**
9810 Bluegrass Parkway
Louisville, KY 40299
502-584-9781, 502-568-1229 (TDD)
http://www.cardinalhill.org
Disability Served: various

Cardinal Hill Specialty Hospital
85 North Grand Avenue
Fort Thomas, KY 41075
859-572-3881
http://www.cardinalhill.org/ltach.html
Disability Served: various

Frazier Rehabilitation Institute
220 Abraham Flexner Way
Louisville, KY 40202
502-582-7400
http://www.jewishHospital.org
Disability Served: various

HealthSouth Northern Kentucky Rehabilitation Hospital
201 Medical Village Drive
Edgewood, KY 41017
859-341-2044
http://www.healthsouth.com
Disability Served: various

HealthSouth Sports Medicine and Rehabilitation Center
1227 Goss Avenue
Louisville, KY 40217
502-636-1200
http://www.healthsouth.com
Disability Served: various

Kentucky Office of Vocational Rehabilitation
209 St. Clair Street
Frankfort, KY 40601
502-564-4440 (Voice/TTY)
wfd.vocrehab@mail.state.ky.us
http://ovr.ky.gov
Disability Served: various

King's Daughter's Medical Center
2201 Lexington Avenue
Ashland, KY 41101
606-327-4000
info@kdmc.net
http://www.kdmc.com
Disability Served: various

Lake Cumberland Regional Hospital Rehabilitation Unit
305 Langdon Street
Somerset, KY 42503

606-679-7441
http://www.lcrh.ky
Disability Served: various

LifeSkills Inc.
922 State Street
Bowling Green, KY 42102
270-901-5000
jmiller@lifeskills.com
http://www.lifeskills.com
Disability Served: various

Park DuValle Community Health Center
3015 Wilson Avenue
Louisville, KY 40211
502-774-4401
http://www.pdchc.org
Disability Served: various

Redwood Rehabilitation Center
71 Orphanage Road
Ft. Mitchell, KY 41017-3099
859-331-0880
http://www.redwoodrehab.org
Disability Served: various

Rehabilitation Hospital of Central Kentucky
134 Heartland Drive
Elizabethtown, KY 42701
270-769-3100
http://www.healthsouth.com
Disability Served: various

Shriners Hospitals for Children
1900 Richmond Road
Lexington, KY 40502
859-266-2101
lexpr@shrinenet.org
http://www.shrinershq.org/shc/lexington
Disability Served: physically disabled

LOUISIANA

The Arc Baton Rouge
8326 Kelwood Avenue
Baton Rouge, LA 70806
225-927-0855
http://www.arcbatonrouge.org
Disability Served: developmentally disabled

The Arc of Caddio-Bossier
351 Jordan Street
Shreveport, LA 71101
318-221-8392
http://www.cbarc.org
Disability Served: developmentally disabled

The Arc of Greater New Orleans
5700 Loyola Avenue
New Orleans, LA 70115
504-897-0134
info@arcgno.org
http://www.arcgno.org
Disability Served: developmentally disabled

The Arc of Iberville
PO Box 201
Plaquemine, LA 70765
225-687-4062
arci@eatel.net
http://www.thearcla.org/chapters/index.php
Disability Served: developmentally disabled

The Arc of Louisiana
365 North 4th Street
Baton Rouge, LA 70802
225-383-1033
arcla@bellsouth.net
http://www.thearcla.org
Disability Served: developmentally disabled

Bancroft Rehabilitation Living Centers
614 West 18th Street
Covington, LA 70433504-232-1905
http://www.bancroftneurohealth.org
Disability Served: traumatic brain injury

CHRISTUS St. Frances Cabrini Hospital
3330 Masonic Drive
Alexandria, LA 71301
318-487-1122
http://www.cabrini.org
Disability Served: various

Deaf Action Center of Greater New Orleans
Catholic Charities
1000 Howard Avenue, Suite 1000
New Orleans, LA 70113-1642
504-310-6869
ccano@archdiocese-no.org

http://www.catholiccharities-no.org
Disability Served: hearing

East Jefferson General Hospital Rehabilitation Center
4200 Houma Boulevard
Matairie, LA 70006
504-456-5000
http://www.eastjeffHospital.com
Disability Served: various

HealthSouth North Louisiana Rehabilitation Hospital
1401 Ezell
Ruston, LA 71270
318-251-3126, 800-548-9157
http://www.healthsouth.com
Disability Served: various

HealthSouth Rehabilitation Hospital of Baton Rouge
8595 United Plaza Boulevard
Baton Rouge, LA 70809
225-927-0567
http://www.healthsouth.com
Disability Served: various

James Association for Retarded Citizens
29150 Health Unit Street
Vacherie, LA 70090
504-265-7910
Disability Served: developmentally disabled, mental retardation

Kenner Regional Medical Center-Rehabilitation Institute of New Orleans
180 West Esplanade Avenue
Kenner, LA 70065
504-468-8600
http://www.kennerregional.com
Disability Served: various

Lighthouse for the Blind in New Orleans
123 State Street
New Orleans, LA 70118
504-899-4501, 888-792-0163
cleee@lhb.org
http://www.lhb.org
Disability Served: vision

Lindy Boggs Medical Center-Rehabilitation Institute of New Orleans
301 North Jefferson Davis Parkway
New Orleans, LA 70119

504-483-5000
http://www.lindyboggsmedctr.com
Disability Served: various

Louisiana Center for the Blind Inc.
101 South Trenton
Ruston, LA 71270
318-251-2891, 800-234-4166
training@lcb-ruston.com
http://www.lcb-ruston.com
Disability Served: vision

Louisiana Rehabilitation Services
755 Third Street
Baton Rouge, LA 70802
225-342-0286, 800-737-2959
http://www.dss.state.la.us/departments/lrs/Vocational_
    Rehabilitation.html
Disability Served: various

Louisiana State University Eye Center
2020 Gravier Street
New Orleans, LA 70112
504-412-1211, 877-304-1104
http://www.lsu-eye.lsuhsc.edu
Disability Served: vision

Louisiana State University Medical Center
Ernest N. Morial Asthma, Allergy, and Respiratory
    Disease Center
New Orleans, LA 70112
888-695-8647
dthoma2@lsumc.edu
http://www.medschool.lsuhsc.edu/asthma_Center
Disability Served: asthma

**Louisiana Tech University Center for Rehabilitation
    Science and Biomedical Engineering**
PO Box 3178
Ruston, LA 71272
318-257-3036
http://www.latech.edu
Disability Served: various

**Meadowcrest Hospital-Rehabilitation Institute
    of New Orleans**
2500 Belle Chasse Highway
Gretna, LA 70056
504-392-3131
http://www.meadowcresthosp.com
Disability Served: various

**Memorial Medical Center-Rehabilitation Institute
    of New Orleans**
2700 Napoleon Avenue
New Orleans, LA 70115
504-899-9311
http://www.memmedctr.com
Disability Served: various

New Orleans Speech and Hearing Center
1639 Toledano Street
New Orleans, LA 70115
504-897-2606 (Voice/TDD)
noshc@hotmail.com
http://www.noshc.org
Disability Served: communication, hearing

Our Lady of Lourdes Rehabilitation Center
611 St. Landry Street
Lafayette, LA 70506
337-289-2859
info@lourdes.net
http://www.lourdes.net
Disability Served: various

TARC
201 East Church Street
Hammond, LA 70401
985-345-8811
http://www.tarc-hammond.com
Disability Served: developmentally disabled

Touro Rehabilitation Center
1401 Foucher Street
New Orleans, LA 70115
504-897-7011
info@touro.com
http://www.touro.com
Disability Served: various

Tulane University Hospital and Clinic
1415 Tulane Avenue
New Orleans, LA 70112
504-988-5800
http://www.tuhc.com
Disability Served: various

**University of New Orleans Training Resource
    and Assistive-Technology Center**
Lake Front Campus, PO Box 1051
New Orleans, LA 70148
504-280-5700 (Voice/TTY)

http://uno.edu
Disability Served: various

MAINE

Addison Point Specialized Services Inc.
PO Box 207
Addison, ME 04606
207-483-6500
Disability Served: developmentally disabled

Charlotte White Center
PO Box 380
Dover-Foxcroft, ME 04426
207-564-2464, 888-440-4158
http://www.charlottewhiteCenter.com
Disability Served: various

Iris Network
189 Park Avenue
Portland, ME 04102
207-774-6273, 800-715-0097
Info@theiris.org
http://www.mcbvi.org
Disability Served: vision

Maine Bureau of Rehabilitation Services
150 State House Station
Augusta, ME 04333-0150
207-624-5950, 888-755-0023 (TTY)
http://www.state.me.us/rehab
Disability Served: various

New England Rehabilitation Hospital of Portland
335 Brighton Avenue
Portland, ME 04102-2374
207-662-8377
paulette.burbank@healthsouth.com
http://www.nerhp.org
Disability Served: various

Roger Randall Center for Developmental Services
48 Green Street
Houlton, ME 04730
207-532-9493
amccarthy@cla-maine.org
http://www.cla-maine.org/RRC.htm
Disability Served: developmentally disabled

Sebasticook Association for Retarded Citizens
Sebasticook Farms
461 Hartland Road

St. Albans, ME 04971
207-938-4615
dju@tdstelme.net
Disability Served: developmentally disabled

**Tri-County Mental Health Services-
Social Learning Center**
80 Strawberry Avenue
Lewiston, ME 04240
207-783-4672
Disability Served: developmentally disabled

MARYLAND

Blind Industries and Services of Maryland
3345 Washington Boulevard
Baltimore, MD 21227
410-737-2600, 888-322-4567
http://bism.org
Disability Served: vision

**Blind Industries and Services of Maryland-
Cumberland**
322 Paca Street
Cumberland, MD 21502
301-724-4111, 888-267-4111
Disability Served: vision

**Blind Industries and Services of Maryland-
Salisbury**
2240 Northwood Drive
Salisbury, MD 21801
Disability Served: vision

Center for Neuro-Rehabilitation
222 Severn Avenue
Annapolis, MD 21403
410-280-8600
sodea@neurorehab.com
Disability Served: traumatic brain injury

Greater Baltimore Medical Center
6701 North Charles Street
Baltimore, MD 21204
443-849-2658
http://www.gbmc.org
Disability Served: various

Kennedy Krieger Institute
707 North Broadway
Baltimore, MD 21205

443-923-9200, 888-554-2080
http://www.kennedykrieger.org
Disability Served: various

Levindale Hebrew Geriatric Center
2434 West Belevedere Avenue
Baltimore, MD 21215
410-601-2100
http://www.lifebridgehealth.org/levindalebody
Disability Served: elderly

Maryland Division of Rehabilitation Services
2301 Argonne Drive
Baltimore, MD 21218-1696
888-554-0334, 410-554-9411 (TTY)
dors@dors.state.md.us
http://www.dors.state.md.us/dors
Disability Served: various

Montebello Rehabilitation Hospital
2201 Argonne Drive
Baltimore, MD 21218
410-554-5200
Disability Served: various

Mount Washington Pediatric Hospital Inc.
1708 West Rogers Avenue
Baltimore, MD 21209-4596
410-578-8600
http://www.mwph.org
Disability Served: various

Rosewood Center
200 Rosewood Lane
Owings Mills, MD 21117
877-4MD-DHMH, 800-735-2258 (TDD)
anzalonej@dhmh.state.md.us
http://ddamaryland.org/rosewood
Disability Served: developmentally disabled

Sinai Rehabilitation Center
2401 West Belvedere Avenue
Baltimore, MD 21215-5271
410-601-9000
http://www.lifebridgehealth.org/sinaiHospital
Disability Served: various

TLC-The Treatment and Learning Centers
9975 Medical Center Drive
Rockville, MD 20850

301-424-5200, ext.152
rpavlin@ttlc.org
http://www.ttlc.org
Disability Served: developmentally disabled, hearing, learning disabled

MASSACHUSETTS

The Arc of Massachusetts
217 South Street
Waltham, MA 02453-2769
781-891-6270
arcmass@arcmass.org
http://www.arcmass.org
Disability Served: developmentally disabled

Baroco Corporation
PO Box 574
Williamsburg, MA 01096
413-584-9978
http://www.baroco.com
Disability Served: developmentally disabled

Berkshire Center
18 Park Street, PO Box 160
Lee, MA 01238
413-243-2576
http://www.berkshireCenter.org
Disability Served: various

Blueberry Hill Healthcare
75 Brimbal Avenue
Beverly, MA 01915
978-927-2020
http://www.blueberryhillrehab.com
Disability Served: various

Boston Center for Blind Children
147 South Huntington Avenue
Boston, MA 02130
617-296-4232
Disability Served: vision

Boston University Center for Psychiatric Rehabilitation
940 Commonwealth Avenue West
Boston, MA 02215
617-353-3549
http://www.bu.edu/cpr
Disability Served: mental health

Carrol Center for the Blind
770 Centre Street
Newton, MA 02458
617-969-6200
dina.rosenbaum@carroll.org
http://www.carroll.org
Disability Served: vision

**Children's Hospital Communication
  Enhancement Center**
300 Longwood Avenue
Boston, MA 02115
617-355-6000
http://www.childrensHospital.org
Disability Served: communication

Clark House of Fox Hill Village
30 Longwood Drive
Westwood, MA 02090
781-326-5652
http://www.clarkhousefhv.com
Disability Served: various

Eagle Pond
One Love Lane
South Dennis, MA 02660
508-385-6034
http://www.eaglepond.com
Disability Served: various

Fairlawn Rehabilitation Hospital Inc.
189 May Street
Worcester, MA 01602
508-791-6351
http://www.fairlawnrehab.org
Disability Served: various

Floating Hospital for Children
755 Washington Street
Boston, MA 02111
617-636-5000
http://www.nemc.org/home/aboutus/childrens.htm
Disability Served: developmentally disabled

**Franciscan Children's Hospital and Rehabilitation
  Center**
30 Warren Street
Boston, MA 02135
617-254-3800
http://www.fch.com
Disability Served: various

Greater Boston Guild for the Blind
1980 Centre Street
West Roxbury, MA 02132
617-323-5111
eyeinfo@gbab.org
http://www.gbab.org
Disability Served: vision

Harrington House
160 Main Street
Walpole, MA 02081
508-660-3080
http://www.harringtonrehab.com
Disability Served: various

HealthAlliance - Burbank Rehabilitation Center
275 Nichols Road
Fitchburg, MA 01420
9788-343-5660
http://www.umassmemorial.org/ummhc/Hospitals/
  alliance/events/carf.cfm
Disability Served: various

HealthSouth Braintree Rehabilitation Hospital
250 Pond Street
Braintree, MA 02184
781-848-5353, 800-99REHAB
http://www.braintreeHospital.org
Disability Served: various

HealthSouth New England Rehabilitation Hospital
2 Rehabilitation Way
Woburn, MA 01801
781-939-1900
http://www.healthsouth.com
Disability Served: various

**HealthSouth Rehabilitation Hospital of Western
  Massachusetts**
14 Chestnut Place
Ludlow, MA 01056
413-589-7581
http://www.healthsouth.com
Disability Served: various

Kolburne School
343 NM Southfield Road
New Marlborough, MA 01230-2199
413-229-8787
kgreco@kolburne.net

http://www.kolburne.net
Disability Served: developmentally disabled, learning disabled, mental health

Massachusetts Eye and Ear Infirmary and Vision Rehabilitation Service
243 Charles Street
Boston, MA 02114
617-523-7900
http://www.meei.harvard.edu
Disability Served: hearing, vision

Massachusetts Rehabilitation Commission
27 Wormwood Street
Boston, MA 02210-1616
800-245-6543 (Voice/TDD)
http://www.mass.gov/mrc
Disability Served: various

New England Sinai Hospital
150 York Street
Stoughton, MA 02072
781-344-0600
http://www.newenglandsinai.org
Disability Served: various

Perkins School for the Blind
175 North Beacon Street
Watertown, MA 02472
617-924-3434
Disability Served: vision

Protestant Guild
411 Waverly Oaks Road, Suite 104
Waltham, MA 02152
781-893-6000
admin@protestantguild.org
http://www.protestantguild.org
Disability Served: developmentally disabled

Rehabilitation Hospital of the Cape and Islands
311 Service Road
East Sandwich, MA 02537
508-833-4000
http://www.rhci.org
Disability Served: various

Shaughnessy-Kaplan Rehabilitation Hospital
Dove Avenue
Salem, MA 01970
978-745-9003

http://www.nsmc.partners.org/skrh/index.html
Disability Served: various

Shriners Burns Institute-Boston Unit
51 Blossom Street
Boston, MA 02114
617-722-3000
http://www.shrinershq.org/shc/boston/index.html
Disability Served: burns

Shriners Hospital for Crippled Children-Springfield
516 Carew Street
Springfield, MA 01104
413-787-2000
http://www.shrinershq.org/shc/springfield/index.html
Disability Served: physically disabled

Southern Worcester County Rehabilitation Center
44 Morris Street
Webster, MA 01570
508-943-0700
http://www.swcrcinc.org
Disability Served: developmentally disabled, physically disabled

Tufts-New England Medical Center
750 Washington Street
Boston, MA 02111
617-636-5000
http://www.nemc.org
Disability Served: various

Vinfen Corporation
950 Cambridge Street
Cambridge, MA 02141-1001
617-441-1800, 617-225-2000 (TTY/TDD)
info@vinfen.org
http://www.vinfen.org
Disability Served: developmentally disabled, mental health

Weldon Rehabilitation Hospital
233 Carew Street
Springfield, MA 01104
413-737-8153
http://www.mercycares.com
Disability Served: various

Whittier Rehabilitation Hospital-Haverhill
76 Summer Street,
Haverhill, MA 01830
978-372-8000

http://www.whittierhealth.com
Disability Served: various

Whittier Rehabilitation Hospital-Westborough
150 Flanders Road, PO Box 1250
Westborough, MA 01581
508-870-2222
http://www.whittierhealth.com
Disability Served: various

Youville Hospital and Rehabilitation Center
1575 Cambridge Street
Cambridge, MA 02138
617-876-4344
admitting@youville.org
http://www.youville.org
Disability Served: various

MICHIGAN
**Botsford General Hospital Inpatient
    Hospitalization Unit**
28050 Grand River Avenue
Farmington Hills, MI 48336-5919
248-471-8000
http://www.botsfordsystem.org
Disability Served: various

Chelsea Community Hospital Rehabilitation Unit
775 South Main Street
Chelsea, MI 48118
734-475-3926
http://www.cch.org
Disability Served: various

Eight CAP Inc.-Head Start
904 Oak Drive-Turk Lake, PO Box 368
Greenville, MI 48834
616-754-9315
nsecor@iserv.net
http://www.mhsa.ws/programs/list.htm
Disability Served: various

Farmington Health Care Center
34225 Grand River Avenue
Farmington, MI 48335
248-477-7373
Disability Served: various

Genesys West Flint Campus
3921 Beecher Road
Flint, MI 48532

810-762-4682
http://www.genesys.org
Disability Served: various

**Greater Detroit Agency for the Blind and
    Visually Impaired**
16625 Grand River Avenue
Detroit, MI 48227
313-272-3900
http://www.gdabvi.org
Disability Served: vision

Hope Network Lansing Rehabilitation Service
2775 East Lansing Drive
East Lansing, MI 48823
517-332-1616
jsiler@hopenetwork.org
http://www.hopenetworkrehab.org
Disability Served: various

Hope Network Rehabilitation Services Big Rapids
Children & Adults Rehabilitation Services
745 Water Tower Road,
Big Rapids, MI 49307
231-592-1061
kfinkbeiner@hopenetwork.org
http://www.hopenetworkrehab.org
Disability Served: various

Hope Network Rehabilitation Services Grand Rapids
1490 East Beltline, SE
Grand Rapids, MI 49506
616-940-0040
Mbailey@hopenetwork.org
http://www.hopenetworkrehab.org
Disability Served: various

Hope Network Rehabilitation Services Mt. Pleasant
601 South Mission Street
Mt. Pleasant, MI 48858
989-779-9988
kfinkbeiner@hopenetwork.org
http://www.hopenetworkrehab.org
Disability Served: various

Hope Network Rehabilitation Services Muskegon
1080 East Sternberg Road
Muskegon, MI 49444-8796
231-799-2200
kfinkbeiner@hopenetwork.org
http://www.hopenetworkrehab.org
Disability Served: various

Mary Free Bed Hospital and Rehabilitation Center
235 Wealthy Street, SE
Grand Rapids, MI 49503
800-528-8989
Info@maryfreebed.com
http://www.maryfreebed.com
Disability Served: various

Mecosta County Medical Center
605 Oak Street
Big Rapids, MI 49307
231-796-8691
http://www.mcghHospital.com
Disability Served: various

Men-O-Mee Activity Center Inc.
607 1st Street
Menominee, MI 49858
906-863-1360
Disability Served: various

Michigan Career and Technical Institute
11611 West Pine Lake Road
Plainwell, MI 49080
877-901-7360
http://www.michigan.gov/mdcd/1,1607,7-122-1681_
    2913---,00.html
Disability Served: various

Michigan Hand Rehabilitation Centers-Dearborn
27321 Newman Street, Suite 100B
Dearborn, MI 48124
313-791-0616
info@michiganhandrehab.com
http://www.michiganhandrehab.com
Disability Served: physically disabled

Michigan Hand Rehabilitation Centers-Detroit
4160 John Road, Suite 1026
Detroit, MI 48201
313-831-1235
info@michiganhandrehab.com
http://www.michiganhandrehab.com
Disability Served: physically disabled

Michigan Hand Rehabilitation Centers-Livonia
15250 Levan Road, Suite A
Livonia, MI 48154
734-464-6311
info@michiganhandrehab.com

http://www.michiganhandrehab.com
Disability Served: physically disabled

Michigan Hand Rehabilitation Centers-Rochester Hills
455 Barclay Circle, Suite B
Rochester Hills, MI 48307
248-853-6965
info@michiganhandrehab.com
http://www.michiganhandrehab.com
Disability Served: physically disabled

Michigan Hand Rehabilitation Centers-Warren
11012 13 Mile, Suite 112A
Warren, MI 48093
586-573-8890
info@michiganhandrehab.com
http://www.michiganhandrehab.com
Disability Served: physically disabled

Michigan Rehabilitation Services
201 North Washington Square, 4th Floor, PO Box 30010
Lansing, MI 48909
800-605-6722, 888-605-6722 (TTY)
http://www.michigan.gov/mdcd/0,1607,7-122-25392---
    ,00.html
Disability Served: various

Mid-Michigan Rehabilitation Center
Head Injury Therapy Services
2707 Ashman Street
Midland, MI 48640-4449
989-631-1100
info@specialtree.com
http://www.specialtree.com
Disability Served: traumatic brain injury

Penrickton Center for Blind Children
26530 Eureka Road
Taylor, MI 48180
734-946-7500
mail@penrickton.com
http://penrickton.com
Disability Served: vision

Rainbow Rehabilitation Centers
5570 Whittaker Road
PO Box 970230
Ypsilanti, MI 48197
734482-1200, 800-968-6644

info@rainbowrehab.com
http://www.rainbowrehab.com
Disability Served: traumatic brain injury

Rehabilitation Institute of Michigan
261 Mack Avenue
Detroit, MI 48201
313-745-1203
http://www.rimrehab.org
Disability Served: various

Saint John Macomb Hospital-Warren
11800 East 12 Mile Road
Warren, MI 48093
586-573-5000
http://www.stjohn.org/Macomb
Disability Served: various

Special Tree Rehabilitation System
39000 Chase Street
Romulus, MI 48174-1303
800-648-6885
info@specialtree.com
http://www.specialtree.com
Disability Served: traumatic brain injury

Special Tree Rehabilitation System Mid-Michigan Rehabilitation Center
Head Injury Therapy Services
2707 Ashman Street
Midland, MI 48640-4449
989-631-1100
info@specialtree.com
http://www.specialtree.com
Disability Served: head/brain injury

Special Tree Rehabilitation System-Special Tree Student Center
16880 Middlebelt Road, Suite 2
Livonia, MI 48154-3366
734-513-5766
info@specialtree.com
http://www.specialtree.com
Disability Served: traumatic brain injury

Special Tree Rehabilitation System-Troy Rehabilitation
1640 Axtell Drive
Troy, MI 48084-4496
800-649-5011

info@specialtree.com
http://www.specialtree.com
Disability Served: head/brain injury

Special Tree Rehabilitation System-Wabash Rehabilitation Center
39010 Wabash Street
Romulus, MI 48174-1148
734-942-0400
info@specialtree.com
http://www.specialtree.com
Disability Served: traumatic brain injury

Three Rivers Area Hospital
701 South Health Parkway
Three Rivers, MI 49093
269-278-1145
info@threerivershealth.org
http://www.threerivershealth.org
Disability Served: various

MINNESOTA
Gillette Children's Specialty Healthcare
200 East University Avenue
St. Paul, MN 55101
651-291-2848
http://www.gillettechildrens.org
Disability Served: various

Mayo Clinic
200 First Street, SW
Rochester, MN 55905
507-284-2511
http://www.mayoclinic.org
Disability Served: various

Minnesota Department of Employment and Economic Development - Rehabilitation Services Branch
332 Minnesota Street, Suite E200
St. Paul, MN 55101
800-328-9095, 800-657-3973 (TTY)
http://www.deed.state.mn.us/rehab/vr/main_vr.htm
Disability Served: various

Minnesota Department of Labor and Industry
Rehabilitation Services Branch
332 Minnesota Street, Suite E200
St. Paul, Minnesota 55101

651-296-5616, 800-328-9095, 651-296-3900 (TTY)
http://www.doli.state.mn.us/vru.html
Disability Served: various

North Memorial Health Care Rehabilitation Center
3300 Oakdale Avenue North
Robbinsdale, MN 55422-2900
76312-520-5200
http://www.northmemorial.com
Disability Served: various

Twin Cities Shriners Hospital
2025 East River Parkway
Minneapolis, MN 55414
612-596-6100, 888-293-2832
http://www.shrinershq.org/shc/twincities
Disability Served: physically disabled

University of Minnesota Children's Hospital
University Campus
420 Delaware Street, SE
Minneapolis, MN 55455
612-273-3000
http://www.fairviewchildrens.org
Disability Served: various

University of Minnesota Children's Hospital
Riverside Campus
2450 Riverside Avenue
Minneapolis, MN 55454
612-273-3000
http://www.fairviewchildrens.org
Disability Served: various

Vision Loss Resources
1936 Lyndale Avenue
Minneapolis, MN 55403-3101
612-871-2222
Kellym@vlrw.org
http://www.visionlossresources.com
Disability Served: vision

MISSISSIPPI
Addie McBryde Rehabilitation Center for the Blind
2550 Peachtree Street, PO Box 5314
Jackson, MS 39296-5314
601-364-2700
http://www.mdrs.state.ms.us/client/addie.html
Disability Served: vision

Mississippi Department of Rehabilitation Services
PO Box 1698
Jackson, MS 39215-1698
http://www.mdrs.state.ms.us/about
Disability Served: various

Mississippi Methodist Rehabilitation Center
1350 East Woodrow Wilson
Jackson, MS 39216
800-223-6672
http://www.mmrcrehab.org
Disability Served: various

MISSOURI
Barnes-Jewish Hospital Department of Rehabilitation
One Barnes-Jewish Hospital Plaza
St. Louis, MO 63110
314-747-3000
http://www.barnesjewish.org
Disability Served: various

Children's Mercy Hospital
2401 Gillham Road
Kansas City, MO 64108-9898
816-234-3000
http://www.childrens-mercy.org
Disability Served: various

Christian Hospital
11133 Dunn Road
St. Louis, MO 63136
314-653-5000
http://www.christianHospital.org
Disability Served: various

Columbia Regional Hospital-
404 Keene Street
Columbia, MO 65201
573-875-9000
http://www.columbiaregional.org
Disability Served: various

Council for Extended Care of Mentally Retarded Citizens
1600 South Hanley, Suite 100A
St. Louis, MO 63144
314-781-4950
Disability Served: developmentally disabled

FACHE, Shriners Hospital for Crippled Children
2001 South Lindbergh Boulevard
St. Louis, MO 63131-3597
314-432-3600
http://www.shrinershq.org/shc/stlouis
Disability Served: physically disabled

Harry S. Truman Children's Neurological Center
15600 Woods Chapel Road
Kansas City, MO 64139
816-373-5060
jlandrum@tnccommunity.com
http://www.tnccommunity.com
Disability Served: various

MERS Goodwill
1727 Locust Street
St. Louis, MO 63103
314-241-3464
http://mersgoodwill.org/charity
Disability Served: various

Missouri Division of Vocational Rehabilitation
3024 Dupont Circle
Jefferson City, MO 65109-0525
877-222-8963, 573-751-0881 (TDD)
http://www.vr.dese.state.mo.us
Disability Served: various

Missouri Rehabilitation Services for the Blind
615 Howerton Court
Jefferson City, MO 65102
573-751-4249, 800-735-2966 (TTD)
http://dss.missouri.gov/fsd/rsb
Disability Served: vision

Poplar Bluff Regional Medical Center-South Campus
621 West Pine Street
Poplar Bluff, MO 63901
573-686-4111
info@pbrmc.hma-corp.com
http://www.poplarbluffregional.com
Disability Served: various

Poplar Bluff Regional Medical Center-North Campus
2620 North Westwood Boulevard
Poplar Bluff, MO 63901-3396
573-785-7721
info@pbrmc.hma-corp.com

http://www.poplarbluffregional.com
Disability Served: various

Rusk Rehabilitation Center
201 Business Loop 70 West
Columbia, MO 65203
573-817-2703
http://www.hsc.missouri.edu/~momscis/rusk.htm
Disability Served: spinal-cord injury, traumatic brain injury

Saint Louis Society for the Blind and Visually Impaired
8770 Manchester Road
Brentwood, MO 63144
314-968-9000
http://www.slsbvi.org
Disability Served: vision

Saint Mary's Hospital of Blue Springs
201 West RD Mize Road
Blue Springs, MO 64014-2533
816-228-5900
Disability Served: various

Service Club for the Blind
4312 Olive Street
St. Louis, MO 63108
314-533-6716, 314-533-6718
Disability Served: vision

SSM Outpatient and Day Institute-Hazelwood
1 Village Square Center
Hazelwood, MO 63043
314-731-4555, 800-258-8988
tasha_lyden@ssmhc.com
http://www.ssmrehab.com
Disability Served: various

MONTANA
Montana Deaconess Medical Center
1101 26th Street South
Great Falls, MT 59405
406-761-1200
Disability Served: various

Montana Department of Social and Rehabilitation Services
111 Sanders, Suite 307, PO Box 4210
Helena, MT 59604-4210

406-444-2590 (Voice/TTY), 877-296-1197
http://www.dphhs.state.mt.us/dsd/index.htm
Disability Served: various

Saint Vincent Hospital and Health Care
1233 North 30th Street
Billings, MT 59101
406-657-7949
http://www.stvincenthealthcare.org
Disability Served: various

NEBRASKA

Madonna Rehabilitation Hospital
5401 South Street
Lincoln, NE 68506
402-489-7102, 800-676-5448
http://www.madonna.org
Disability Served: various

Martin Luther Homes of Beatrice Inc.
722 South 12th Street, PO Box 607
Beatrice, NE 68310
402-223-4066
jcampbell@mlhs.com
Disability Served: various

Martin Luther Homes of Nebraska Inc.
220 West South 21st Street
York, NE 68467
402-362-2180
jschoepf@mlhs.com
Disability Served: various

**Munroe-Meyer Institute for Genetics
     and Rehabilitation**
985450 Nebraska Medical Center
Omaha, NE 68198-5450
402-559-6460
http://www.unmc.edu/mmi
Disability Served: developmentally disabled

Nebraska Vocational Rehabilitation
PO Box 94987
Lincoln, NE 68509
402-471-3644, 877-637-3422
s_chapin@vocrehab.state.ne.us
http://www.vocrehab.state.ne.us
Disability Served: various

NEVADA
Las Vegas Healthcare and Rehabilitation Center
2832 South Maryland Parkway
Las Vegas, NV 89109
702-735-5848
http://www.lasvegaskindred.com
Disability Served: various

Nevada Division of Rehabilitation
505 East King Street, Room 502
Carson City, NV 89701-3705
775-684-4040, 775-684-8400 (TTY)
detrvr@nvdetr.org
http://www.detr.state.nv.us/rehab/reh_index.htm
Disability Served: various

University Medical Center
1800 West Charleston Boulevard
Las Vegas, NV 89102
702-383-2239
http://www.umcsn.com
Disability Served: various

NEW HAMPSHIRE
Crotched Mountain Rehabilitation Center
One Verney Drive
Greenfield, NH 03047
603-547-3311, ext. 235
http://www.crotchedmountain.org
Disability Served: various

**Exeter Hospital Department of Physical Medicine
     and Rehabilitation**
5 Alumni Drive
Exeter, NH 03833
603-778-7311
http://www.foreveryday.com
Disability Served: various

Hackett Hill Nursing Center and Integrated Care
191 Hackett Hill Road
Manchester, NH 03102
603-668-8161
Disability Served: various

**HealthSouth New Hampshire Rehabilitation
     and Sports Medicine**
Building 2, 8025 South Willow Street, Suite 209
Manchester, NH 03103

603-668-5748
http://www.healthsouth.com
Disability Served: various

Lakeview Neuro Rehabilitation Center Inc.
101 Highwatch Road
Effingham Falls, NH 03814
603-539-7451, 800-478-1045
admitnh@lakeviewsystem.com
http://www.lakeviewsystem.com
Disability Served: traumatic brain injury

**New Hampshire Bureau of Vocational Rehabilitation
     Services**
21 South Fruit Street
Concord, NH 03301
603-271-3471 (Voice/TTY), 800-299-1647
http://www.ed.state.nh.us/VR
Disability Served: various

Northeast Rehabilitation Hospital
70 Butler Street
Salem, NH 03079
603-893-2900
http://www.northeastrehab.com
Disability Served: various

**Northern New Hampshire Mental Health
     and Developmental Services**
87 Washington Street
Conway, NH 03818
603-447-3347
http://www.nnhmhds.org
Disability Served: developmentally disabled, mental health

Saint Joseph New England Rehabilitation Center
172 Kinsley Street
Nashua, NH 03061-2013
603-882-3000
scaron@sjh-nh.org
http://www.stjosephHospital.com/rehab
Disability Served: various

NEW JERSEY
Atlantic Coast Rehabilitation and Healthcare Center
485 River Avenue
Lakewood, NJ 08701
732-364-7100
info@atlanticcoastrehab.com

http://www.atlanticcoastrehab.com
Disability Served: various

Bancroft NeuroHealth
425 Kings Highway East
Haddonfield, NJ 08033-0018
856-429-0010
http://www.bancroftneurohealth.org
Disability Served: developmentally disabled

Betty Bacharach Rehabilitation Hospital
61 West Jim Leeds Road
Pomona, NJ 08240-0723
609-748-5460
Disability Served: traumatic brain injury

**Cerebral Palsy of Monmouth and Ocean County
     Schroth School & Technical Education Center**
1701 Kneeley Boulevard
Wanamassa, NJ 07712
732-493-5900
http://www.monmouth-oel.org/cerebralpalsy.htm
Disability Served: cerebral palsy

Children's Specialized Hospital
150 New Providence Road
Mountainside, NJ 07092-2590
888-CHILDREN
http://www.childrens-specialized.org
Disability Served: various

Daughters of Miriam Center for the Aged
155 Hazel Street
Clifton, NJ 07015
201-772-3700
Disability Served: elderly

Devereux New Jersey Treatment Network
901 Mantua Pike
Woodbury, NJ 08096
856-384-9680
http://www.devereuxnj.org
Disability Served: behavioral disorders, developmentally
     disabled

JFK Johnson Rehabilitation Institute
65 James Street
Edison, NJ 08818
732-321-7000
http://www.njrehab.org
Disability Served: various

JFK Medical Center Pediatric Rehabilitation Department
2050 Oak Tree Road
Edison, NJ 08818
732-548-7610
http://www.njrehab.org
Disability Served: various

Kessler Institute for Rehabilitation
1199 Pleasant Valley Way
West Orange, NJ 07052
973-731-3600, 800-248-3221
http://www.kessler-rehab.com
Disability Served: physically disabled

Lourdes Regional Rehabilitation Center
1600 Haddon Avenue
Camden, NJ 08103
609-757-3500
http://www.lourdesnet.org/lourdes/rehab.php
Disability Served: various

Matheny Hospital and School
Highland Avenue, PO Box 339
Peapack, NJ 07977
908-234-0011
developmeny@matheny.org
http://www.matheny.org
Disability Served: developmentally disabled

New Jersey Division of Vocational Rehabilitation Services
135 East State Street, PO Box 398
Trenton, NJ 08625-0398
609-292-5987, 609-292-2919 (TTY)
http://www.nj.gov/labor/dvrs/vrsindex.html
Disability Served: various

Riverview Rehabilitation Center
Meridian Health
1350 Campus Parkway
Neptune, NJ 07753
800-560-9990
http://www.meridianhealth.com/rmc.cfm/Services/
    OrthopedicRehab/rehab.cfm?PrintablePage=Yes
Disability Served: physically disabled

Somerset Valley Nursing Home
1621 Route 22 West
Bound Brook, NJ 08805

908-469-2000
Disability Served: various

NEW MEXICO

Abrazos Family Support Services
PO Box 788
Bernalillo, NM 87004
505-867-3396
info@abrazosnm.org
http://www.swcr.org/early_intervention.htm
Disability Served: developmentally disabled

HealthSouth Rehabilitation Hospital
7000 Jefferson, NE
Albuquerque, NM 87109
505-344-9478
http://www.infoimagination.org/test/healthsouthnm
Disability Served: various

New Mexico Division of Vocational Rehabilitation
435 St. Michael's Drive, Building D
Santa Fe, NM 87505
505-954-8500, 800-224-7005
http://www.state.nm.us/dvr
Disability Served: various

Rehabilitation Hospital of New Mexico
505 Elm Street, NE
Albuquerque, NM 87102
505-727-4700
http://www.albuquerqueHospital.com
Disability Served: various

San Juan Regional Medical Center Rehabilitation Services
525 South Schwartz Street
Farmington, NM 87401
505-327-3422
http://www.sanjuanregional.com/network/rehab_ctr/
    index.html
Disability Served: various

NEW YORK

Association for the Blind and Visually Impaired Goodwill Industries of Greater Rochester
422 South Clinton Avenue
Rochester, NY 14620-1198
585-232-1111, 585-232-6707

info@abvi-goodwill.com
http://www.ibnys.org/affiliates.asp?act=1&affID=2
Disability Served: vision

Association for Vision Rehabilitation and Employment
55 Washington Street
Binghamton, NY 13901
607-724-2428, 607-771-8045
http://www.ibnys.org/affiliates.asp?act=1&affID=3
Disability Served: vision

Brooklyn Bureau of Community Service
285 Schermerhorn Street
Brooklyn, NY 11217
718-310-5600
info@bbcs.org
http://www.bbcs.org
Disability Served: various

Buffalo Hearing and Speech Center
50 East North Street
Buffalo, NY 14203
716-885-8318
info@askbhsc.org
http://www.askbhsc.org
Disability Served: communication, hearing

Burke Rehabilitation Hospital
785 Mamaroneck Avenue
White Plains, NY 10605
914-597-2500
web@burke.org
http://www.burke.org
Disability Served: various

Central Association for the Blind and Visually Impaired
507 Kent Street
Utica, NY 13501
315-797-2233
info@cabvi.org
http://www.ibnys.org/affiliates.asp?act=1&affID=6
Disability Served: vision

Elmhurst Hospital Center
79-01 Broadway
Elmhurst, NY 11373
718-334-4000
http://www.nyc.gov/html/hhc/qhn/html/ehc.html
Disability Served: various

Flushing Hospital
4500 Parsons Boulevard
Flushing, NY 11355
718-670-5515
http://www.flushingHospital.org
Disability Served: various

Helen Hayes Hospital
Route 9W
West Haverstraw, NY 10993
845-786-4225, 888-707-3422, 845-947-3187 (TTY)
http://www.helenhayeshospital.org
Disability Served: physically disabled

Helen Keller Services for the Blind-Brooklyn
57 Willoughby Street
Brooklyn, NY 11201
718-522-2122
info@helenkeller.org
http://www.helenkeller.org
Disability Served: vision

Helen Keller Services for the Blind-Nassau
One Helen Keller Way
Hempstead, NY 11550
516-485-1234
info@helenkeller.org
http://www.helenkeller.org
Disability Served: vision

Helen Keller Services for the Blind-National Center
141 Middle Neck Road
Sands Point, NY 11050
516-944-8900
hkncinfo@hknc.org
http://www.helenkeller.org
Disability Served: vision

Helen Keller Services for the Blind-Suffolk
40 New York Avenue
Huntington, NY 11743
631-424-0022
info@helenkeller.org
http://www.helenkeller.org
Disability Served: vision

Lighthouse International Headquarters
111 East 59th Street
New York, NY 10022-1202
212-821-9200

visionrehab@lighthouse.org
http://www.lighthouse.org
Disability Served: vision

New York-Presbyterian/Columbia
622 West 168th Street
New York, NY 10032
212-305-2500
http://www.nyp.org
Disability Served: various

New York State Office of Vocational and Educational Services for Individuals with Disabilities
99 Washington Avenue
Albany, NY 12234
518-474-2714
http://www.vesid.nysed.gov
Disability Served: various

Norman Marcus Pain Institute
30 East 40th Street
New York, NY 10016
212-532-7999
http://www.backpainusa.com
Disability Served: back pain, chronic pain

Northeastern Association of the Blind at Albany
301 Washington Avenue
Albany, NY 12206
518-463-1211
info@naba-vision.org
http://www.ibnys.org/affiliates.asp?act=1&affID=11
Disability Served: vision

Pain Alleviation Center
125 South Service Road
Jericho, NY 11753
516-997-PAIN
http://www.painCenter.com
Disability Served: chronic pain

Pilot Industries-Ellenville
48 Canal Street
Ellenville, NY 12428
914-647-7711
Disability Served: various

Rusk Institute of Rehabilitation Medicine
400 East 34th Street
New York, NY 10016
212-263-6034

http://www.med.nyu.edu/rusk
Disability Served: various

Skills Unlimited Inc.
405 Locust Avenue
Oakdale, NY 11769
631-567-3320
skillsunlimited2002@yahoo.com
http://www.skillsunlimited.org
Disability Served: various

NORTH CAROLINA
Academy Eye Associates
3115 Academy Road
Durham, NC 27707
919-493-7456
http://www.academyeye.com
Disability Served: vision

Clinical Center for the Study of Development and Learning
University of North Carolina-Chapel Hill
Biological Science Research Center, CB #7255
Chapel Hill, NC 27599-7255
919-966-5171
Stephen.hooper@cdl.unc.edu
http://cdl.unch.unc.edu
Disability Served: developmentally disabled

Forsyth Medical Center
3333 Silas Creek Parkway
Winston-Salem, NC 27103
336-718-5780
http://www.forsythmedicalCenter.org
Disability Served: various

Horizon Rehabilitation Center
3100 Ervin Road
Durham, NC 27705
919-383-1546, 800-541-7750
Disability Served: various

Industries of the Blind Inc.
914-920 West Lee Street
Greensboro, NC 27403
336-274-1591
sales@iob-gso.com
http://www.industriesoftheblind.com
Disability Served: vision

Learning Services-Carolina
707 Moorhead Avenue
Durham, NC 27707
888-419-9955, ext. 12
http://www.learningservices.com/durham.htm
Disability Served: traumatic brain injury

Lions Industries for the Blind Inc.
4126 Berkeley Avenue
Kinston, NC 28504
252-523-1019
http://www.lionsindustries.org
Disability Served: vision

Lions Services Inc.
4600-A North Tryon Street
Charlotte, NC 28213
704-921-1527
lionsinc@aol.com
http://www.lionsservices.org
Disability Served: vision

**North Carolina Division of Vocational
Rehabilitation Services**
803 Mail Service Center 27699
Raleigh, NC 27611
919-733-7807, 800-215-7227
http://dvr.dhhs.state.nc.us
Disability Served: various

Pitt County Memorial Hospital
2100 Stantonsburg Road
Greenville, NC 27834
252-847-4837
http://www.uhseast.com
Disability Served: various

Thoms Rehabilitation Hospital
68 Sweeten Creek Road, PO Drawer 15025
Asheville, NC 28803
828-277-4800
info@carepartners.org
http://www.carepartners.org
Disability Served: various

Winston-Salem Industries for the Blind
7730 North Point Drive
Winston-Salem, NC 27106
336-759-0551, 800-242-7726
info@wsifb.com
http://www.wsifb.com
Disability Served: vision

NORTH DAKOTA

Altru Health System
1200 South Columbia Road
Grand Forks, ND 58206
701-780-5000
http://www.altru.org
Disability Served: various

MedCenter One Rehabilitation Center
300 North Seventh Street
Bismarck, ND 58501
701-323-6000
http://www.medCenterone.com
Disability Served: various

MeritCare Hospital Rehabilitation Services
1720 South University Avenue
Fargo, ND 58122
701-280-4611
http://www.meritcare.com
Disability Served: various

North Dakota Vocational Rehabilitation Agency
600 East Boulevard Avenue, Department 325
Bismarck, ND 58505
701-328-2310
http://www.state.nd.us/humanservices/services/
  disabilities/vr
Disability Served: various

**Saint Alexius Medical Center Inpatient
Rehabilitation Unit**
900 East Broadway
Bismarck, ND 58506-5510
701-530-4890
http://www.st.alexius.org
Disability Served: various

Trinity RehabCare Center
407 Third Street, SE
Minot, ND 58701
701-857-5616
Disability Served: various

OHIO

Bellefaire/JCB
22001 Fairmount Boulevard
Shaker Heights, OH 44118
216-932-2800, 800-879-2522
http://www.bellefairejcb.org
Disability Served: various

Cleveland Sight Center
1909 East 101st Street, PO Box1988
Cleveland, OH 44106-8696
216-791-8118
info@clevelandsightCenter.org
http://www.clevelandsightcenter.org/about/history.htm
Disability Served: vision

Clovernook-Cincinnati
7000 Hamilton Avenue
Cincinnati, OH 45231-5297
513-522-3860 (Voice/TDD)
http://www.clovernook.org
Disability Served: vision

Clovernook-Dayton
111 West First Street, Suite 515
Dayton, OH 45402-1105
937-223-2059
http://www.clovernook.org
Disability Served: vision

Columbus Speech and Hearing Center
510 East North Broadway
Columbus, OH 43214
614-263-5151, 614-263-2299 (TTY)
http://www.columbusspeech.org
Disability Served: communication, hearing

Columbus Speech and Hearing Center-Satellite
10567 Sawmill Parkway, Suite 105
Powell, OH 43065
614-793-2250, 614-263-2299 (TTY)
http://www.columbusspeech.org
Disability Served: communication, hearing

**CommuniCare at Waterford Commons Skilled
    Nursing and Rehabilitation Center**
955 Garden Lake Parkway
Toledo, OH 43614
419-382-2200
http://communicarehealth.com/solution.asp?locid=50
Disability Served: various

**CommuniCare of Clifton Postacute and
    Rehabilitation Center**
625 Probasco Street
Cincinnati, OH 45220
513-281-2464

http://communicarehealth.com/solution.asp?locid=14
Disability Served: various

Doctors Hospital
5100 West Broad Street
Columbus, OH 43228
614-544-1000
http://www.ohiohealth.com/facilities/doctors
Disability Served: various

**Easter Seals of Mahoning, Trumbull, and
    Columbiana Counties-Boardman Office**
721 Boardman-Poland Road, Suite 104
Boardman, OH 44512
330-758-5503
http://mtc.easterseals.com
Disability Served: various

**Easter Seals of Mahoning, Trumbull, and
    Columbiana Counties-Warren Office**
155 South Park
Warren, OH 44481
330-399-1001
http://mtc.easterseals.com
Disability Served: various

**Easter Seals of Mahoning, Trumbull, and
    Columbiana Counties-Youngstown Office**
299 Edwards Street
Youngstown, OH 44502
330-743-1168
http://mtc.easterseals.com
Disability Served: various

Fairfield Regional Vision Rehabilitation Center Inc.
784 East Main Street, Suite D
Lancaster, OH 43130
614-687-4785
frvrc@greenapple.com
http://www.uwayfairfieldco.org/center.html
Disability Served: vision

Four Oaks School
623 Dayton-Xenia Road
Xenia, OH 45385
513-562-7535
mconrad@co.greene.oh.us
http://www.co.greene.oh.us/fcf/parenteducation.htm
Disability Served: developmentally disabled

Genesis-Good Samaritan
800 Forest Avenue
Zanesville, OH 43701
740-454-5000
http://www.genesishcs.org
Disability Served: various

Grady Memorial Hospital
561 West Central Avenue
Delaware, OH 43015
740-369-8711
info@gradyHospital.com
http://www.gradyHospital.com
Disability Served: various

Great Lakes Regional Rehabilitation Center
3700 Kolbe Road
Lorain, OH 44053
216-960-3400
http://www.ehealthconnection.com/regions/Lorain/
    content/show_facility.asp?facility_id=56
Disability Served: various

HCR Manor Care Foundation
PO Box 10086
Toledo, OH 48699-0086
419-252-5989
foundation@hcr-manorcare.com
http://www.hcr-manorcare.org
Disability Served: various

Heather Hill Rehabilitation Hospital
12340 Bass Lake Road
Chardon, OH 44024
440-285-4040
info@heatherhill.org
http://www.heatherhill.org
Disability Served: various

Holzer Medical Center
385 Jackson Pike
Gallipolis, OH 45631
614-446-5905
Disability Served: various

Live Oaks Career Development Campus
5956 Buckwheat Road
Milford, OH 45150-2287
513-575-1900
Disability Served: various

Medical University of Ohio
3000 Arlington Avenue
Toledo, OH 43614
419-383-4000
http://www.mco.edu
Disability Served: various

Medical University of Ohio Rehabilitation Hospital
3065 Arlington Avenue
Toledo, OH 43614
419-383-6529, 800-323-8383
http://www.meduohio.edu
Disability Served: various

MetroHealth Medical Center
2500 MetroHealth Drive
Cleveland, OH 44109
216-778-7800
http://www.metrohealth.org
Disability Served: various

Newark Healthcare Center
75 McMillen Drive
Newark, OH 43055
740-344-0357
http://www.newarkhealthcare.com
Disability Served: various

Ohio Rehabilitation Services Commission
400 East Campus View Boulevard
Columbus, OH 43235-4604
614-438-1200 (Voice/ TTY), 800-282-4536 (Voice/ TTY)
http://www.state.oh.us/rsc
Disability Served: various

Ohio State University Hospitals Dodd Hall
380 West 9th Avenue
Columbus, OH 43210
614-293-3800
http://medicalCenter.osu.edu/patientcare/
    hospitalsandservices/programs/services/?ID=219
Disability Served: traumatic brain injury

Philomatheon Society of the Blind
2701 West Tuscarawas Street
Canton, OH 44708
330-453-9157
http://my.raex.com/~philo
Disability Served: vision

Rehabilitation Institute of Ohio at Miami Valley Hospital
1 Wyoming Street
Dayton, OH 45409-2793
937-208-8000
http://www.miamivalleyHospital.com/rehab.htm
Disability Served: various

Saint Francis Health Care Center
401 North Broadway Street
Green Springs, OH 44836
419-639-2626, 800-248-2552
plantops@sfhcc.org
http://www.sfhcc.org
Disability Served: various

Saint Rita's Medical Center
730 West Market Street
Lima, OH 45801
419-227-3361, 800-232-7762
http://www.stritas.org
Disability Served: various

Samuel W. Bell Home for the Sightless Inc.
3775 Muddy Creek Road
Cincinnati, OH 45238
513-241-0720
Disability Served: vision

Shriners Burn Institute-Cincinnati Unit
3229 Burnet Avenue
Cincinnati, OH 45229-3095
513-872-6000, 800-875-8580
http://www.shrinershq.org/shc/cincinnati
Disability Served: burns

Six County Inc.
2845 Bell Street
Zanesville, OH 43701-1794
740-454-9766
info@sixcounty.org
http://www.sixcounty.org
Disability Served: mental health

TAC Industries Inc.
110 West Leffel Lane
Springfield, OH 45505
937-328-5200
http://www.tacind.com
Disability Served: developmentally disabled

OKLAHOMA

Dean A. McGee Eye Institute
608 Stanton L. Young Drive
Oklahoma City, OK 73104
405-271-6060
http://www.dmei.org
Disability Served: vision

Integris Jim Thorpe Rehabilitation Center at Southwest Medical Center
4219 South Western Avenue
Oklahoma City, OK 73109
405-644-5200
http://www.integris-health.com/INTEGRIS
Disability Served: various

Kaiser Rehabilitation Center
1125 South Trenton Avenue
Tulsa, OK 74120
918-579-7100
http://www.hillcrest.com/kaiser
Disability Served: various

Jane Phillips Rehab Services
3500 Southeast Frank Phillips Boulevard
Bartlesville, OK 74006
918-333-7200
http://www.jpmc.org
Disability Served: various

McAlester Regional Health Center
One Clark Bass Boulevard
McAlester, OK 74501
918-426-1800
http://www.mrhcok.com
Disability Served: various

Oklahoma Department of Rehabilitation Services
3535 Northwest 58th Street, Suite 500
Oklahoma City, OK 73112
405-951-3400, 800-845-8476
http://www.okrehab.org
Disability Served: various

Oklahoma League for the Blind
501 North Douglas Avenue
Oklahoma City, OK 73106
405-232-4644
info@olb.org
http://www.olb.org
Disability Served: vision

Saint Anthony Hospital Rehabilitation Center
1000 North Lee Street, Box 205
Oklahoma City, OK 73101
405-272-7386
St_Anthony@ssmhc.com
http://www.saintsok.com
Disability Served: various

Saint Mary's Regional Medical Center
Rehab Care Program
305 South 5th Street
Enid, OK 73701
580-249-5533
http://www.stmarysregional.com
Disability Served: various

OREGON

The Arc of Oregon
1745 State Street
Salem, OR 97301
503-581-2726
info@arcoregon.org
http://www.arcoregon.org
Disability Served: developmentally disabled

Casey Eye Institute
3375 Southwest Terwilliger Boulevard
Portland, OR 97239-4197
503-494-3000
http://www.ohsuhealth.com/cei
Disability Served: vision

Douglas Community Medical Center
738 West Harvard Boulevard
Roseburg, OR 97470
541-673-6641
Disability Served: various

Garten Foundation
3334 Industrial Way, NE
Salem, OR 97303
503-581-4472
garten@garten.org
http://www.garten.org
Disability Served: various

Legacy Emanuel Rehabilitation Outpatient Center
Emanuel Specialty Center
3025 North Vancouver Avenue

Portland, OR 97227
503-413-1500
http://www.legacyhealth.org/body.cfm?id=1037
Disability Served: various

Legacy Good Samaritan Hospital and Medical Center
1015 Northwest 22nd Avenue
Portland, OR 97210
503-229-7711
http://www.legacyhealth.org/body.
   cfm?id=35&oTopID=0
Disability Served: various

Oakhill-Senior Program
1190 Oakhill Avenue, SE
Salem, OR 97302
503-364-9086
Disability Served: elderly

Oregon Health Sciences University
3181 Southwest Sam Jackson Park Road
Portland, OR 97239
503-494-8311
http://www.ohsuhealth.com
Disability Served: various

Oregon Office of Vocational Rehabilitation Services
500 Summer Street, NE, E-87
Salem, OR 97310-1018
877-277-0513, 503-945-5894 (TTY)
vrinfo@state.or.us
http://www.oregon.gov/DHS/vr
Disability Served: various

Salem Hospital Regional Rehabilitation Center
2561 Center Street, NE
Salem, OR 97301
503-561-5967
http://www.salemHospital.org
Disability Served: various

Shriner's Hospital Portland
3101 Southwest Sam Jackson Park Road
Portland, OR 97239
503-241-5090
http://www.shcc.org
Disability Served: physically disabled

PENNSYLVANIA

Allied John Heinz Institute of Rehabilitation Medicine
150 Mundy Street
Wilkes-Barre, PA 18702
570-826-3800
tpugh@allied-services.org
http://www.allied-services.org/aboutalliedrehabhosp.
    html
Disability Served: various

Beechwood Rehabilitation Services
469 East Maple Avenue
Langhorne, PA 19047
215-750-4299, 800-782-3299
dcerra-tyl@woods.org
http://www.beechwoodrehab.com
Disability Served: chemical dependency

Blind and Vision Rehabilitation Services of Pittsburgh
1800 West Street
Homestead, PA 15120
412-368-4400, 412-368-4095 (TDD)
http://www.pghvis.org
Disability Served: vision

Bryn Mawr Rehabilitation Hospital
414 Paoli Pike, PO Box 3007
Malvern, PA 19355
610-251-5400, 888-REHAB-41
rehabinfo@mlhs.org
http://www.mainlinehealth.org/br
Disability Served: various

Chestnut Hill Rehabilitation Hospital
8601 Stenton Avenue
Wyndmoor, PA 19038
215-233-6200
http://www.chh.org
Disability Served: various

Devereux Beneto
655 Sugartown Road
Malvern, PA 19355
800-935-6789
http://www.devereuxbeneto.org
Disability Served: behavioral disorders, mental retardation

Devereux Kanner CARES
620 Boot Road
Downington, PA 19335

610-873-4930
http://www.devereuxcares.org
Disability Served: autism

Devereux National
444 Devereux Drive, PO Box 638
Villanova, PA 19085
800-345-1292
http://www.devereux.org
Disability Served: various

Devereux Pocono Center
RR 1, Box 27-A Junction, Routes 191 & 507 South
Newfoundland, PA 18445
570-676-3237
http://www.devereuxpocono.org
Disability Served: various

Devereux Whitlock
139 Leopard Road
Berwyn, PA 19312
610-296-6800
http://www.devereuxwhitlock.org
Disability Served: developmentally disabled

Doylestown Hospital Rehabilitation Center
595 West State Street
Doylestown, PA 18901
215-345-2200
http://www.dh.org
Disability Served: various

Erie Shriners Hospital for Crippled Children
1645 West 8th Street
Erie, PA 16505
814-875-8700
http://www.shrinershq.org/shc/erie
Disability Served: physically disabled

Fox Subacute at Clara Burke
251 Stenton Avenue
Plymouth Meeting, PA 19462
610-828-2272
Disability Served: various

Fox Subacute Center
2644 Bristol Road
Warrington, PA 18976
215-343-2700
Disability Served: various

Good Samaritan Hospital-Robert L. Miller Rehab Center
4th and Walnut Streets
Lebanon, PA 17042
717-270-7729
http://www.gshleb.org
Disability Served: various

Good Shepherd Rehabilitation Hospital
543 Saint John Street
Allentown, PA 18103
610-776-3100
info@goodshepherdrehab.org
http://www.goodshepherdrehab.org
Disability Served: various

Good Shepherd Rehabilitation Hospital at Pocono Medical Center
206 East Brown Street
East Stroudsburg, PA 18301
570-476-3302
info@goodshepherdrehab.org
http://www.goodshepherdrehab.org
Disability Served: various

HealthSouth Altoona Pain Management
2005 Valley View Boulevard
Altoona, PA 16602
814-944-3535
http://www.healthsouth.com
Disability Served: chronic pain

HealthSouth Harmarville Rehabilitation Center
Guys Run Road, PO Box 11460
Pittsburgh, PA 15238
412-828-1300
http://www.healthsouth.com
Disability Served: various

HealthSouth Nittany Valley Rehabilitation Hospital
550 West College Avenue
Pleasant Gap, PA 16823
814-359-3421
http://www.healthsouth.com
Disability Served: various

HealthSouth Rehabilitation Hospital of Erie
143 East 2nd Street
Erie, PA 16507
814-878-1200

http://www.healthsouth.com
Disability Served: various

HealthSouth Rehabilitation Hospital of Greater Pittsburgh
2380 McGinley Road
Monroeville, PA 15146
412-856-2400
http://www.healthsouth.com
Disability Served: various

HealthSouth Rehabilitation Hospital of Mechanicsburg
175 Lancaster Boulevard
Mechanicsburg, PA 17055
717-691-3700
http://www.healthsouth.com
Disability Served: various

Magee Rehabilitation Hospital
1513 Race Street
Philadelphia, PA 19102-1177
800-96-MAGEE
magee@mageerehab.org
http://www.mageerehab.org
Disability Served: various

MossRehab
60 East Township Line Road
Elkins Park, PA 19027
215-663-6000
http://www.einstein.edu/facilities/mossrehab
Disability Served: various

MossRehab
1200 West Tabor Road
Philadelphia, PA 19141
215-456-9900
http://www.einstein.edu/facilities/mossrehab
Disability Served: various

Pennsylvania Office of Vocational Rehabilitation
Seventh and Forster Streets, Labor and Industry Building
Harrisburg, PA 17120
800-442-6351, 800-233-3008 (TTY)
ovr@dli.state.pa.us
http://www.dli.state.pa.us/ovr
Disability Served: various

Philadelphia Shriners Hospital
3551 North Broad Street
Philadelphia, PA 19140
215-430-4000, 800-281-4050
http://www.shrinershq.org/shc/philadelphia
Disability Served: various

Success Rehabilitation Inc.
5666 Clymer Road
Quakertown, PA 18951
215-538-3488
success@successrehab.com
http://www.successrehab.com
Disability Served: traumatic brain injury

Wills Eye Hospital
840 Walnut Street
Philadelphia, PA 19107
215-928-3000
http://www.willseye.org
Disability Served: vision

RHODE ISLAND
Hasbro Children's Hospital
593 Eddy Street
Providence, RI 02903
401-444-4000
http://www.lifespan.org/partners/hch
Disability Served: various

Rhode Island Office of Rehabilitation Services
40 Fountain Street
Providence, RI 02903
401-421-7005, 401-421-7016 (TTY)
http://www.ors.state.ri.us
Disability Served: various

Shake-A-Leg
PO Box 1264
Newport, RI 02840
401-849-8898
timf@shakealeg.org
http://www.shakealeg.org
Disability Served: various

Vanderbilt Rehabilitation Center in Bristol
450 Hope Street, 3rd Floor
Bristol, RI 02809
401-254-2828, 800-984-6043

http://www.lifespan.org/Services/Rehab/VRC
Disability Served: various

Vanderbilt Rehabilitation Center in Newport
20 Powel Avenue
Newport, RI 02840
401-845-1605
http://www.lifespan.org/Services/Rehab/VRC
Disability Served: various

SOUTH CAROLINA
The Arc of Anderson County
1105 Hanover Road
Anderson, SC 29621
864-224-2667
http://www.arcsc.org
Disability Served: developmentally disabled

Association for the Blind Inc.
2209 Mechanic Street
Charleston, SC 29405
843-723-6915
Disability Served: vision

Colleton Regional Hospital
501 Robertson Boulevard
Waterboro, SC 29488
843-549-2000
http://www.colletonmedical.com
Disability Served: various

Greenville Shriners Hospital
950 West Faris Road
Greenville, SC 29605-4277
864-271-3444
http://www.shrinershq.org/shc/greenville
Disability Served: physically disabled

HealthSouth Charleston Outpatient Services
9181 Medcom Street
Charleston, SC 29406
843-820-7777
http://www.healthsouth.com
Disability Served: various

HealthSouth Rehabilitation Hospital
2935 Colonial Drive
Columbia, SC 29203
803-254-7777

http://www.healthsouth.com
Disability Served: various

HealthSouth Spine and Rehabilitation Center
1245 Savannah Highway
Charleston, SC 29407
843-852-3479
http://www.healthsouth.com
Disability Served: various

Hitchcock Rehabilitation Center
690 Medical Park Drive
Aiken, SC 29801
803-648-8344, 800-207-6924
mail@hitchcock.aiken.net
http://www.hitchcockrehab.com
Disability Served: various

South Carolina Association of the Deaf Inc.
437 Center Street
West Columbia, SC 29169
803-794-3175, 803-794-7059 (TTY)
info@scadservices.org
http://www.scadservices.org
Disability Served: hearing

South Carolina School for the Deaf and Blind
355 Cedar Springs Road
Spartanburg, SC 29302-4699
864-585-7711 (Voice/TTY)
cmabry@scsdb.k12.sc.us
http://www.scsdb.k12.sc.us
Disability Served: hearing, vision

South Carolina Vocational Rehabilitation Department
1410 Boston Avenue, PO Box 15
West Columbia, SC 29171
803-896-6500
info@scvrd.state.sc.us
http://www.scvrd.net
Disability Served: various

SOUTH DAKOTA
Avera McKennan Hospital and University Health Center
800 East 21st Street
Sioux Falls, SD 57117-5045
605-322-5050

http://www.averamckennan.org
Disability Served: various

Avera Sacred Heart Hospital Medical Rehabilitation Unit
501 Summit
Yankton, SD 57078
605-668-8297
http://www.averasacredheart.com
Disability Served: various

Avera St. Luke's Hospital Rehabilitation Center
305 South State Street
Aberdeen, SD 57401
605-622-5857
http://www.averastlukes.org
Disability Served: various

Black Hills Rehabilitation Hospital
2908 Fifth Street
Rapid City, SD 57701
605-719-1212
http://www.rcrh.org
Disability Served: various

Children's Care Hospital and School
2501 West 26th Street
Sioux Falls, SD 57105
605-782-2300
http://www.cchs.org
Disability Served: various

Children's Care Hospital and School Rehabilitation Center
1100 West 41st Street
Sioux Falls, SD 57105
605-782-2400
Disability Served: various

Sioux Valley Hospital and University Medical Center
1305 West 18th Street
Sioux Falls, SD 57117-5039
605-333-1000
http://www.siouxvalley.org
Disability Served: various

South Dakota Division of Rehabilitation Services
500 East Capitol
Pierre, SD 57501-5070
605-773-3195

eric.weiss@state.sd.us
http://www.state.sd.us/dhs/drs
Disability Served: various

South Dakota Rehabilitation Center for the Blind

800 West Avenue North
Sioux Falls, SD 57104
605-367-5260, 800-658-5441
dawn.backer@state.sd.us
http://www.state.sd.us/dhs/sbvi/SDRC.htm
Disability Served: vision

TENNESSEE

Baptist Hospital Of East Tennessee

137 Blount Avenue
Knoxville, TN 37920
865-632-5011
http://www.baptistoneword.org
Disability Served: various

Clovernook-Memphis

346 St. Paul Avenue
Memphis, TN 38126
901-523-9590
http://www.clovernook.org
Disability Served: vision

HealthSouth Cane Creek Rehabilitation Hospital

180 Mount Pelia Road
Martin, TN 38237
731-587-4231
http://www.healthsouth.com
Disability Served: various

Nashville Rehabilitation Hospital

610 Gallatin Road
Nashville, TN 37206
615-226-4330
admin@nrhcares.com
http://www.nrhcares.com
Disability Served: various

Patricia Neal Rehab Center-Ft. Sanders Regional Medical Center

1901 Clinch Avenue
Knoxville, TN 37916
865-541-1446
http://www.patneal.org/pnrc-home.cfm
Disability Served: various

Patrick Rehab Wellness

Lincoln County Health Facilities
1001 Huntsville Highway
Fayetteville, TN 37334
931-433-0273
yrussell@lchealthsystem.com
http://www.lchealthsystem.com/lchs.nsf/View/
    PatrickCenter
Disability Served: various

Siskin Hospital for Physical Rehabilitation

One Siskin Plaza
Chattanooga, TN 37403
423-634-1200
info@siskinrehab.org
http://www.siskinrehab.org
Disability Served: physically disabled

Tennessee Vocational Rehabilitation Services

Citizens Plaza Building, 400 Deaderick Street, Room 1100
Nashville, TN 37248-0001
615-313-4714
Disability Served: various

TEXAS

Baptist St. Anthony's Health System Rehabilitation Center

1600 Wallace Boulevard
Amarillo, TX 79106
806-212-3141
http://www.bsahs.org
Disability Served: various

Baylor Institute for Rehabilitation

3505 Gaston Avenue
Dallas, TX 75246
214-820-9300
http://baylorhealth.com
Disability Served: various

Bayshore Medical Center-

4000 Spencer Highway
Pasadena, TX 77504
713-359-2000
http://www.bayshoremedical.com
Disability Served: various

Brown-Karhan Health Care

3035 Highway 290 West
Dripping Springs, TX 78620

512-894-0701
info@brown-karhan.com
http://www.brown-karhan.com
Disability Served: mental health, traumatic brain injury

Brown Schools Rehabilitation Center
1106 West Dittmar Road
Austin, TX 78745
512-444-4835
Disability Served: various

Callier Center for Communication Disorders-Dallas
1966 Inwood Road
Dallas, TX 75235
214-905-3000
http://www.callier.utdallas.edu
Disability Served: communication

Callier Center for Communication Disorders-Richardson
811 Synergy Park Boulevard
Richardson, TX 75080
972-883-3630
http://www.callier.utdallas.edu
Disability Served: communication

Centre for Neuro Skills
1320 West Walnut Hill
Irving, TX 75038
972-580-8500, 800-554-5448
texas@neuroskills.com
http://www.neuroskills.com
Disability Served: traumatic brain injury

Clear Lake Rehabilitation Hospital
655 East Medical Center Boulevard
Webster, TX 77598
713-286-1500
Disability Served: various

Covenant Medical Center
3615 19th Street
Lubbock, TX 79410
806-725-1011
http://www.covenanthealth.org/frontpage/Default.htm
Disability Served: various

Dallas Lighthouse for the Blind
4245 Office Parkway
Dallas, TX 75204

214-821-2375
http://www.dallaslighthouse.org
Disability Served: vision

Dallas/Tarrant Services for Visually Impaired Children
4242 Office Parkway
Dallas, TX 75204
214-828-9900
Disability Served: vision

Easter Seals San Antonio, Texas
2203 Babcock Road
San Antonio, TX 78229
210-614-3911
http://www.easterseals.com
Disability Served: various

El Paso Lighthouse for the Blind
200 Washington Street
El Paso, TX 79905
915-532-4495
htyler@elp.rr.com
http://www.lighthouse-elpaso.com
Disability Served: vision

Galveston Shriners Hospital
815 Market Street
Galveston, TX 77550-2725
409-770-6600
http://www.shrinershq.org/shc/galveston
Disability Served: burns

Good Shepherd Medical Center-
700 East Marshall Avenue
Longview, TX 75601
903-315-2000
http://www.gsmc.org
Disability Served: various

HealthSouth Plano Rehabilitation Hospital
2800 West 15th Street
Plano, TX 75075
972-612-9000
http://www.healthsouth.com
Disability Served: various

HealthSouth Rehabilitation Center-Beaumont
3395 Plaza Ten Boulevard, Suite A
Beaumont, TX 77707
409-839-3460

http://www.healthsouth.com
Disability Served: various

HealthSouth Rehabilitation Hospital
19002 McKay Drive
Humble, TX 77338
713-446-6148
http://www.healthsouth.com
Disability Served: various

HealthSouth Rehabilitation Hospital-of Arlington
3200 Matlock Road
Arlington, TX 76015
817-468-4000
http://www.healthsouth.com
Disability Served: various

HealthSouth Rehabilitation Hospital of Austin
1215 Red River
Austin, TX 78701
512-474-5700
http://healthsouth.com
Disability Served: various

HealthSouth Riosa Outpatient Services
9119 Cinnamon Hill
San Antonio, TX 78240
210-691-0737
http://www.healthsouth.com
Disability Served: various

Hillcrest Baptist Medical Center
3000 Herring Avenue
Waco, TX 76708
254-202-2577
http://www.hillcrest.net
Disability Served: various

Houston Shriners Hospital
6977 Main Street
Houston, TX 77030
713-797-1616
http://www.shrinershq.org/shc/houston
Disability Served: physically disabled

IHS Hospital-Dallas
7955 Harry Hines Boulevard
Dallas, TX 75235
214-637-0000

tim.lozier@ihs-inc.com
Disability Served: various

IHS of Dallas-Treemont
5550 Harvest Hill Road
Dallas, TX 75230
972-661-1862
Disability Served: various

Institute for Rehabilitation and Research
1333 Moursund
Houston, TX 77030-3405
713-799-5000, 713-797-5790 (TDD)
Disability Served: various

Integrated Health Services of Amarillo
5601 Plum Creek Drive
Amarillo, TX 79124
806-351-1000, 800-419-2100
http://www.medCenter.org
Disability Served: various

Lighthouse of Houston
PO Box 130345
Houston, TX 77019
713-527-9561
jblando@houstonlighthouse.org
http://www.houstonlighthouse.org
Disability Served: vision

Mabee Rehabilitation Center
1325 Pennsylvania Avenue
Ft. Worth, TX 76104
817-882-2022
Disability Served: various

Medical Center of Arlington-Rehabilitation Services
3301 Matlock Road
Arlington, TX 76015
817-472-4906
http://www.medicalCenterarlington.com
Disability Served: physically disabled

Memorial Rehabilitation Hospital
207 Tradewinds Boulevard
Midland, TX 79706
432-520-2333
http://www.midland-memorial.com
Disability Served: physically disabled

Nacogdoches Memorial Hospital Cecil R. Bomar Rehabilitation Center
1204 Mound Street
Nacogdoches, TX 75961
936-564-4611
info@nacmem.org
http://www.nacmem.org
Disability Served: various

Navarro Regional Hospital-Rehabilitation Unit
3201 West Highway 22
Corsicana, TX 75110
903-654-6800
Disability Served: various

North Texas Rehabilitation Center
1005 Midwestern Parkway
Wichita Falls, TX 76302
940-322-0771
ntrc@ntrehab.org
http://www.ntrehab.org/index.htm
Disability Served: various

Productive Rehabilitation Institute of Dallas for Ergonomics
5701 Maple Avenue, Suite 100
Dallas, TX 75235
214-351-6600
pride@airmail.net
http://www.pridedallas.com
Disability Served: spinal-cord injury

Rio Vista Physical Rehabilitation Hospital
1740 Curie Drive
El Paso, TX 79935
915-591-1479
http://www.sphn.com
Disability Served: physically disabled

Saint David's Rehabilitation Center
1005 East 32nd Street
Austin, TX 78705
512-476-7111
http://www.stdavidsrehab.com
Disability Served: spinal-cord injury, traumatic brain injury

San Antonio Lighthouse
2305 Roosevelt Avenue
San Antonio, TX 78210
210-533-5195, 800-362-4335
http://www.salighthouse.org
Disability Served: vision

Shannon Medical Center-Rehabilitation Unit
120 East Harris Street
San Angelo, TX 76903
325-657-5617
http://www.shannonhealth.com
Disability Served: various

South Texas Lighthouse for the Blind
PO Box 9697
Corpus Christi, TX 78469
512-883-6553
Disability Served: vision

South Texas Rehabilitation Hospital
425 East Alton Gloor Boulevard
Brownsville, TX 78526
956-554-6000
http://strh.ernesthealth.com
Disability Served: various

Texas Department of Assistive and Rehabilitative Services
4800 North Lamar Boulevard, 3rd Floor
Austin, TX 78756
800-628-5115
DARS.Inquiries@dars.state.tx.us
http://www.dars.state.tx.us
Disability Served: various

Transitional Learning Center
1528 Postoffice Street
Galveston, TX 77550
409-762-6661, 800-TLC-GROW
http://tlcrehab.org
Disability Served: various

Travis Association for the Blind
PO Box 3297
Austin, TX 78764-3297
512-442-2329
http://www.austinlighthouse.org
Disability Served: vision

Valley Regional Medical Center
100 A.E. Alton Gloor
Brownsville, TX 78526

956-350-7000
http://www.valleyregionalmedicalCenter.com
Disability Served: various

Warm Springs Rehabilitation Hospital San Antonio
5101 Medical Drive
San Antonio, TX 78229
210-616-0100
sleblanc@wssahosp.org
http://www.warmsprings.org
Disability Served: various

West Texas Lighthouse for the Blind
2001 West Austin Street
San Angelo, TX 76903
325-653-4231
wtlb@wcc.net
http://www.lighthousefortheblind.org
Disability Served: vision

UTAH

The Arc of Utah
155 South 300 West, Suite 201
Salt Lake City, UT 84101
801-364-5060, 800-371-5060
thearc@arcutah.org
http://www.arcutah.org
Disability Served: developmentally disabled

HealthSouth Rehabilitation Hospital of Utah
8074 South 1300 East
Sandy, UT 84094
801-561-3400
http://www.healthsouth.com
Disability Served: various

Intermountain Shriners Hospital
Fairfax Road at Virginia Street
Salt Lake City, UT 84103
801-532-5307, 800-237-5055
http://www.shrinershq.org/shc/intermountain
Disability Served: physically disabled

LDS Hospital Rehabilitation Center
8th Avenue & C Street
Salt Lake City, UT 84143
801-408-5400
http://www.ihc.com
Disability Served: physically disabled

Mc Kay-Dee Stewart Rehabilitation Services
4401 Harrison Boulevard
Ogden, UT 84403-3195
801-387-2100
http://www.ihc.com/xp/ihc/mckaydee
Disability Served: various

Primary Children's Medical Center
100 North Medical Drive
Salt Lake City, UT 84113-1100
801-588-2000
http://www.ihc.com/xp/ihc/primary
Disability Served: various

**Robert G. Sanderson Community Center of the Deaf
and Hard of Hearing**
5709 South 1500 West
Taylorsville, UT 84123
801-263-4860 (Voice/TTY), 800-860-4860
Disability Served: hearing

University Health Care Rehabilitation Center
50 North Medical Drive
Salt Lake City, UT 84132
801-581-2121
hscwebmaster@hsc.utah.edu
http://uuhsc.utah.edu/uuhsc/patient/Hospital.htm
Disability Served: various

Utah State Office of Rehabilitation
250 East 500 South
Salt Lake City, UT 84114-4200
801-538-7530
http://www.usor.state.ut.us
Disability Served: various

Utah State Office of Rehabilitation
Division of Services for the Blind and Visually Impaired
PO Box 144200
Salt Lake City, UT 84114-4200
800-473-7530
http://www.usor.utah.gov/dsbvi.htm
Disability Served: vision

Wasatch Valley Rehabilitation
2200 East 3300 South
Salt Lake City, UT 84109
801-486-2096
http://www.wasatchvalleyrehab.com
Disability Served: various

VERMONT

Rutland Regional Medical Center
160 Allen Street
Rutland, VT 05701
802-775-7111
http://www.rrmc.org
Disability Served: various

Vermont Achievement Center
88 Park Street
Rutland, VT 05702-6283
802-775-2395
tmoore@vac-rutland.com
http://www.vacvt.org
Disability Served: various

Vermont Division of Vocational Rehabilitation
Osgood II Building,103 South Main Street
Waterbury, VT 05671-2303
866-879-6757 (Voice/TTY)
janetr@dad.state.vt.us
http://www.vocrehabvermont.org
Disability Served: various

VIRGINIA

Carilion Roanoke Memorial Hospital
1906 Belleview Avenue, PO Box 13367
Roanoke, VA 24033
540-981-7000
http://www.carilion.com/crmh
Disability Served: various

Children's Hospital
2924 Brook Road
Richmond, VA 23220
804-321-7474
 http://www.childrenshosp-richmond.org/
Disability Served: various

Faith Mission Home
3540 Mission Home Lane
Free Union, VA 22940
804-985-2294
Disability Served: developmentally disabled, traumatic brain injury

Inova Mount Vernon Hospital
2501 Parker's Lane
Alexandria, VA 22306

703-664-7190, 800-554-REHAB
http://www.inova.org/inovapublic.srt/imvh/index.jsp
Disability Served: various

Kluge Children's Rehabilitation Center
Route 250 West, Ivy Road
Charlottesville, VA 22901
434-924-KCRC
http://www.healthsystem.virginia.edu/internet/
        pediatrics/Facilities/Outpatient.cfm#Kluge_outpt
Disability Served: various

Pines Residential Treatment Center
825 Crawford Parkway
Portsmouth, VA 23704
877-227-7000
http://www.absfirst.com/facilities_pines.html
Disability Served: behavioral disorders

Sheltering Arms Physical Rehabilitation Hospital
8254 Atlee Road
Richmond, VA 23116
804-764-7054
http://www.shelteringarms.com/facRehabHospital.html
Disability Served: various

Southside Virginia Training Center
26317 West Washington Street, PO Box 4110
Petersburg, VA 23803
804-524-7000
http://www.svtc.dmhmrsas.virginia.gov
Disability Served: developmentally disabled

Virginia Department of Rehabilitative Services
8004 Franklin Farms Drive
Richmond, VA 23288
800-552-5019, 800-464-9950 (TTY)
800-552-5019 (Voice/TTY)
drs@drs.virginia.gov
http://vadrs.org
Disability Served: various

WASHINGTON

Arden Rehabilitation and Health Care Center
16357 Aurora Avenue North
Seattle, WA 98133
206-542-3103
http://www.ardenrehab.com
Disability Served: various

Community Services for the Blind and Partially Sighted
9709 Third Avenue, NE, Suite 100
Seattle, WA 98115-2027
206-525-5556, 800-458-4888
csbps@csbps.com
http://www.csbps.com
Disability Served: vision

First Hill Care Center
1334 Terry Avenue
Seattle, WA 98101-2796
206-624-1484
Disability Served: various

Good Samaritan Hospital-
407 14th Avenue, SE
Puyallup, WA 98372
253-697-4000
info@goodsamhealth.org
http://www.goodsamhealth.org
Disability Served: various

Harborview Medical Center
325 Ninth Avenue
Seattle, WA 98104
206-731-3000
http://www.uwmedicine.org/Facilities/Harborview
Disability Served: various

Lakeside–Milam Recovery Centers Inc.
535 Dock Street, Suite 104
Tacoma, WA 98402
253-272-2242
http://www.lakesidemilam.com
Disability Served: chemical dependency

ManorCare Health Services-Gig Harbor
3309 45th Street Center, NW
Gig Harbor, WA 98335
253-858-8688
gigharbor@manorcare.com
http://www.hcr-manorcare.com
Disability Served: various

ManorCare Health Services-Lynnwood
3701 188th Street, SW
Lynnwood, WA 98037
206-775-9222
lynnwood@manorcare.com

http://www.hcr-manorcare.com
Disability Served: various

ManorCare Health Services-Spokane
North 6025 Assembly
Spokane, WA 99205
509-326-8282
http://www.hcr-manorcare.com
Disability Served: various

ManorCare Health Services-Tacoma
5601 South Orchard Street
Tacoma, WA 98409
253-474-8421
tacoma@manorcare.com
http://www.manorcare.com
Disability Served: various

Northwest Hospital Center for Medical Rehabilitation
1550 North 115th Street
Seattle, WA 98133-9733
206-368-1794
http://www.nwHospital.org/services/rehab_main.asp
Disability Served: various

Park Manor Convalescent Center
1710 Plaza Way
Walla Walla, WA 99362
509-529-4218
Disability Served: various

Providence Everett Medical Center
Providence Hospital
916 Pacific Avenue
Everett, WA 98201
425-258-7123
http://www.providence.org/Everett
Disability Served: various

Rainier Vista Care Center
920 12th Avenue, SE
Puyallup, WA 98372
253-841-3422
http://www.rainiervistacc.com
Disability Served: various

Rehabilitation Enterprises of Washington
490 Tyee Drive, Suite 104
Olympia, WA 98512
360-943-7654

http://www.halcyon.com/cei/rew.htm
Disability Served: various

Seattle Medical and Rehabilitation Center
555 16th Avenue
Seattle, WA 98122
206-324-8200
Disability Served: various

Seattle Spine and Rehabilitation Medicine
3213 Eastlake Avenue East, Suite A1
Seattle, WA 98102
206-861-8200
http://www.ssarm.yourmd.com
Disability Served: spinal-cord injury

Swedish Medical Center/Providence
500 17th Avenue
Seattle, WA 98122-5711
206-320-2000
http://www.swedish.org
Disability Served: various

Washington Division of Vocational Rehabilitation
PO Box 45340
Olympia, WA 98504-5340
800-637-5627, 360-438-8000
http://www1.dshs.wa.gov/dvr
Disability Served: various

WEST VIRGINIA
Children's Therapy Clinic Inc.
317 Washington Street West
Charleston, WV 25302
304-342-9515
jennifer@childrenstherapyclinic.com
http://www.childrenstherapyclinic.com
Disability Served: various

**HealthSouth Mountain View Regional Rehabilitation
Hospital**
1160 Van Voorhis Road
Morgantown, WV 26505
304-598-1100, 800-388-2451
http://www.healthsouth.com
Disability Served: various

HealthSouth Western Hills Rehabilitation Hospital
3 Western Hills Drive
Parkersburg, WV 26105

304-420-1300
http://www.healthsouth.com
Disability Served: various

West Virginia Division of Rehabilitation Services
State Capitol, PO Box 50890
Charleston, WV 25305-0890
304-766-4601, 800-642-8207
http://www.wvdrs.org
Disability Served: various

WISCONSIN
Colonial Manor Medical and Rehabilitation Center
1010 East Wausau Avenue
Wausau, WI 54403
715-842-2028
http://www.colonialmanormrc.com
Disability Served: various

Columbia St. Mary's Columbia Campus
2025 East Newport Avenue
Milwaukee, WI 53211
414-298-6750
http://www.columbia-stmarys.com/body.cfm?id=53
Disability Served: traumatic brain injury

**Continuing Education Center for Community-Based
Rehabilitation Programs**
University of Wisconsin-Stout
214 10th Avenue East, 101 VRB
Menomonie, WI 54751
715-232-2236
http://cec.uwstout.edu
Disability Served: various

Curative at Isaac Coggs Community Health Center
2770 North Fifth Street
Milwaukee, WI 53212
414-286-8835
http://www.curative.org
Disability Served: physically disabled

Curative-Cudahy
5071 South Lake Drive
Cudahy, WI 53110
414-744-7630
http://www.curative.org
Disability Served: physically disabled

Curative -92nd Street
1000 North 92nd Street
Milwaukee, WI 53226
414-259-1414
http://www.curative.org
Disability Served: physically disabled

Eastview Medical and Rehabilitation Center
729 Park Street
Antigo, WI 54409
715-623-2356
http://www.eastviewmedrehab.com
Disability Served: various

Extendicare Health Services Inc.
111 West Michigan Street
Milwaukee, WI 53203-2903
800-395-5000
http://www.extendicare.com
Disability Served: various

Lakeview Medical Center Rehabilitation Services
1100 North Main Street
Rice Lake, WI 54868
715-236-6408
http://www.lakeviewmedical.com
Disability Served: various

Middleton Village Nursing and Rehabilitation Center
6201 Elmwood Avenue
Middleton, WI 53562
608-831-8300
http://www.middletonvillage.com
Disability Served: various

Midwest Neurological Rehabilitation Center
1701 Sharp Road
Waterford, WI 53185
414-534-2301, 800-697-5380
Disability Served: traumatic brain injury

Mount Carmel Medical and Rehabilitation Center
677 East State Street
Burlington, WI 53105
262-763-9531
http://www.mtcarmelrehab.com
Disability Served: various

Sacred Heart Hospital
900 West Clairemont Avenue
Eau Claire, WI 54701

715-839-4121
http://www.sacredheartHospital-ec.org
Disability Served: various

Saint Catherine's Hospital
3556 Seventh Avenue
Kenosha, WI 53140
414-656-3361
Disability Served: various

Saint Joseph's Hospital
611 St. Joseph Avenue
Marshfield, WI 54449
715-387-1713
sjhweb@stjosephs-marshfield.org
http://www.ministryhealth.org
Disability Served: various

Wisconsin Division of Vocational Rehabilitation
2917 International Lane, Suite 300, PO Box 7852
Madison, WI 53707
608-243-5600, 608-243-5601 (TTY)
http://www.dwd.state.wi.us/dvr
Disability Served: various

Woodstock Health and Rehabilitation Center
3415 Sheridan Road
Kenosha, WI 53140
262-657-6175
http://www.woodstockhealth.com
Disability Served: various

WYOMING

The Arc of Laramie County
1616 East 19th Street, Suite 7, PO Box 1812
Cheyenne, WY 82003
307-632-1209
arc-lc@trib.com
Disability Served: developmentally disabled

The Arc of Natrona County
318 West B Street
Casper, WY 82602
307-577-4913
arc_nc@trib.com
Disability Served: developmentally disabled

The Arc of Uinta and Lincoln Counties
917 Main Street
Evanston, WY 82930

307-789-7679
thearc@vcn.com
Disability Served: developmentally disabled

The Arc of Wyoming
PO Box 2161
Casper, WY 82601
307-237-9110
thearc@vcn.com
Disability Served: developmentally disabled

Ivinson Memorial Hospital
255 North 30th Street
Laramie, WY 82072
307-742-2141
gregk@ivinsonHospital.org
http://www.ivinsonHospital.org
Disability Served: various

Wyoming Division of Vocational Rehabilitation
1100 Herschler Building
Cheyenne, WY 82002
307-777-7389
http://wyomingworkforce.org/how/vr.aspx
Disability Served: various

PUERTO RICO
Puerto Rico Division of Vocational Rehabilitation
PO Box 191118
Hato Rey, PR 00919
787-728-6550
Disability Served: various

CANADA
Bloorview MacMillan Children's Centre
25 Buchan Court
Toronto, ON M2J 4S9
Canada
416-425-6220, 800-363-2440
info@bloorviewmacmillan.on.ca
http://www.bloorviewmacmillan.on.ca
Disability Served: various

Bloorview MacMillan Children's Centre
150 Kilgour Road
Toronto, ON M4G 1R8
Canada
416-425-6220, 800-363-2440
info@bloorviewmacmillan.on.ca
http://www.bloorviewmacmillan.on.ca
Disability Served: various

Vocational and Rehabilitation Research Institute
3304 - 33 Street, NW
Calgary, AB T2L 2A6
Canada
http://www.vrri.org
Disability Served: various

SELF-HELP AND ADVOCACY ORGANIZATIONS

These organizations are dedicated to providing self-help and advocacy services to persons with disabilities.

Advocacy Center for Persons with Disabilities
2671 Executive Center Circle West, Suite 100
Tallahassee, FL 32301-5092
850-488-9071, 800-342-0823, 800-346-4127 (TDD)
info@advocacycenter.org
http://www.advocacycenter.org
Disability Served: various
The Advocacy Center for Persons with Disabilities is a nonprofit organization that provides protection and advocacy services in the state of Florida. The center's mission is to advance the dignity, equality, self-determination, and expressed choices of individuals with disabilities.

Advocacy Inc.
7800 Shoal Creek Boulevard, Suite 171E
Austin, TX 78757
512-454-4816
http://www.advocacyinc.org
Disability Served: various
This organization provides protection and advocacy assistance for people with disabilities who live in Texas.

Advocates in Action
Box 41528
Providence, RI 02940-1528
401-785-2028
aina@aina.org
http://www.aina-ri.org
Disability Served: various
This organization provides advocacy, public education, support groups, and conferences for people with disabilities.

Alabama Disabilities Advocacy Program
Box 870395
Tuscaloosa, AL
35487-0395
205-348-4928, 800-826-1675
adap@adap.ua.edu
http://www.adap.net
Disability Served: various

The mission of this organization is to provide quality, legally based advocacy services to people with disabilities in order to protect, promote, and expand their rights.

American Self-Help Group Clearinghouse
100 East Hanover Avenue, Suite 202
Cedar Knolls, NJ 07297
973-326-6789, 800-367-6274
http://www.njgroups.org
Disability Served: various
This clearinghouse helps people find and form self-help groups.

Association of Self Advocates of North Carolina
PO Box 17271
Raleigh, NC 27609
800-662-8706 ext. 120
http://www.cdl.unc.edu/stir/asanc
Disability Served: developmentally disabled
The mission of this organization is to enable, encourage, and empower people with developmental disabilities to become more independent and make their own decisions, and to educate the community, government leaders, families, guardians and service providers about self-advocacy and the abilities of people with disabilities.

Autism Society of America
7910 Woodmont Avenue, Suite 300
Bethesda, MD 20814-3067
301-657-0881, 800-3AUTISM
http://www.autism-society.org
Disability Served: autism
This organization provides information and referral, advocacy, and education regarding autism.

Center on Human Policy
805 South Crouse Avenue
Syracuse, NY 13244-2280
315-443-3851, 800-894-0826, 315-443-4355 (TTY)
thechp@syr.edu
http://thechp.syr.edu

Disability Served: various

This organization is a Syracuse University–based policy, research, and advocacy organization involved in the national movement to ensure the rights of people with disabilities.

Commission on Accreditation of Rehabilitation Facilities

4891 East Grant Road
Tucson, AZ 85712
520-325-1044, 888-281-6531 (Voice/TTY)
http://www.carf.org
Disability Served: various

This nonprofit organization advocates for the improvement of services for the disabled.

Council of Parent Attorneys and Advocates

7484 Candlewood Road, Suite R
Hanover, MD 21076
http://www.copaa.net
Disability Served: various

This organization advocates in order to secure high-quality educational services for children with disabilities.

Deafpride

1350 Potomac Avenue, SE
Washington, DC 20003
202-675-6700 (Voice/TDD)
Disability Served: hearing

Deafpride is a nonprofit advocacy organization that works for the rights of deaf people and their families. It assists groups with organizing and working together for change throughout the United States.

Disabilities Advocacy and Support Network

1515 East Pythian, PO Box 5030
Springfield, MO 65801-5030
417-895-7464, 888-549-6635
SDASN@aol.com
http://disabilitiesnetwork.org
Disability Served: developmentally disabled

The network provides educational support and guidance, encourages awareness within the community, and offers a therapeutic social outlet for individuals with development disabilities and their families.

Disabilities Rights Center

18 Low Avenue
Concord, NH 03301-4971

603-228-0432, 800-834-1721 (Voice/TDD)
advocacy@drcnh.org
http://www.drcnh.org
Disability Served: various

This statewide organization works on behalf of people with disabilities to pursue total civil and legal rights.

disABILITY LINK

755 Commerce Drive, Suite 415
Decatur, GA 30030
404-687-8890, 404-687-9175 (TTY), 800-239-2507 (Voice/TTY)
hilarye@disabilitylink.org
http://www.disabilitylink.org/docs/voices/voices.html
Disability Served: various

This organization is committed to promoting the rights of all people with disabilities. Among its many programs are People First of Atlanta and the Georgia Peer Support Project.

Disability Rights Education and Defense Fund Inc.

2212 Sixth Street
Berkeley, CA 94710
510-644-2555 (Voice/TTY)
dredf@dredf.org
http://www.dredf.org
Disability Served: various

This group acts as a national law and policy center dedicated to protecting and advancing the civil rights of people with disabilities. This goal is achieved through legislation, litigation, advocacy, technical assistance, and education and training of attorneys, advocates, persons with disabilities, and parents of children with disabilities.

Federation of Families for Children's Mental Health

1101 King Street, Suite 420
Alexandria, VA 22314-2971
703-684-7710
ffcmh@ffcmh.org
http://www.ffcmh.org
Disability Served: mental health

This national, parent-run advocacy organization focuses on the needs of children with emotional, behavioral, or mental disorders.

HEATH Resource Center

2121 K Street, NW, Suite 220
Washington, DC 20037

202-973-0904 (Voice/TTY), 800-544-3284
askheath@gwu.edu
http://www.heath.gwu.edu/aboutus.htm
Disability Served: various
This federally supported clearinghouse provides information on postsecondary education for individuals with disabilities.

Judge David L. Bazelon Center for Mental Health Law

1101 15th Street, NW, Suite 1212
Washington, DC 20005
202-467-5730
http://www.bazelon.org
Disability Served: developmentally disabled, mental health
The mission of the center is to protect and advance the rights of adults and children who have mental health issues and developmental disabilities.

Marion Indiana Self Advocates

Carey Services
2724 South Carey Street, Building B
Marion, IN 46953
765-668-8961
selfadvocate04@yahoo.com
http://www.geocities.com/selfadvocate04/intro.html
Disability Served: various
This organization helps educate persons with disabilities, their families, and the community on their rights and responsibilities.

Mosaic

650 J Street, Suite 305
Lincoln, NE 68508-2220
800-443-4899
integrity@mosaicinfo.org
http://www.mosaicinfo.org
Disability Served: developmentally disabled
This organization offers services to people with developmental disabilities and other special needs.

National Alliance of Blind Students

1155 15th Street, NW, Suite 1004
Washington, DC 20005
202-467-5081, 800-424-8666
info@acb.org
http://www.blindstudents.org
Disability Served: vision
The alliance advocates for the rights of high school and college students with visual impairments.

National Association of the Deaf

814 Thayer Avenue, Suite 250
Silver Spring, MD 20910
301-587-1788
nadinfo@nad.org
http://www.nad.org
Disability Served: hearing
This organization safeguards the civil rights of the deaf and hard of hearing in education, employment, health care, and telecommunications.

National Disability Rights Network

900 Second Street, NE, Suite 211
Washington, DC 20002
202-408-9514, 202-408-9521 (TTY)
info@ndrn.org
http://www.ndrn.org
Disability Served: various
The network serves individuals with a wide range of disabilities. It advocates for basic rights and equality in health care, education, employment, housing, transportation, and within the juvenile and criminal justice systems.

National Organization on Disability

910 Sixteenth Street, NW, Suite 600
Washington, DC 20006
202-293-5960, 202-293-5968
ability@nod.org
http://www.nod.org
Disability Served: various
This organization's mission is to raise disability awareness through programs and information, and to expand the participation and contribution of adults and children with disabilities in all aspects of life.

North Dakota Disabilities Advocacy Consortium

400 East Broadway, Suite 402
Bismarck, ND 58501
701-223-0347, 877-766-6709
http://www.nddac.org
Disability Served: various
The consortium is an independent group of North Dakota organizations that in advocate for public policy that will benefit people with disabilities and their families who reside in the state. Its goal is to educate policymakers and others on the needs of people with disabilities using research and a grass-roots campaign.

Northeast Independent Living Program Inc.
20 Ballard Road
Lawrence, MA 01843
978-687-4288, 800-845-6457, 978-687-4288 (TDD)
MWalker@nilp.org
http://www.nilp.org
Disability Served: various
This organization serves people ages 14 and up with all types of disabilities. It provides information and referral, advocacy, peer counseling, and skills training.

People First International
PO Box 12642
Salem, OR 97309
503-362-0336
people1@people1.org
http://www.open.org/~people1/index.htm
Disability Served: developmentally disabled
People First is a self-help organization of persons with developmental disabilities. There are People First chapters worldwide.

People First of Anchorage Alaska
Center for Human Development
2702 Gambell Street
Anchorage, AK 99503
907-272-8270, 800-243-2199, 907-264-6206 (TTY)
info@alaskachd.org
http://www.alaskachd.org/peoplefirst
Disability Served: various
People First of Alaska is a local self-advocacy group that teaches its members to defend their rights and to be understood by service providers.

People First of California Inc.
1225 Eighth Street, Suite 210
Sacramento, CA 95814
916-552-6625
info@peoplefirstca.org
http://www.peoplefirstca.org
Disability Served: developmentally disabled
The mission of this organization is to help start, inform, and support local chapters so that people with developmental disabilities residing in California are able to speak for themselves, know their rights and responsibilities, and are treated as respected, valued members of the community.

People First of Illinois
PO Box 4294
Bloomington, IL 61702-4294

309-820-8844
ppl1st@peoplefirstofillinois.org
http://www.peoplefirstofillinois.org
Disability Served: various
People First of Illinois is comprised of people with various types of disabilities. This group is committed to empowering people with disabilities to make their own decisions and choices, and to speak for themselves.

People First of Missouri
Institute for Human Development
2220 Holmes, 3rd Floor
Kansas City, MO 64108
816-235-1770, 800-444-0821, 800-452-1185 (TTY)
peoplefirstofmissouri@mail.com
http://www.missouripeoplefirst.org/index.html
Disability Served: developmentally disabled
This is a self-advocacy and self help organization for persons with developmental disabilities residing in the state of Missouri.

People First of New Hampshire
4 Park Street, Suite #201
Concord, NH 03301
603-568-2128, 800-566-2128
peoplefirstnh@verizon.net
http://www.peoplefirstofnh.org
Disability Served: various
This organization is comprised of people with disabilities who reside in New Hampshire working together to take charge of their lives. This is done by members learning how to make decisions, understand their rights and responsibilities, and speak up for themselves.

People First of Northwest Louisiana
c/o Arc of Caddo-Bossier
351 Jordan Street
Shreveport, LA 71101
318-221-8392
http://www.cbarc.org
Disability Served: various
The northwest Louisiana chapter of People First is an organization of adults who are self-advocates and consumers of disability services. This group meets monthly and shares civic information and objectives as well as social and recreational activities. It is supported by the Arc of Caddo-Bossier.

People First of Ohio
PO Box 988
Mt. Vernon, OH 43050
740-397-6100, 888-959-8838
PeopleFirst@ecr.net
http://www.peoplefirstofohio.org
Disability Served: developmentally disabled
This organization helps people with disabilities be
treated as equals in society.

People First of Oregon
PO Box 12642
Salem, OR 97309
503-362-0336
people1@people1.org
http://www.open.org/people1/index.htm
Disability Served: developmentally disabled
People First of Oregon is committed to empowering
people with disabilities to make their own decisions
and choices, and to speak for themselves.

People First of South Florida
5555 Biscayne Boulevard
Miami, FL 33137
http://www.encore4.net/peoplefirst
Disability Served: various
This South Florida organization teaches people with
disabilities how to protect their rights and live
as productive and respected members of the
community.

People First of Tennessee Inc.
855 West College Street
Murfreesboro, TN 37129
615-898-0075
peoplefirst@geocities.com
http://www.geocities.com/nashville/opry/3843
Disability Served: various
People First of Tennessee is a local self-advocacy group
that teaches its members to defend their rights and
to be understood by service providers.

People First of Virginia Beach
c/o Foundry United Methodist Church
2801 Virginia Beach Boulevard
Virginia Beach, VA 23450
757-437-6100
pfvbeach@hotmail.com
http://www.geocities.com/pfvbeach/page3.html
Disability Served: developmentally disabled

This is an organization that promotes the self-advocacy
of adults with developmental disabilities living in the
state of Virginia.

People First of Wisconsin
Rosary Hall Marion Center
3195 South Superior Street, Room 113
Milwaukee, WI 53207
414-483-2546, 888-270-5352
http://www.peoplefirstwi.org
Disability Served: various
People First of Wisconsin is a statewide, grassroots
advocacy organization run by and for people
with disabilities. Among its many projects are:
self-advocacy training workshops, outreach to
employers on the benefits of hiring people with
disabilities, and publication of a newsletter, On The
Move.

People First of Wyoming
c/o The Governor's Planning Council on Developmental
Disabilities
Herschler Building, 122 West 25th Street, Room 1608
Cheyenne, WY 82002
307-777-7230 (Voice/TDD), 800-438-5791
http://ddcouncil.state.wy.us/peoplefirst.htm
Disability Served: various
People First of Wyoming believes that individuals with
disabilities and their families should have access to a
wide range of supports and services that allow them
choices about how they work, live and play in their
community.

Self Advocates Becoming Empowered
PO Box 104
Northport, AL 35473
http://www.sabeusa.org
Disability Served: various
The mission of this organization is to ensure that people
with disabilities are treated as equals in society.

Self-Advocacy Network
c/o STCC 1 Armory Square
Springfield, MA 01009
413-536-2401, ext. 3026
san@aol.com
http://www.peoplefirst.org.uk/san.html
Disability Served: various
The network is comprised of people with disabilities who
live in the Springfield-Westfield, Massachusetts area.

It promotes self-advocacy through community and political involvement and education.

Self-Advocacy Association of NYS Inc.
Capital District DSO
500 Balltown Road
Schenectady, NY 12304
518-382-1454
http://www.sanys.org
Disability Served: various
This is an organization formed and led by people with disabilities. The association accomplishes its goal of equality by educating the public, advocacy, networking, sharing information and resources, and promoting respect and dignity for those who are disabled.

Self Help for Hard of Hearing People
7910 Woodmont Avenue, Suite 1200
Bethesda, MD 20814
301-657-2248, 301-657-2249 (TTY)
http://www.shhh.org
Disability Served: hearing
This nonprofit, educational organization is dedicated to the well-being of people of all ages who do not hear well. The largest international consumer organization of its kind, SHHH has a national office, an international membership, and a nationwide support network of chapters and groups.

Son-Rise Program at the Option Institute
2080 South Undermountain Road
Sheffield, MA 01257-9643
413-229-2100
http://www.autismtreatmentcenter.org
Disability Served: various
This organization is a teaching center dedicated to educating parents and assisting professionals to design and implement parent-directed, child-centered, home-based programs for children with special needs.

Speaking For Ourselves
502 West Germantown Pike, Suite 550
Plymouth Meeting, PA 19462
610-825-4592
http://www.speaking.org
Disability Served: various
The mission of this organization is to teach the public about the needs, goals, and potential of people with disabilities.

Statewide Parent Advocacy Network of New Jersey
35 Halsey Street, 4th Floor
Newark, NJ 07102
973-642-8100, 800-654-SPAN
http://www.spannj.org
Disability Served: various
The goal of the network is to empower families, and inform and involve professionals and other interested individuals, about the developmental and educational rights of children, including those with disabilities.

United Cerebral Palsy of Minnesota
1821 University Avenue West, Suite 219 South
St Paul, MN 55104-2801
800-328-4827, ext. 1437
Disability Served: cerebral palsy
This organization provides advocacy, public education, support groups, and workshops for people with disabilities.

WeCAHR
211 Main Street
Danbury, CT 06810
http://www.wecahr.org
Disability Served: various
WeCAHR advocates for the civil and human rights of people with disabilities residing in Connecticut's Housatonic Valley region.

West Coast Disabilities Advocacy Center
6742 Western Avenue, Suite 14
Buena Park, CA 90621
http://www.wcdisabilityadvocacy.org
Disability Served: various
The center offers information, advocacy, and referrals for people with disabilities. Its services include transportation assistance, employment counseling, credit counseling, workshops, and recreational activities.

Wheelweb.com
comments@wheelweb.com
http://www.wheelweb.com
Disability Served: spinal-cord injury
This Web site offers information about spinal cord injuries and treatment options. It also has a chat room and a bulletin board.

STATE TECH ACT PROGRAMS AND ORGANIZATIONS

The Technology-Related Assistance for Individuals with Disabilities Act provides funding to states to assist them in developing easily accessible, consumer-responsive systems of access to assistive technology, technology services, and information. These organizations provide training, information, and advocacy, as well as product loans. State programs vary widely.

ALABAMA

Alabama STAR System for Alabamians with Disabilities
2129 East South Boulevard
Montgomery, AL 36116-2455
334-281-8780, 800-441-7607
http://www.rehab.state.al.us/star
Disability Served: various
The mission of the STAR program is to enhance independence, productivity and quality of life for all Alabamians with disabilities through access to assistive technology devices and services.

ALASKA

Assistive Technologies of Alaska
3600 Bragaw
Anchorage, AK 99508
907-261-8233, 800-478-4467 (Voice/TDD)
kent_ireton@labor.state.ak.us
http://www.labor.state.ak.us/at/index.htm
Disability Served: various
The purpose of the Assistive Technologies Project is to ensure all Alaskans have the assistive technology and related services needed to live, work, and participate in their community.

ARIZONA

Arizona Technology Access Program (AzTAP)
2400 North Central Avenue, Suite 300
Phoenix, AZ 85004
602-728-9534, 800-477-9921
Jill.sherman@nau.edu
http://www.nau.edu/ihd/aztap
Disability Served: various
The mission of the AzTAP is to increase access to assistive technology (AT) devices and services for individuals with disabilities and their families, and facilitate the development of a consumer-responsive AT service

delivery system. Program staff members work with consumers, service providers, state agencies, private industry, legislators, and other interested individuals to facilitate the development of a statewide system to provide AT services.

ARKANSAS

Arkansas Increasing Access Capabilities Network (ICAN)
2201 Brookwood Drive, Suite 117
Little Rock, AR 72201
501-666-8868 (Voice/TDD), 800-828-2799 (Voice/TDD)
bmvuletich@ars.state.ar.us
http://www.arkansas-ican.org
Disability Served: various
The Increasing Capabilities Access Network (ICAN), a federally funded program of Arkansas Rehabilitation Services, is designed to make technology available and accessible for all who need it. ICAN is a funding information resource and provides information on new and existing technology free to any person regardless of age or disability.

CALIFORNIA

California Assistive Technology System (CATS)
California Department of Rehabilitation
Assistive Technology Systems Change Unit
2000 Evergreen Street
Sacramento, CA 95815
916-274-6325, 916-263-8685 (TDD)
atinfo@dor.ca.gov
http://www.atnet.org/resources/about_cats.htm
Disability Served: various
CATS is a statewide project that promotes access to assistive technologies, related services, and information to enable people with disabilities to be successful, independent and productive.

COLORADO

Colorado Assistive Technology Project (CATP)
1245 East Colfax Avenue, Suite 200
Denver, CO 80218
303-315-1280, 800-255-3477
jim.sandstrum@uchsc.edu
http://www.uchsc.edu/atp/projects/catp/catp.htm
Disability Served: various
CATP has four major areas of focus: public awareness, training and technical assistance, interagency coordination, and outreach to rural and underrepresented populations.

CONNECTICUT

Connecticut Tech Act Project
Bureau of Rehabilitation Services
25 Sigourney Street, 11th Floor
Hartford, CT 06106
203-298-2042
Techact@UConnvm.uconn.edu
http://www.techactproject.com
Disability Served: various
The Connecticut Tech Act Project provides information and advocacy services regarding assistive technology issues. The project's goal is to make sure that Connecticut's residents with disabilities get access to assistive technology.

DELAWARE

Delaware Assistive Technology Initiative (DATI)
PO Box 269
Wilmington, DE 19899-0269
302-651-6790, 800-870-DATI, 302-651-6794 (TDD)
dati@asel.udel.edu
http://www.dati.org
Disability Served: various
DATI focuses on improving public awareness, public access to information, training, technical assistance, and funding for assistive technology devices and services. The project maintains three resource centers that house assistive technology devices and materials available for demonstration and short-term loan.

FLORIDA

Florida Assistive Technology Project
325 John Knox Road, Building 400, Suite 402
Tallahassee, FL 32303
850-487-3278, 888-788-9216
faast@faast.org
http://www.faast.org
Disability Served: various
The project works with consumers, family members, caregivers, providers, and agencies to ensure that individuals with disabilities benefit from assistive technology as they move between home, school, work, and the community.

GEORGIA

Georgia Tools for Life
Georgia Department of Labor
Division of Rehabilitation Services
VR Tools for Life Program
1700 Century Circle
Atlanta, GA 30345
800-497-8665
http://www.gatfl.org
Disability Served: various
Services include consumer intake, assistive technology scholarships, assistive technology training through hands-on assistive technology demonstrations and educational workshops, Touch the Future Expo, and the Microsoft Life Long Learning lab.

HAWAII

Assistive Technology Resource Centers of Hawaii
414 Kuwili Street, Suite 104
Honolulu, HI 96817
808-532-7110 (Voice/TTY)
atrc-info@atrc.org
http://www.atrc.org
Disability Served: various
The centers provide information and training on devices, services, and funding resources. They also increase assistive technology awareness and promote advocacy among persons with disabilities.

IDAHO

Idaho Assistive Technology Project
129 West Third Street
Moscow, ID 83843-4401
208-885-6949, 208-885-9429
rseiler@uidaho.edu
http://www.educ.uidaho.edu/idatech

Disability Served: various

This organization assists individuals with disabilities to achieve a higher quality of life and greater independence through increased access to assistive technology.

ILLINOIS

Illinois Assistive Technology Project (IATP)
1 West Old State Capitol Plaza, Suite 100
Springfield, IL 62701
217-522-7985, 217-522-9966 (TTY)
wgunther@iltech.org
http://www.iltech.org
Disability Served: various

The IATP's mission is to break down barriers that prevent people with disabilities from accessing the assistive technology that lets them learn, work, play, and live in the community. The IATP's major programs include: information and assistance through 800 lines; an assistive technology demonstration center; an assistive technology device loan program; a low-interest cash loan program; a quarterly newsletter that is distributed to 7,500 individuals; assistive technology trainings which focuses primarily on capacity-building and train-the-trainer programs; publication of TechNotes on a variety of topics; and a policy change program which monitors hundreds of bills which affect people with disabilities and informs consumers about these and other state and federal initiatives.

INDIANA

ATTAIN
32 East Washington Street, Suite 1400
Indianapolis, IN 46204
317-486-8808, 800-528-8246
attain@attaininc.org
http://www.attaininc.org
Disability Served: various

Attain provides direct service programs promotes the availability and use of assistive technology. This is achieved through consumer-driven programs that promote community-based services. Attain is the only statewide technology program in Indiana that serves people of all ages and all disabilities.

IOWA

Iowa Program for Assistive Technology (IPAT)
Center for Disabilities and Development
100 Hawkins Drive, Room S295

Iowa City, IA 52242-1011
319-356-0550, 800-331-3027, 877-686-0032 (TTY)
http://www.uiowa.edu/infotech/
Disability Served: various

IPAT works with consumers and family members, service providers, and state and local agencies and organizations to promote assistive technology through awareness, training, and policy work.

KANSAS

Assistive Technology for Kansans
2601 Gabriel
Parsons, KS 67357
620-421-8367 (Voice/TTD)
ssimmons@ku.edu
http://www.atk.ku.edu
Disability Served: various

The Assistive Technology for Kansans project provides information and referral, advocacy, acquisition and maintenance of devices, peer counseling, and public awareness services. These services are offered at five regional sites throughout Kansas.

KENTUCKY

Kentucky Assistive Technology Services
8412 Westport Road
Louisville, KY 40242
502-429-4484, 800-327-5287
Chase.Forrester@mail.state.ky.us
http://www.katsnet.org
Disability Served: various

KATS is a statewide network of organizations and individuals improving the productivity and quality of life for individuals with disabilities by enhancing the availability of assistive technology devices and services. Through advocacy activities and capacity building efforts, the mission of this collaborative system is to make assistive technology information, devices, and services easily obtainable for people of any age and any disability.

LOUISIANA

Louisiana Assistive Technology Access Network (LATAN)
3042 Old Forge Drive, Suite B
Baton Rouge, LA 70808
225-925-9500, 800-270-6185
jnesbit@latan.org

http://www.latan.org
Disability Served: various
LATAN assists individuals with disabilities to achieve
a higher quality of life and greater independence
through increased access to assistive technology.

MAINE
Maine CITE Coordinating Center
University of Maine
46 University Drive
Augusta, ME 04330
207-621-3195, 207-621-3482 (TDD)
iweb@doe.k12.me.us
http://www.mecite.doe.k12.me.us
Disability Served: various
Maine CITE is a statewide project to help make assistive
and universally designed technology more available
to Maine residents who have disabilities.

MARYLAND
Maryland Technology Assistance Program
2301 Argonne Drive, Room T-17
Baltimore, MD 21218
800-832-4827, 866-881-7488 (TTY)
mdtap@mdod.state.md.us
http://www.mdtap.org
Disability Served: various
This organization provides a wide range of services
including disseminating information to individuals
with disabilities, working to change perceptions
about individuals with disabilities, and promoting
change in Maryland laws.

MASSACHUSETTS
**Massachusetts Assistive Technology Partnership
(MATP)**
Children's Hospital
1295 Boylston Street, Suite 310
Boston, MA 02215
617-735-7153, 617-355-7301 (TTY)
http://www.matp.org
Disability Served: various
The goal of MATP is to empower people to find the
best assistive technology (AT) and training, explore
funding options, and get educated about AT issues.
MATP serves people who need assistive devices,
parents or caregivers of people who need AT,
professionals who need AT information, employees
and employers, and students and educators.

MICHIGAN
Michigan Assistive Technology Project
780 West Lake Lansing Road, Suite 200
East Lansing, MI 48823
517-333-2477, 800-760-4600
sysop@match.org
http://www.match.org
Disability Served: various
The project is a centralized, integrated, statewide
assistive technology information system for use by
participants in the Michigan Assistive Technology
Project including Community Assistive Technology
Councils, information and referral services, assistive
technology providers, consumers, families, and
employers.

MINNESOTA
Minnesota STAR Program
50 Sherburne Avenue, Room 309
Saint Paul, MN 55155
651-296-2771, 800-657-3862
chuck.rassbach@state.mn.us
http://www.admin.state.mn.us/assistivetechnology
Disability Served: various
The STAR Program informs Minnesotans about issues of
assistive technology, promotes assistive technology
for the citizens of Minnesota through state and
federal legislation, works with state agencies, and
builds community collaborative and communication
efforts.

MISSISSIPPI
Mississippi Project START
PO Box 1698
Jackson, MS 39406-5163
601-987-4872, 800-852-8328 (Voice/TTY)
contactus@msprojectstart.org
http://www.msprojectstart.org
Disability Served: various
The mission of Project START is to ensure the provision of appropriate technology-related services for
Mississippians with disabilities by increasing the
awareness of and access to assistive technology, and
by helping the existing service systems to become
more consumer responsive so that all Mississippians
with disabilities will receive appropriate technology-
related services and devices.

MISSOURI

Community Rehabilitation Program-Regional Continuing Education Program
University of Missouri-Columbia
601 West Nifong Boulevard, Suite 1C
Columbia, MO 65203
573-884-3473
crprcep7@crprcep7.org
http://www.crprcep7.org
Disability Served: various
This is an educational resource at the University of Missouri for community rehabilitation programs in Iowa, Kansas, Missouri, and Nebraska.

Missouri Assistive Technology
4731 South Cochise, Suite 114
Independence, MO 64055-6975
816-373-5193, 800-647-8557, 800-647-8558 (TTY)
matpmo@swbell.net
http://www.at.mo.gov
Disability Served: various
This agency is responsible for the service delivery, policy implementation, and funding of assistive technology to people with disabilities living in the state of Missouri.

Show-Me Tech
Services for Independent Living
1401 Hathman Place
Columbia, MO 65201
573-874-1646
sil@silcolumbia.org
http://www.silcolumbia.org/smt.htm
Disability Served: various
This is an assistive-technology demonstration center where persons with disabilities, family members, service providers, schools, and businesses can receive information on adaptive devices, as well as hands-on demonstrations.

MONTANA

MonTECH
The University of Montana
Rural Institute on Disabilities
634 Eddy Avenue, CHS 009
Missoula, MT 59812-6696
406-243-5676, 800-732-0323
montech@ruralinstitute.umt.edu
http://montech.ruralinstitute.umt.edu
Disability Served: various
MonTech provides free, confidential information about assistive technology devices and services for Montanans of all ages.

NEBRASKA

Nebraska Assistive Technology Partnership
5143 South 48th Street, Suite C
Lincoln, NE 68516
402-471-0734, 888-806-6287
http://www.nde.state.ne.us/ATP
Disability Served: various
The Assistive Technology Partnership is dedicated to helping Nebraskans with disabilities obtain assistive technology devices and services.

NEVADA

Nevada Assistive Technology Project
Rehabilitation Division
Office of Community-Based Services
711 South Stewart Street
Carson City, NV 89710
775-687-4452, 775-687-3388 (TTY)
pgowins@govmail.state.nv.us
http://hr.state.nv.us/directors/disabilitysvcs/dhr_odsprog.htm#State%20Assistive%20Technology%20Act%20Program
Disability Served: various
The project helps Nevada residents obtain and use assistive technology.

NEW HAMPSHIRE

New Hampshire Technology Partnership Project
The Concord Center
10 Ferry Street, Unit 14
Concord, NH 03301
603-228-2084, 800-238-2048
Disability Served: various
The goal of the New Hampshire Technology Partnership Project is to increase access to assistive technology for citizens with disabilities in the state of New Hampshire. This is accomplished through the creation and support of consumer-driven systems for the provision of state-of-the-art assistive technology products and services.

NEW JERSEY

New Jersey Technology Assistive Resource Program

New Jersey Protection and Advocacy Inc.

210 South Broad Street, 3rd Floor

Trenton, NJ 08608

609-292-9742, 800-922-7233, 609-633-7106 (TTY)

advocate@njpanda.org

http://www.njpanda.org

Disability Served: various

This consumer-directed, nonprofit organization helps people with disabilities get access to assistive technology.

NEW MEXICO

New Mexico Technology Assistance Program (NMTAP)

435 Saint Michael Drive, Building D

Sante Fe, NM 87505

800-866-2253, 800-659-4915 (TTY)

awinnegar@state.nm.us

http://www.nmtap.com

Disability Served: various

NMTAP offers free services to New Mexicans with disabilities to help them obtain assistive technology.

NEW YORK

New York State TRAID Project

New York State Office of Advocate for Persons with Disabilities

One Empire State Plaza, Suite 1001

Albany, NY 12223-1150

518-473-4609, 800-522-4369

oapwdinfo@oapwd.org

http://www.oapwd.org

Disability Served: various

The TRAID project undertakes a variety of educational and outreach programs to better equip individuals with disabilities to secure the assistive technology services, equipment, and support that they require to lead more independent and productive lives.

NORTH CAROLINA

North Carolina Assistive Technology Project

Division of Vocational Rehabilitation Services

1110 Navaho Drive, Suite 101

Raleigh, NC 27609-7322

919-850-2787

jmedlicott@ncatp.org

http://www.ncatp.org

Disability Served: various

The project provides a statewide, consumer-responsive system of assistive technology services for all North Carolinians with disabilities.

NORTH DAKOTA

North Dakota Interagency Program for Assistive Technology

IPAT Technology Access Center

3509 Interstate Boulevard

Fargo, ND 58103

701-365-4729

jlee@polarcomm.com

http://www.ndipat.org

Disability Served: various

The project's services include an assistive technology senior safety program, regional technical assistance, and an equipment loan library.

OHIO

Ohio Assistive Technology Project

445 East Dublin-Granville Road, Building L

Worthington, OH 43085

614-293-9134, 800-784-3425

spetka.1@osu.edu

http://www.atohio.org

Disability Served: various

The project's mission is to help Ohio residents with disabilities acquire assistive technology. It offers several different programs to accomplish that goal.

OKLAHOMA

Oklahoma ABLE Tech

Oklahoma State University Wellness Center

1514 West Hall of Fame

Stillwater, OK 74078-0618

405-744-9748 (Voice/TDD), 800-257-1705

blunruh@okstate.edu

http://okabletech.okstate.edu/overview

Disability Served: various

The purpose of Oklahoma ABLE Tech is to increase access to assistive technology for people of all ages and all disabilities through a variety of consumer responsive activities. ABLE Tech is a statewide program.

OREGON

Oregon Technology Access for Life Needs Project
Access Technologies Inc.
3070 Lancaster Drive, NE
Salem, OR 97305-1396
503-361-1201, 800-677-7512
laurie@accesstechnologiesinc.org
http://www.accesstechnologiesinc.org
Disability Served: various
The project helps the disabled access and use assistive technology.

PENNSYLVANIA

Pennsylvania's Initiative on Assistive Technology (PIAT)
1301 Cecil B Moore Avenue, 423 Ritter Annex
Philadelphia, PA 19122
215-204-1356 (Voice/TTY), 800-204-PIAT (Voice/TTY)
piat@temple.edu
http://disabilities.temple.edu/programs/assistive/piat/index.htm
Disability Served: various
PIAT's priority activities include the development, implementation, and monitoring of laws, policies, practices, and organizational structures to improve access to assistive technology for all Pennsylvanians with disabilities, as well as older Pennsylvanians.

RHODE ISLAND

Rhode Island Assistive Technology Access Project
40 Fountain Street
Providence, RI 02903
401-421-7005, 401-421-7016 (TDD)
reginac@ors.ri.gov
http://www.atap.state.ri.us
Disability Served: various
The Rhode Island Assistive Technology Access Project is designed as a statewide partnership of organizations and agencies, each with a targeted assistive technology focus, working together to provide information and improve access to assistive technology for individuals with disabilities.

SOUTH CAROLINA

South Carolina Assistive Technology Project (SCATP)
University of South Carolina School of Medicine Center for Disability Resources
Columbia, SC 29208

803-935-5263
jjendron@usit.net
http://www.sc.edu.scatp
Disability Served: various
SCATP's goal is to enhance independence, productivity, and quality of life for all South Carolinians through access to assistive technology devices and services. SCATP provides training and technical assistance, and works with consumers, service providers, state agencies, and policy makers to support children and adults with disabilities in their efforts to acquire and use technology as a routine part of day-to-day living.

SOUTH DAKOTA

DakotaLink
1161 Deadwood Avenue, Suite 5
Rapid City, SD 57702
605-394-6742 (Voice/TDD), 800-645-0673 (Voice/TDD)
info@dakotalink.net
http://www.dakotalink.net
Disability Served: various
DakotaLink is a statewide program of resources and supports that enable individuals in South Dakota to have greater access to assistive technology devices and services, to maintain independence, to explore funding options, and to become educated about assistive technology issues.

TENNESSEE

Tennessee Technology Access Project (TTAP)
Citizens Plaza Office Building, 400 Deadrick Street, 14th Floor
Nashville, TN 37248
615-313-5183, 800-732-5059, 615-741-4566 (TDD)
TN.TTAP@state.tn.us
http://www.tennessee.gov/humanserv/ttap_index.htm
Disability Served: various
TTAP's mission is to maintain a statewide program of technology-related assistance that is timely, comprehensive, and consumer driven in order to ensure that all Tennesseans with disabilities have the information, services, and devices that they need.

TEXAS

Texas Technology Access Project
University of Texas at Austin
Building 2, 4030 West Braker Lane, Suite 220, Mail Code L4000

Austin, TX 78759
512-232-0740, 800-828-7839
http://tatp.edb.utexas.edu
Disability Served: various
The Texas Technology Access Project provides information, offers training and technical assistance, and works with policy makers to support children and adults with disabilities in their efforts to acquire and use technology as a routine part of day-to-day living.

UTAH

Utah Assistive Technology Program
6588 Old Main Hill
Logan, UT 84322-6588
435-797-3824, 800-524-5152
http://www.uatpat.org
Disability Served: various
The Utah Assistive Technology Program is designed to help individuals know what assistive technology is available, understand how to receive funding, and to find links and resources.

VERMONT

Vermont Assistive Technology Program
103 South Main Street, Osgood II Building
Waterbury, VT 05671-2303
866-879-6757 (Voice/TTY), 802-241-1455
http://www.vocrehabvermont.org
Disability Served: various
The Vermont Assistive Technology Program provides outreach, resources, information and referral, assessment, equipment tryout, and training and support to individuals with disabilities, their families, and service providers.

VIRGINIA

Virginia Assistive Technology System (VATS)
Department of Rehabilitative Services
8004 Franklin Farms Drive, PO Box K-300
Richmond, VA 23288-0300
804-662-9990, 800-435-8490
knorrkh@drs.state.va.us
http://www.vats.org
Disability Served: various
VATS has developed a statewide comprehensive system of assistive technology, and works to assist Virginians

with disabilities in accessing assistive and information technology devices and services.

WASHINGTON

Washington Assistive Technology Alliance
University of Washington
Box 357920
Seattle, WA 98195-7920
206-685-4181, 800-841-8345 (Voice/TTY)
uwctds@u.washington.edu
http://wata.org
Disability Served: various
The alliance's activities include information and referral; consultation and training related to selection of assistive technology devices, services, and funding; legal advice and advocacy; policy development; and legislative action.

The Washington Assistive Technology Foundation
1823 East Madison, Suite 1000
Seattle, WA 98122
206-328-5116, 800-214-8731 (Voice/TTY)
info@watf.org
http://www.watf.org
Disability Served: various
The Washington Assistive Technology Foundation is a nonprofit organization dedicated to improving the socio-economic circumstances of people with disabilities through access to technology.

WEST VIRGINIA

West Virginia Assistive Technology System
Center for Excellence in Disabilities
959 Hartman Run Road
Morgantown, WV 26505
304-766-4698, 800-841-8436
contact@cedwvu.org
http://cedwvu.org
Disability Served: various
The West Virginia Assistive Technology System is dedicated to increasing awareness of and accessibility to assistive technology for West Virginians of all ages and all types of disabilities.

WISCONSIN

Wisconsin Assistive Technology Initiative
Polk Library
800 Algoma Boulevard

Oshkosh, WI 54901
920-424-2247, 800-991-5576
info@wati.org
http://www.wati.org
Disability Served: various
The mission of the Wisconsin Assistive Technology
Initiative is to ensure that every child in Wisconsin
who needs assistive technology (AT) will have equal
and timely access to an appropriate evaluation and
the provision and implementation of any needed
AT devices and services. The project is designed to
increase the capacity of school districts to provide
assistive technology services by making training and
technical assistance available to teachers, therapists,
administrators, and parents throughout Wisconsin.

Wisconsin Assistive Technology Program (WisTech)
1 West Wilson Street, Room 1151, PO Box 7851
Madison, WI 53707-7851
608-266-8905, 608-267-9880 (TTY)
lauxhm@dhfs.state.wi.us
http://dhfs.wisconsin.gov/disabilities/wistech
Disability Served: various
WisTech provides information on selecting, funding,
installing, and using assistive technology.

WYOMING
**Wyoming's New Options In Technology
(WYNot Program)**
University of Wyoming
1000 East University Avenue, Department 4298
Laramie, WY 82071
307-766-2084, 800-861-4312
wynot.uw@uwyo.edu
http://wind.uwyo.edu/wynot
Disability Served: various
The WYNot Program connects individuals with
disabilities and other Wyoming residents to
information, training, and technical assistance
about assistive technology equipment and services.

NORTHERN MARIANA ISLANDS
**Northern Mariana Islands Assistive Technology
Project-STRAID**
1312 Anatahan Drive, PO Box 502565
Saipan, MP 96950-2565
670-664-7000
gddc@cnmiddcouncil.org
http://www.cnmiddcouncil.org
Disability Served: various
The mission of the STRAID project is to enhance the
quality of life and opportunities for individuals with
disabilities in the Commonwealth, enabling them to
become independent, productive, integrated, and
fully included in the community through the use of
assistive technology devices and services.

PUERTO RICO
Puerto Rico Technology Act Program
Universidad de Puerto Rico
Administración Central
Instituto FILIUS
PO Box 364984
San Juan, PR 00936-4984
787-767-8642 (Voice/TTY)
pratp@pratp.upr.edu
http://www.pratp.upr.edu
Disability Served: various
The program helps residents of Puerto Rico to access
assistive technology.

SUPPORT GROUPS AND HOTLINES

These organizations provide such services as information and referral, advocacy, support services, education, brochures and publications, rehabilitation services, independent living services, and more.

Ability Society of Alberta
906 Eighth Avenue, SW, Suite 600
Calgary, AB T2P 1H9
Canada
403-262-9445
info@abilitysociety.org
http://www.abilitysociety.org
Disability Served: various
This organization provides information, education, and access to assistive technology, including computers. There is a fee for some services. Subsidies are available to Calgary residents only.

Academy of Dispensing Audiologists
401 North Michigan Avenue, Suite 2200
Chicago, IL 60611
866-493-5544
http://www.audiologist.org
Disability Served: hearing
This organization supports the dispensing of hearing aids by qualified audiologists.

Adaptive Environments Center
374 Congress Street, Suite 301
Boston, MA 02210
617-695-1225
info@AdaptiveEnvironments.org
http://www.adaptenv.org
Disability Served: various
The center promotes accessibility as well as universal design through education programs, technical assistance, training, consulting, publications, and public advocacy.

Alexander Graham Bell Association for the Deaf
3417 Volta Place, NW
Washington, DC 20007
202-337-5220
info@agbell.org
http://www.agbell.org
Disability Served: hearing
This association is an international organization dedicated to improving opportunities for people with hearing impairments. Scholarships, financial aid, and publications are available.

Amateur Athletic Foundation of Los Angeles (AAF)
2141 West Adams Boulevard
Los Angeles, CA 90018
323-730-4600
info@aafla.org
http://www.aafla.org
Disability Served: various
The AAF offers information, research, and education on sports and coaching. The foundation also houses the largest sports research library in North America.

**American Academy of Otolaryngology—
   Head and Neck Surgery**
One Prince Street
Alexandria, VA 22314-3357
703-836-4444
http://www.entnet.org
Disability Served: various
This organization offers resources, publications, and continuing medical education courses on otolaryngology-head and neck surgery.

American Academy of Pediatrics
141 Northwest Point Boulevard
Elk Grove Village, IL 60007-1098
847-434-4000
commun@aap.org
http://www.aap.org
Disability Served: various
This organization provides information and support for children with disabilities.

American Action Fund for Blind Children and Adults
1800 Johnson Street, Suite 100
Baltimore, MD 21230
410-659-9315
actionfund@nfb.org
http://www.actionfund.org
Disability Served: vision
This organization provides support services to persons who are blind.

American Association of the Deaf-Blind
8630 Fenton Street
Silver Spring, MD 20910

301-495-4403
info@aadb.org
http://www.aadb.org
Disability Served: hearing, vision
This organization is dedicated to improving services for deaf-blind people.

American Back Society
2647 International Boulevard, Suite 401
Oakland, CA 94601
510-536-9929
info@americanbacksoc.org
http://www.americanbacksoc.org
Disability Served: back injury, spinal-cord injury
This membership organization is dedicated to finding cures and remedies for spinal injuries.

American Cancer Society Inc.
2200 Century Parkway, Suite 950
Atlanta, GA 30345
404-315-1123
http://www.cancer.org
Disability Served: cancer patients and survivors
This national organization provides a number of services and programs through thousands of local chapters.

American Council of the Blind
1155 15th Street, NW, Suite 1004
Washington, DC 20005
202-467-5081, 800-424-8666
support@acb.org
http://www.acb.org
Disability Served: vision
The council is a national membership organization dedicated to promoting the independence and well being of blind and visually impaired people. Services include a monthly magazine, a hotline, student scholarships, and information and referral.

American Deafness and Rehabilitation Association
PO Box 480
Myersville, MD 21773
ADARAorgn@aol.com
http://www.adara.org
Disability Served: hearing
The association is dedicated to improving services for persons with hearing impairments.

American Diabetes Association
1701 North Beauregard Street
Alexandria, VA 22311

800-342-2383
AskADA@diabetes.org
http://www.diabetes.org
Disability Served: diabetes
This association provides general information about diabetes to patients and professionals.

American Hearing Research Foundation
8 South Michigan Avenue, Suite 814
Chicago, IL 60603-4539
312-726-9670
lkoch@american-hearing.org
http://www.american-hearing.org
Disability Served: hearing
The foundation provides support for medical research into the causes, prevention, and care of deafness.

American Heart Association
7272 Greenville Avenue
Dallas, TX 75231
800-553-6321
http://www.amhrt.org
Disability Served: various
The association provides support, information, education, publications, seminars, and conferences through local state chapters.

American Institute of Architects (AIA)
Information Center
1735 New York Avenue, NW
Washington, DC 20006-5292
202-626-7300, 800-AIA-3837
infocentral@aia.org
http://www.aia.org
Disability Served: various
The AIA's information center offers publications and materials on adapted buildings and architecture.

American Lung Association
61 Broadway, 6th Floor
New York, NY 10006
212-315-8700, 800-586-4872
http://www.lungusa.org
Disability Served: various
The association disseminates and provides seminars, and other informational programs to increase awareness of lung cancer and disease. It has more than 200 affiliate groups across the nation, Puerto Rico, and the U.S. Virgin Islands.

American Paraplegia Society
75-20 Astoria Boulevard
Jackson Heights, NY 11370
718-803-3782
aps@unitedspinal.org
http://www.apssci.org
Disability Served: spinal-cord injury
The society promotes research of the causes, cure,
and prevention of spinal cord injury.

American Red Cross
2025 East Street, NW
Washington, DC 20006
202-303-4498
http://www.redcross.org
Disability Served: various
This organization provides support services, information,
seminars, conferences, and publications and has
about 1,000 chapters nationwide.

American Society for Deaf Children
PO Box 3355
Gettysburg, PA 17325
717-334-7922 (Voice/TTY), 800-942-2732
asdc1@aol.com
http://deafchildren.org
Disability Served: hearing
This membership organization of parents and families
offers counseling services and educational materials
on the subject of deaf children.

American Sudden Infant Death Syndrome Institute
509 Augusta Drive
Marietta, GA 30067
770-426-8746, 800-232-SIDS
http://www.sids.org
Disability Served: various
This organization is dedicated to the prevention of
sudden infant death and the promotion of infant
health through research, clinical services, education,
and family support.

American Tinnitus Association
PO Box 5
Portland, OR 97207-0005
503-248-9985, 800-634-8978
tinnitus@ata.org
http://www.ata.org
Disability Served: hearing
This membership organization has a goal of silencing
tinnitus through education, advocacy, research,
and support.

American Wheelchair Bowling Association
PO Box 69
Clover, VA 24534-0069
434-454-2269
bowlawba@aol.com
http://www.awba.org
Disability Served: physically disabled
This association promotes wheelchair bowling
and leagues, and regulates wheelchair-bowling
tournaments.

Amytrophic Lateral Sclerosis Association
27001 Agoura Road, Suite 150
Calabasas Hills, CA 91301-5104
818-880-9007, 800-782-4747
http://www.alsa.org
Disability Served: physically disabled
The association is dedicated to finding the cause
and cure for Amytrophic Lateral Sclerosis.

The Arc of the United States
1010 Wayne Avenue, Suite 650
Silver Spring, MD 20910
301-565-3842
info@thearc.org
http://www.thearc.org
*Disability Served: developmentally disabled, mental
retardation*
This nonprofit organization provides services to
those with mental retardation. Services include
employment, training, education, and independent
living. Research grants are also available.

Arthritis Foundation
1330 West Peachtree Street, Suite 100
Atlanta, GA 30357-0669
404-872-7100, 800-568-4045
http://www.arthritis.org
Disability Served: physically disabled
This national organization provides information, support
services, educational materials, fund raising activities,
and seminars on arthritis.

Aspire of WNY
2356 North Forest Road
Getzville, NY 14068
716-505-5500

info@aspirewny.org
http://www.aspirewny.com
Disability Served: communication, developmentally disabled
This organization offers assessment and training in the use of augmentative or alternative communication systems for those with a developmental or acquired disability that impacts their speech or intelligibility. They assist in obtaining funding for communication aids and also offer short-term loans of communication aids and devices.

Assistance Dogs of America Inc.

8806 State Route 64
Swanton, OH 43558
419-825-3622
http://www.adai.org
Disability Served: various
This organization trains dogs to assist the mobility handicapped.

Assistive Device Center

California State University
School of Engineering and Computer Sciences
6000 J Street
Sacramento, CA 95819
916-924-0280
Disability Served: communication
The center focuses on augmentative communication aids and offers assistance in product evaluation and training.

Assistive Technology Clinic

University of Washington Medical Center
Department of Rehabilitative Medicine
1959 Northeast Pacific
Seattle, WA 98195-6490
206-598-4830
http://www.uwmedicine.org
Disability Served: various
This clinic provides evaluations and prescriptions for wheelchair seating, augmentative communication, computer interfaces, and more.

Assistive Technology Educational Network of Florida

434 North Tampa Avenue
Orlando, FL 32805
407-317-3504, 800-328-3678
http://www.aten.scps.k12.fl.us
Disability Served: various

This statewide center serves students ages three to 21 with assistive technology needs. Services include a resource lab, loan library, training, and technical support.

Associated Blind Inc.

315 Fifth Avenue, Suite 807
New York, NY 10016
212-683-4950
http://www.tabinc.org
Disability Served: physically disabled, vision
This organization provides programs and services to persons who are blind, visually impaired, or physically disabled so that they may achieve economic and social independence.

Association for Children's Mental Health

2465 Woodlake Circle, Suite 140
Okemos, MI 48864
517-381-5125, 888-ACMH-KID
http://www.acmh-mi.org
Disability Served: behavioral disorders, developmentally disabled, mental health
This organization provides support services, advocacy, resources, and more to parents of children with emotional, behavioral, or mental health disorders.

Association for Children with Down Syndrome Inc.

4 Fern Place
Plainview, NY 11779
516-221-4700
information@acds.org
http://www.acds.org
Disability Served: Down Syndrome
This organization provides support services, educational programs, and information for children with Down Syndrome, and other developmental disabilities, and their families.

Association for Macular Diseases Inc.

210 East 64th Street
New York, NY 10021
212-605-3719, 800-MACULA4
association@retinal-research.org
http://www.macula.org
Disability Served: vision
This volunteer organization provides information and support to those suffering from macular degeneration.

Auditory-Verbal Center of Atlanta Inc.
1750 Century Circle, Suite 16
Atlanta, GA 30345
404-633-8911
avc1@bellsouth.net
http://www.avc-atlanta.org
Disability Served: hearing
The center provides programs for infants and children
who are hearing impaired, as well as audiological
services and the sale of hearing aids and assistive
devices.

Auditory-Verbal International
1390 Chain Bridge Road, Suite 100
McLean, VA 22101
703-739-1049, 703-739-0874 (TDD)
audiverb@aol.com
http://www.auditory-verbal.org
Disability Served: hearing
This organization focuses on children with hearing
impairments and provides training and education
to help them learn to communicate.

Augmentative and Alternative Communication Clinic
University of Wisconsin-Eau Claire
Department of Communication Disorders
113 HSS Building
Eau Claire, WI 54702-4004
715-836-3980
http://www.uwec.edu
Disability Served: communication
The clinic provides assessment and evaluation for those
with limited ability to speak, write, type, or dial.

**Augmentative Communication and Technology
  Services**
350 Santa Ana Avenue
San Francisco, CA 94127-1953
415-333-7739
mjbuz@aol.com
http://www.acts-at.com
Disability Served: severe communication disorders
This organization provides augmentative
communication assessment and intervention to
infants, children, and adults in the San Francisco
Bay area. Other services include training to
families and staff and assisting school districts in
meeting the needs of students using augmentative
communication and assistive technology in the
school setting.

Augmentative Communication Center
Queen's College
65-30 Kissena Boulevard
Flushing, NY 11367
718-997-5000
http://www.qc.cuny.edu
Disability Served: communication
The center provides evaluations and treatment for
augmentative communication as well as speech/
language therapy.

Augmentative Communication Program
Heartspring
8700 East 29th Street North
Wichita, KS 67226
316-634-8700, 800-835-1043
Disability Served: communication
The program provides assessment, consultation,
and treatment of communication disabilities.

Autism Services Center
PO Box 507
Huntington, WV 25710-0507
304-525-8014
http://www.autismservicescenter.org
*Disability Served: autism, developmentally disabled,
  mental retardation*
This center provides various services, including case
management, residential, day programs, personal
care, assessments and evaluations, supported
employment, independent living, and family
support. The center has a national autism hotline
and distributes information regarding autism and
related disabilities to callers.

Autism Society of America
7910 Woodmont Avenue, Suite 300
Bethesda, MD 20814
301-657-0881, 800-3-AUTISM
http://www.autism-society.org
Disability Served: autism, developmentally disabled
This organization provides information and referral,
advocacy, and education, as well as newsletters
and publications regarding autism.

AVKO Educational Research Foundation
3084 West Willard Road
Clio, MI 48420-7801
810-686-9283
http://www.avko.org

Disability Served: dyslexic, learning disabled
This foundation maintains a free daily reading clinic
and develops and publishes materials for teachers,
home schoolers, and parents to use with persons
who are dyslexic or have spelling and/or reading
problems.

Barkley Speech-Language and Hearing Clinic
University of Nebraska-Lincoln
253 Barkley Memorial Center, PO Box 830731
Lincoln, NE 68583-0731
402-472-2071
http://www.unl.edu/barkley/spath/clinic.shtml
Disability Served: hearing
The clinic provides evaluations for augmentative
communication speech-language therapy and
is primarily concerned with the academic and
psychological aspects of speech-language and
hearing.

Barron Collier Jr. Foundation
2600 Golden Gate Parkway, Suite 200
Naples, FL 33105
239-262-2600
Disability Served: various
This organization works to support and fund the
Special Olympics.

Beach Center on Families and Disability
University of Kansas
Haworth Hall, 1200 Sunnyside Avenue, Room 3136
Lawrence, KS 66045-7534
785-864-7600, 785-864-3434
beachcenter@ku.edu
http://www.beachcenter.org
Disability Served: various
This organization conducts research and provides
training for families and persons with disabilities.

Better Hearing Institute
515 King Street, Suite 420
Alexandria, VA 22314
703-684-3391
mail@betterhearing.org
http://www.betterhearing.org
Disability Served: hearing
This nonprofit organization offers public information
programs and educational services with the goal
of increasing awareness about hearing loss.

Blind Babies Foundation
1814 Franklin Street, 11th Floor
Oakland, CA 94612
510-446-2229
bbfinfo@blindbabies.org
http://www.blindbabies.org
Disability Served: vision
This organization provides services and programs for
infants and preschool aged children who are visually
impaired.

Blind Children's Center
4120 Marathon Street
Los Angeles, CA 90029
323-664-2153, 800-222-3566
info@blindchildrenscenter.org
http://www.blindchildrenscenter.org
Disability Served: vision
The center offers a number of services for blind children,
including research programs, support services,
evaluations, educational programs, and parent
support groups.

Blind Children's Fund
311 West Broadway, Suite 1
Mt. Pleasant, MI 48858
989-779-9966
karla@blindchildrensfund.org
http://www.blindchildrensfund.org
Disability Served: vision
This organization provides information and early
intervention services for pre-school children who
are blind, or visually or multi-impaired.

Blissymbolics Communication International
Canada
705-762-0028
info@blissymbolics.org
http://www.blissymbolics.org
Disability Served: hearing
This support and educational organization designs
computer programs using Blissymbols and acts
as a resource center for the use of Blissymbols.

Brain Injury Association of America
8201 Greensboro Drive, Suite 611
McLean, VA 22102
800-444-6443
FamilyHelpline@biausa.org

http://www.biausa.org/Pages/home.html
Disability Served: traumatic brain injury
The association provides information, support services, referrals, and publications concerning head injury.

Breaking New Ground
Purdue University, 1146 ABE Building
West Lafayette, IN 47907-1146
765-494-5088, 800-825-4264
bng@ecn.purdue.edu
http://www.breakingnewground.info
Disability Served: various
This organization serves farmers and rural families in Indiana who have been impacted by disabilities.

Buckmasters Disabled Sportsmen Resources
10540 Daystar Drive
Tuscaloosa, AL 35405
205-366-8415
dsullivan@buckmasters.com
http://www.badf.org/DisabledHunters.html
Disability Served: various
This organization offers information and links to adaptive equipment, state laws/regulations, hunting opportunities, and local and national disabled groups for disabled hunters.

Cancer Care Inc.
275 7th Avenue
New York, NY 10001
800-813-HOPE
http://www.cancercare.org
Disability Served: cancer patients and survivors
This volunteer organization provides information, educational materials, seminars, and more for persons with cancer, their families, friends, and caregivers.

Cancer Information Service (CIS)
Building 31, 31 Center Drive, MSC 2580, Room 10A07
Bethesda, MD 20892-2580
800-4CANCER, 800-332-8615 (TTY)
http://cis.nci.nih.gov
Disability Served: cancer patients and survivors
The CIS is the voice of the National Cancer Institute. Through 19 regional offices, which serve all 50 states and Puerto Rico, the service provides the latest, most accurate cancer information for patients, their families, the general public, and health professionals.

CIS information specialists provide thorough, personalized attention to each caller on cancer issues that include prevention, screening and early detection, diagnosis, treatment, and research. Calls can be answered in English and Spanish, and all calls are kept confidential.

Candlelighters Childhood Cancer Foundation
PO Box 498
Kensington, MD 20895-0498
301-962-3520, 800-366-2223
staff@candlelighters.org
http://www.candlelighters.org
Disability Served: cancer patients and survivors
This organization provides support, information, and social activities for children and adolescents with cancer.

The Capper Foundation
3500 Southwest 10th Avenue
Topeka, KS 66604-1995
785-272-4060
abilities@capper.org
http://www.capper.org
Disability Served: physically disabled
This foundation provides services in early intervention, education, pediatric therapy, and assistive technology. The mission of the Capper Foundation is to enhance the independence of people with physical disabilities, primarily children.

Caption Center
125 Western Avenue
Boston, MA 02134
617-300-3600
http://main.wgbh.org/wgbh/access
Disability Served: hearing
The Caption Center provides closed-captioning and subtitling services for television, videos, DVDs, CD-ROMs, the Web, and first-run and specialty movie theaters. The center also publishes a consumer information series (distributed free) on topics ranging from getting local news captions to an explanation of recent federal captioning mandates, which will increase the percentage of captioned television to almost 100 percent by 2006.

Center for Adaptive Technology
Southern Connecticut State University
501 Crescent Street, Engleman B17

New Haven, CT 06515
203-392-5799
cat@southernct.edu
http://www.southernct.edu/departments/cat
Disability Served: various
The center provides computer access, evaluations, and
training services for persons with learning, visual, and
physical disabilities.

The Center for Best Practices in Early Childhood
32 Horrabin, 1 University Circle
Macomb, IL 61455
309-298-1634
http://www.wiu.edu/thecenter
Disability Served: various
This organization encourages the integration of
technology in the preschool curriculum. Training is
offered to early childhood professionals and their
families. Curriculum materials, books, and videotapes
are available.

Center for Children
6100 Radio Station Road, PO Box 2924
La Plata, MD 20646
301-609-9887
kolesar@center-for-children.org
http://www.center-for-children.org
Disability Served: mental health
The Center for Children is a private, nonprofit organization
that provides comprehensive mental health services to
children and their families.

Center for Independent Living
2539 Telegraph Avenue
Berkeley, CA 94704
510-841-4776
http://www.cilberkeley.org
Disability Served: various
The center provides information on programs that
serve residents of Alameda County, California, with
disabilities. Call for details on assistance offered.

Center for Mental Health Services
U.S. Substance Abuse and Mental Health Services
Administration
PO Box 42557
Washington, DC 20015
800-789-2647
http://www.mentalhealth.samhsa.gov/cmhs
Disability Served: mental health

This government organization advocates for mental
health policies and sets national standards for mental
health services and programs.

Center for Understanding Aging
200 Executive Boulevard, Suite 201
Sothington, CT 06489
718-824-4004
coer.natal@snet.net
http://www.ucp.org/ucp_channelres.cfm/1/16/100/1132
Disability Served: elderly
This organization serves as a clearinghouse of
information on aging issues.

Center for Universal Design
North Carolina State University
College of Design
Campus Box 8613
Raleigh, NC 27695-8613
919-515-3082, 800-647-6777
cud@ncsu.edu
http://www2.ncsu.edu/ncsu/design/cud
Disability Served: various
This organization promotes and develops universal
design in housing, commercial environments,
products, and landscapes by conducting research and
training, providing design development, consulting,
technical assistance, and information services.

Cerebral Palsy Association of Middlesex County
10 Oak Drive
Edison, NJ 08837
732-549-1687
info@cpamc.org
http://www.cpamc.org
Disability Served: cerebral palsy
The association provides augmentative communication
evaluation and seating assessment, as well as
a private school, adult programs, and an infant
program.

Cerebral Palsy Inc.
2801 South Webster Avenue
Green Bay, WI 54301
920-337-1122
info@cp-center.org
http://www.cp-center.org
Disability Served: various
Cerebral Palsy Inc. provides a wide range of therapy
for children and adults with varied diagnoses.

Cerebral Palsy Research Foundation
5111 East 21st Street North, PO Box 8217
Wichita, KS 67208-0217
316-688-5201
infor@cprf.org
http://www.cprf.org
Disability Served: various
This organization assists persons with disabilities to be
more independent in the workplace, at home, and on
the road by providing all types of assistive technology.

Challenge Unlimited/Ironstone Therapy
450 Lowell Street
Andover, MA 01810
978-475-4056
info@ChallengeUnlimited.org
http://www.challengeunlimited.org
Disability Served: various
Challenge Unlimited Inc., serves individuals with and
without disabilities using therapeutic riding.

Charcot-Marie-Tooth Association (CMTA)
2700 Chestnut Street
Chester, PA 19013-4867
800-606-2682
info@charcot-marie-tooth.org
http://www.charcot-marie-tooth.org
Disability Served: Charcot-Marie-Tooth Disease
The CMTA offers patient support, public education,
promotion of research for the treatment and cure
of Charcot-Marie-Tooth Disease.

**Chicago Lighthouse for People Who Are Blind
or Visually Impaired**
1850 West Roosevelt Road
Chicago, IL 60608-1298
312-666-1331, 312-666-8874 (TDD)
support@chicagolighthouse.org
http://www.thechicagolighthouse.org
Disability Served: vision
This organization provides health evaluations,
counseling, education, professional training,
rehabilitation teaching, computer training, and
employment services for persons who are blind
or visually impaired.

Children of Aging Parents
PO Box 167
Richboro, PA 18954
800-227-7294

info@caps4caregivers.org
http://www.caps4caregivers.org
Disability Served: elderly
This organization provides information and support
to caregivers of the elderly.

Children's Adaptive Technology Service
Children's Hospital and Medical Center
PO Box 5371
Seattle, WA 98105-0371
206-987-2000
http://www.seattlechildrens.org
Disability Served: various
This organization provides adaptive technology services
for children, including augmentative communication,
power mobility, and computer access.

Children's Tumor Foundation
95 Pine Street, 16th Floor
New York, NY 10005
212- 344-6633, 800-323-7938
info@ctf.org
http://www.ctf.org
Disability Served: physically disabled
This organization provides information to patients with
neurofibromatosis and raises funds for medical
research.

Christian Record Services Inc.
4444 South 52nd Street
Lincoln, NE 68516
402-488-0981
info@christianrecord.org
http://www.christianrecord.org
Disability Served: hearing, vision
The foundation offers a lending library, produces Braille
and large print publications, and hosts programs and
summer camps for persons with hearing and vision
impairments. Limited scholarships are available to
full-time college students who are blind or visually
impaired.

Clearinghouse on Disability Information
550 12th Street, SW, Room 5133
Washington, DC 20202-2550
202-245-7307, 202-205-5637 (TTD)
http://www.ed.gov/about/offices/list/osers
Disability Served: various
This national clearinghouse offers information on all
disabilities.

Cleft Palate Foundation
1504 East Franklin Street, Suite 102
Chapel Hill, NC 27514-2820
919-933-9044, 800-24-CLEFT
info@cleftline.org
http://www.cleft.org
Disability Served: physically disabled
The foundation provides information and referral,
   publications, and educational materials on cleft
   palates and other craniofacial anomalies. The
   foundation offers a hotline service as well.

Cleveland FES Center
11000 Cedar Avenue, Suite 230
Cleveland, OH 44106-3052
216-231-3257, 800-666-2353
jag8@case.edu
http://fescenter.case.edu
Disability Served: physically disabled
This research and development center develops
   functional electrical stimulation (FES) systems
   to restore function for individuals with paralysis.

Cleveland Sight Center
1909 East 101st Street, PO Box 1988
Cleveland, OH 44106-8696
216-791-8118
http://www.clevelandsightcenter.org
Disability Served: hearing, vision
The center provides social, rehabilitation, education,
   and support services for blind and visually impaired
   children and adults; early intervention programs for
   children birth to age six; low vision clinic; aids and
   appliances shop; Braille and taping transcription;
   rehabilitation training; orientation and mobility
   training; computer access training; employment
   services and job placement; recreation program;
   resident camping; talking books; radio reading
   services; food service training; and snack-bar
   employment. It also serves deaf-blind persons
   and offers free vision screenings.

Closing the Gap
526 Main Street, PO Box 68
Henderson, MN 56044
507-248-3294
ckneip@closingthegap.com
http://www.closingthegap.com
Disability Served: various
This organization is an informal source of information

on how computer technology can be used to help
   people with disabilities. It publishes a newspaper
   and sponsors an annual conference.

Coalition on Sexuality and Disability Inc.
122 East 23rd Street
New York, NY 10010
212-242-3900
Disability Served: various
This organization provides information, resources,
   and materials for persons with disabilities regarding
   sexual issues.

Collier County Association for the Blind
850 6th Avenue North
Naples, FL 33940
941-649-1122
ccab@juno.com
http://gator.naples.net/social/ccab
Disability Served: vision
The association provides a number of services to blind
   citizens of Collier County, Florida, including support
   services, recreational activities, independent living
   skills training, and more.

Communication Enhancement Center
2111 Pontiac Lake Road
Waterford, MI 48328
248-209-2000
http://www.oakland.k12.mi.us
Disability Served: communication
The center provides evaluations, demonstrations,
   and augmentative communication services.

Communication Service for the Deaf
102 North Krohn Place
Sioux Falls, SD 57103
605-367-5760, 605-367-5761 (TTY), 800-642-6410
http://www.c-s-d.org
Disability Served: hearing
This organization offers information and referral,
   advocacy services, and peer counseling.

Community Connections
801 Pennsylvania Avenue, SE, Suite 201
Washington, DC 20003-2152
202-546-1512
info@ccdc1.org
http://www.communityconnectionsdc.org
Disability Served: mental health

This organization offers support services for persons with mental health problems living in the District of Columbia and Montgomery County, Maryland.

The Compassionate Friends
PO Box 3696
Oak Brook, IL 60522-3696
630-990-0010, 877-969-0010
nationaloffice@compassionatefriends.org
http://www.compassionatefriends.org
Disability Served: various
This is a nonprofit, self-help organization offering friendship and understanding to families who have experienced the death of a child of any age, from any cause. It provides support for bereaved parents, grandparents, and siblings. The Compassionate Friends also publish a catalog of printed resources and a national magazine for parents, grandparents, siblings, and professionals. The group also hosts an annual national conference and various regional conferences.

Council for Exceptional Children (CEC)
1110 North Glebe Road, Suite 300
Arlington, VA 22201
703-620-3660, 866-915-5000 (TTY)
service@cec.sped.org
http://www.cec.sped.org
Disability Served: various
This nonprofit membership association is dedicated to improving educational outcomes for students with disabilities and/or the gifted. The association advocates for governmental policies, sets professional standards, provides continuing professional development, publishes newsletters and journals, and more. Departments include the following: the Association for the Gifted, Technology and Media Division, Council for Children with Behavioral Disorders, Council for Educational Diagnostic Services, Division for Children's Communication Development, Division on Career Development and Transition, Division for Culturally and Linguistically Diverse Exceptional Learners, Division for Early Childhood, Division of International Special Education and Services, Division for Learning Disabilities, Division for Physical and Health Disabilities, Division on Visual Impairments, and the Division on Mental Retardation and Developmental Disabilities.

Council of Better Business Bureaus Foundation
4200 Wilson Boulevard, Suite 800
Arlington, VA 22203
703-276-0100
http://www.bbb.org
Disability Served: various
The foundation provides publications on ADA requirements for businesses.

Council of Citizens with Low Vision
1155 15th Street, NW
Washington, DC 20005
800-733-2258
http://www.cclvi.org
Disability Served: vision
This membership organization is dedicated to increasing the awareness of professionals and other interested persons of the capabilities, potential, and special needs of persons with low vision.

Cystic Fibrosis Foundation
6931 Arlington Road
Bethesda, MD 20814
301-951-4422, 800-FIGHT-CF
info@cff.org
http://www.cff.org
Disability Served: cystic fibrosis
This foundation supports a nationwide network of care centers, offers general information publications, and funds research centers, research grants, and clinical trials. Visit its Web site for information regarding specific grants.

D.E.A.F. Inc.
215 Brighton Avenue
Allston, MA 02134
617-254-4041 (Voice/TTY), 800-886-5195 (Voice/TTY)
info@deafinconline.org
http://www.deafinconline.org
Disability Served: hearing
This organization provides information and referral, educational programs, advocacy, skills assessment, and training for people who are deaf and hard of hearing.

Dallas Lighthouse for the Blind Inc.
4245 Office Parkway
Dallas, TX 75204
214-821-2375
http://www.dallaslighthouse.org
Disability Served: vision
This organization provides blind and visually impaired citizens in Dallas, Texas, with a number of services,

such as vocational rehabilitation, independent living skills training, counseling and support services, education.

Deaf REACH

3521 12th Street, NE
Washington, DC 20017
202-832-6681 (Voice/TTY)
http://www.deaf-reach.org
Disability Served: hearing
This organization provides information and referral, advocacy, counseling services, and more, for persons with hearing impairments in the Washington, D.C., area.

The Denver Foundation

950 South Cherry Street, Suite 200
Denver, CO 80246
303-300-1790
mwayoeoe@denverfoundation.org
http://www.denverfoundation.org
Disability Served: various
This community foundation supports nonprofit organizations in the six-county metropolitan Denver area.

Depression and Bipolar Support Alliance (DBSA)

730 North Franklin Street, Suite 501
Chicago, IL 60610-7224
312-642-0049, 800-826-3632
programs@dbsalliance.org
http://www.ndmda.org
Disability Served: mental health
The DBSA provides educational resources about depressive illnesses and advocates for improved treatment and access to care through distribution of free informational brochures, a bookstore, peer-led support groups, and membership and volunteer opportunities.

Descriptive Video Service (DVS)

DVS/WGBH Educational Foundation
125 Western Avenue
Boston, MA 02134
617-300-3600 (Voice/TTY)
access@wgbh.org
http://main.wgbh.org/wgbh/pages/mag/resources/ dvs-home-video-catalogue.html
Disability Served: vision
This organization provides narrated descriptions of television programs. The narration describes visual elements such as actions, body language, settings, and graphics. DVS is available on a number of popular public television series and movies on home video.

Developmental Services of Northwest Kansas Inc.

PO Box 1016
Hays, KS 67601
785-625-5678
comments@notes1.dsnwk.org
http://www.dsnwk.org
Disability Served: developmentally disabled
This organization provides services to children, youth, and adults in Northwest Kansas with mild to severe developmental disabilities.

Direct Link for the disABLED

PO Box 1036
Solvang, CA 93464
805-688-1603
Disability Served: various
This nonprofit group maintains a database of organizations and resources for persons with disabilities.

Disabled and Alone/Life Services for the Handicapped Inc.

61 Broadway
New York, NY 10006
212-532-6740, 800-995-0066
info@disabledandalone.org
http://www.disabledandalone.org
Disability Served: various
This national nonprofit organization helps families plan for the future of a family member with a disability and carries out the lifetime care plan (according to the family member's instructions and the person's special needs) after the family is no longer around. The organization also publishes a newsletter, *LifeLines.*

Disabled/Special Needs Users' Group (D/SNUG)

Boston Computer Society
One Kendall Square
Cambridge, MA 01239
617-252-0600
Disability Served: various
D/SNUG is a special interest group of the Boston Computer Society. A quarterly newsletter is available.

Dogs for the Deaf Inc.
10175 Wheeler Road
Central Point, OR 97502
541-826-9220 (Voice/TDD)
http://www.dogsforthedeaf.org
Disability Served: hearing
This organization trains dogs to serve those who are
deaf or hard of hearing.

**DO-IT (Disabilities, Opportunities, Internetworking
and Technology)**
PO Box 355670
Seattle, WA 98195-5670
206-685-DOIT
doit@u.washington.edu
http://www.washington.edu/doit
Disability Served: various
DO-IT's goal is to increase the participation of people
with disabilities in challenging postsecondary
programs and careers. High school and college
students with disabilities who are pursuing college
and careers may participate in the DO-IT program.

DREAMMS for Kids Inc.
273 Ringwood Road
Freeville, NY 13068-5606
607-539-3027
janet@dreamms.org
http://www.dreamms.org
Disability Served: developmentally disabled
This service agency advocates for the use of technology
by students with special needs.

Ear Foundation
PO Box 330867
Nashville, TN 37203
615-627-2724 (Voice/TDD), 800-545-HEAR (Voice/TDD)
info@earfoundation.org
http://www.earfoundation.org
Disability Served: hearing
The foundation works to enrich the lives of the hearing
and balance impaired through public awareness and
continuing medical education.

Easter Seals
230 West Monroe Street, Suite 1800
Chicago, IL 60606
312-726-6200, 312-726-4258 (TTY)
http://www.easterseals.com
Disability Served: various

This national organization provides a number of services
and programs for persons with disabilities or special
needs and their families, including advocacy,
rehabilitation services, publications and materials,
education, and more.

Easter Seals North Georgia Inc.
5600 Roswell Road, Prado North, Suite 100
Atlanta, GA 30342
404-943-1070
http://northgeorgia.easterseals.com
Disability Served: various
Easter Seals provides services including therapeutic
rehabilitation, childcare, Head Start, and childcare
training.

Enabled Online.com
321 Wilton Circle
Sanford, FL 32773
407-474-3841
info@EnabledOnline.com
http://enabledonline.com
Disability Served: various
This Web site is an online meeting place for persons
with disabilities, their loved ones, and caregivers.

Family Resource Associates
35 Haddon Avenue
Shrewsbury, NJ 07702
732-747-5310
http://www.familyresourceassociates.org
Disability Served: developmentally disabled
This organization provides information and referrals,
advocacy, support services, recreational activities,
workshops, educational materials, and more for children with developmental disabilities and their families.

Federal Citizens Information Center
18th & F Street, NW
Washington, DC 20405
888-878-3256
http://www.pueblo.gsa.gov
Disability Served: various
The center, which is provided by the U.S. General
Services Administration, offers free print and online
resources relating to health, family, employment, and
other topics.

Federation for Children with Special Needs
1135 Tremont Street, Suite 420
Boston, MA 02120

617-236-7210
fcsninfo@fcsn.org
http://www.fcsn.org
Disability Served: various
This organization provides information and referral as well as technical assistance and training to parents and families of children with disabilities.

Federation of Families for Children's Mental Health
1101 King Street, Suite 420
Alexandria, VA 22314
703-684-7710
ffcmh@ffcmh.org
http://ffcmh.org
Disability Served: mental health
This national family-run organization provides information and support to children with mental health needs, as well as to their families and caregivers.

Fidelco Guide Dog Foundation Inc.
103 Old Iron Ore Road
Bloomfield, CT 06002
860-243-5200
gjskarl@fidelco.org
http://www.fidelco.org
Disability Served: vision
This organization breeds, raises, and trains German Shepherd guide dogs.

Fight for Sight
381 Park Avenue South, Suite 809
New York, NY 10016
212-679-6060
info@fightforsight.com
http://www.fightforsight.com
Disability Served: vision
This health organization supports research on blindness and helps support pediatric eye centers.

Florida Diagnostic and Learning Resources Systems (FDLRS)
5555 Southwest 93rd Avenue
Miami, FL 33165
305-274-3501
http://www.paec.org/fdlrsweb/index.htm
Disability Served: various
This organization is a special education support system for educators and other professionals who work with exceptional children. FDLRS operates through the Dade County Public Schools Office of Exceptional Student Education.

Foundation Center Library Services
The Foundation Center
79 Fifth Avenue, Department ZE
New York, NY 10003
212-620-4230, 800-424-9836
http://fdncenter.org/newyork
Disability Served: various
This organization provides information on foundations and corporate giving programs.

Friends of Libraries for Deaf Action
2930 Craiglawn Road
Silver Spring, MD 20904-1816
301-572-5168 (Voice/TTY)
folda86@aol.com
http://www.folda.net
Disability Served: hearing
This organization promotes library access and quality resources for the deaf community wherever they live, work, attend school, or visit.

Girls Incorporated
120 Wall Street
New York, NY 10005-3902
800-374-4475
http://www.girlsinc.org
Disability Served: various
This youth organization helps girls, particularly those in high-risk, underserved areas, through research, advocacy, and program development. They provide informal education programs that encourage girls to take risks and master challenges. Operation SMART is a current program focused on girls with disabilities.

Goodwill Industries International Inc.
15810 Indianola Drive
Rockville, MD 20855
800-741-0186
contactus@goodwill.org
http://www.goodwill.org
Disability Served: various
This association provides training and employment services for people with disabilities.

Guide Dogs for the Blind Inc.
PO Box 151200
San Rafael, CA 94915-1200

415-499-4000, 800-295-4050
http://www.guidedogs.com
Disability Served: *vision*
This organization trains guide dogs to assist visually
impaired persons in safe travel. It also trains visually
impaired people on how to interact with and use the
dogs for enhanced mobility and travel.

Guide Dog Foundation for the Blind Inc.
371 East Jericho Turnpike
Smithtown, NY 11787-2976
631-930-9000, 800-548-4337
info@guidedog.org
http://www.guidedog.org
Disability Served: *vision*
This organization provides rehabilitation to the visually
impaired through the use of guide dogs to enhance
mobility and independence.

H.E.A.R.-Hearing Education and Awareness for Rockers
PO Box 460847
San Francisco, CA 94102
415-409-3277
http://www.hearnet.com
Disability Served: *hearing*
This organization's mission is the prevention of hearing
loss and tinnitus among musicians and music fans
(especially teens) through education awareness and
grassroots outreach advocacy.

Head Injury Hotline
212 Pioneer Building
Seattle, WA 98104-2221
206-621-8558
brain@headinjury.com
http://www.headinjury.com
Disability Served: *traumatic brain injury*
This organization is a nonprofit clearinghouse founded
and operated by head-injury survivors since 1985.
Services include advice, handbooks, seminars, and
advocacy.

Health Resources and Services Administration
HRSA Information Center
PO Box 2910
Merrifield, VA 22116
888-ASK-HRSA, 877-4TY-HRSA (TTY)
ask@hrsa.gov
http://www.ask.hrsa.gov/Feedback.cfm

Disability Served: *various*
This clearinghouse provides publications and
information to parents, children, and professionals
concerned with disabilities or related health issues.

Helen Keller National Center for Deaf-Blind Youth and Adults
57 Willoughby Street
Brooklyn, NY 11201
718-522-2122
info@helenkeller.org
http://www.helenkeller.org
Disability Served: *hearing, vision*
This nonprofit agency assists those who are deaf-blind
in gaining skills needed to live independent lives. It
provides comprehensive evaluation and vocational
rehabilitation training, as well as job and residential
placement assistance to students.

Hospitalized Veterans Writing Project
5920 Nall, Room 105
Mission, KS 66202
913-432-1214
http://www.veteransvoices.org
Disability Served: *various*
This project urges hospitalized veterans to write about
their rehabilitation and publishes their work in a
64-page magazine, *Veterans' Voices* that is published
three times annually in the spring, summer, and fall.

House Ear Institute
2100 West Third Street, 5th Floor
Los Angeles, CA 90057
213-483-4431, 800-388-8612, 213-484-2642 (TDD)
http://www.hei.org
Disability Served: *hearing*
Through research and education, the institute aims
to improve the quality of life of those with an ear
disease, or hearing or balance disorder. It also offers
outreach programs that focus on families with
hearing-impaired children.

Independent Living Research Utilization
The Institute for Rehabilitation and Research
2323 South Shepherd, Suite 1000
Houston, TX 77019
713-520-0232 (Voice/TTY)
http://ilru@ilru.org
Disability Served: *various*
This organization provides information, resources,
and independent living consultations.

Industry-Labor Council
National Center for Disability Services
201 IU Willets Road
Albertson, NY 11507
516-465-3737
Disability Served: various
The council promotes the integration of persons with
disabilities in the work force and provides assistance
to businesses to meet these goals.

Infinitec
160 North Wacker Drive
Chicago, IL 60606
312-368-0380
ldyer@ucpnet.org
http://www.ucpnet.org
Disability Served: various
This division of the United Cerebral Palsy Association
of Greater Chicago provides assistive technology
information, employment training, adult
developmental training, and workshops for
educators, parents, and professionals. A library and
resource center and technology exchange network
are also available.

International Dyslexia Association
Chester Building, 8600 La Salle Road, Suite 382
Baltimore, MD 21286-2044
410-296-0232, 800-ABCD-123
info@interdys.org
http://www.interdys.org
Disability Served: dyslexia
This nonprofit scientific and educational organization
focuses on dyslexia. Free information and referral for
testing, tutoring, and effective teaching approaches
are provided.

International Foundation for Stutterers
304 Hampshire Drive
Plainsboro, NJ 08502
609-275-3806
Disability Served: communication
This organization provides speech therapy, information,
and resources for people who stutter and their
families.

International Hearing Dog Inc.
5901 East 89th Avenue
Henderson, CO 80640-8315
303-287-3277

ihdi@aol.com
http://www.ihdi.org
Disability Served: hearing
This organization trains dogs to assist persons who
are deaf or hard of hearing.

John Milton Society for the Blind
475 Riverside Drive, Room 455
New York, NY 10115
212-870-3335
Disability Served: vision
This organization provides free Christian literature, in
Braille, in large print, and on audiocassettes, to the
blind and visually impaired. Publications include
magazines for adults and youth, Bible studies,
calendars, and a directory of resources.

**Johns Hopkins University Center for Technology
in Education**
6740 Alexander Bell Drive, Suite 302
Columbia, MD 21046
410-312-3800
cte@jhu.edu
http://cte.jhu.edu
Disability Served: various
The center conducts research and provides information
regarding assistive technology and disability for
children and youth.

Junior Blind of America
5300 Angeles Vista Boulevard
Los Angeles, CA 90043
323-295-4555, 800-352-2290
info@fjb.org
http://www.fjb.org
Disability Served: vision
The foundation is a private, nonprofit agency that
provides a wide range of programs and services
for blind, visually impaired, and multiply disabled
blind children, youths, and adults, as well as their
families. Programs offered include the infant-family
program, children's special education school,
children's residential program, Davidson Program
for Independence (for adults), and a year-round
recreation program that includes a summer
residential camp, Camp Bloomfield.

Just One Break
120 Wall Street, 20th Floor
New York, NY 10005

212-785-7300, 212-785-4515 (TTY)
jobs@justonebreak.com
http://www.justonebreak.com
Disability Served: various
This unique organization serves job seekers with
physical, emotional, or developmental disabilities.
Full evaluation of applicants includes ability to
work, type of work possible, and type of physical
environment required. Job placement is provided to
suitable applicants. There is no charge for the service.

Juvenile Diabetes Research Foundation International

120 Wall Street, 19th Floor
New York, NY 10005-4001
800-533-2873
info@jdrf.org
http://www.jdf.org
Disability Served: diabetes
The foundation's mission is to find a cure for diabetes
and its complications through the support of
research.

Laradon

5100 Lincoln Street
Denver, CO 80216
303-296-2400
http://www.laradon.org
Disability Served: developmentally disabled
This organization provides education, training, and
support services to children and adults with
developmental disabilities.

Laurent Clerc National Deaf Education Center

800 Florida Avenue, NE
Washington, DC 20002-3695
202-651-5051
http://clerccenter.gallaudet.edu/InfoToGo/index.html
Disability Served: hearing
The center provides information on topics dealing with
deafness and hearing loss. It responds to questions
from the general public and deaf and hard of hearing
people, their families, and professionals who work
with them.

Learning Disabilities Association of Arkansas

7509 Cantrell Road, Suite 103C
Little Rock, AR 72207
501-666-8777
info@ldaarkansas.org
http://www.ldaarkansas.org

Disability Served: learning disabled
This organization provides information, has a lending
library of books and tapes, and assists in increasing
awareness and improving education and vocational
opportunities for people with learning disabilities in
Arkansas.

Learning Disabilities Association of New York State

1202 Troy-Schenectady Road
Latham, NY 12210
518-608-8992
hal@associationresources.com
http://www.ldanys.org
Disability Served: learning disabled
This association provides education, support services,
and rehabilitative and vocational assistance to
persons with learning disabilities in New York State.

Life Development Institute

18001 North 79th Avenue, E-71
Glendale, AZ 85308
623-773-2774
http://www.life-development-inst.org
Disability Served: attention deficit order, learning disabled
This organization offers support, information, vocational
training, and independent living skills training
to adults and older adolescents with learning
disabilities, attention deficit disorders, and other
related conditions.

Lighthouse International

111 East 59th Street
New York, NY 10022-1202
212-821-9200, 800-829-0500
http://www.lighthouse.org
Disability Served: vision
This organization provides information to professionals
and to people of all ages with impaired vision,
and their families, about vision loss and vision
rehabilitation. It also provides a nationwide listing
of low-vision services, vision rehabilitation services,
support groups, and other related organizations.

Little People of America Inc.

5289 Northeast Elam Young Parkway, Suite F-100
Hillsboro, OR 97124
503-846-1562, 888-572-2001
info@lpaonline.org
http://www.lpaonline.org
Disability Served: various

This organization provides support services and networking programs for people of short stature.

Lowe Syndrome Association
18919 Voss Road
Dallas, TX 75287-2766
612-869-5693
info@lowesyndrome.org
http://www.lowesyndrome.org
Disability Served: Lowe Syndrome
The association provides information, fosters communication among families, and sponsors medical research related to Lowe Syndrome.

MAB Community Services
200 Ivy Street
Brookline, MA 02146
617-738-5110
Disability Served: mental retardation, traumatic brain injury, vision
MAB is an organization that serves individuals who are blind and visually impaired, adults with mental retardation, and adolescents who have sustained brain injuries.

March of Dimes Birth Defects Foundation
1275 Mamaroneck Avenue
White Plains, NY 10605
914-428-7100, 888-MO-DIMES
http://www.modimes.org
Disability Served: various
This resource center provides information and referral services to the public on pregnancy and birth defects.

Marin Puzzle People Inc.
17 Buena Vista Avenue
Mill Valley, CA 94941
415-383-8763
Disability Served: learning disabled
Marin Puzzle People assists adults with learning disabilities to reach their potential for social and vocational success through educational, social, and vocational experiences.

Mott Children's Health Center
806 Tuuri Place
Flint, MI 48503
810-767-5750
CHSInfo@mottchc.org
http://www.mottchc.org

Disability Served: communication
The center provides comprehensive health care services for at risk children of Genesee County. Their programs include medical and dental services, speech and vision screenings and therapies, and early intervention programs.

Mount Vernon Center for Community Mental Health
8119 Holland Road
Alexandria, VA 22306
703-360-6910
Disability Served: mental health
The center is dedicated to providing education, counseling, and advocacy services to mentally ill people in the Mount Vernon area of Fairfax County, Virginia.

Multiple Sclerosis Foundation Inc.
6350 North Andrews Avenue
Ft. Lauderdale, FL 33309-2130
954-776-6805, 800-225-6495
admin@msfocus.org
http://www.msfacts.org
Disability Served: multiple sclerosis
The Multiple Sclerosis Foundation Inc. is a nonprofit organization that provides traditional and alternative health care options and home care assisted programs. It also publishes a newsletter, provides phone support, an in-house library, information and referrals, and networking with regional support groups. The foundation awards grants to universities for research on the cause, cure, prevention, and treatment of multiple sclerosis. Temporary custodial home care, home renovations, used medical equipment, and summer camp programs are also offered.

Muscular Dystrophy Association
3300 East Sunrise Drive
Tucson, AZ 85718-3208
520-529-2000, 800-572-1717
mda@mdausa.org
http://www.mdausa.org
Disability Served: physically disabled
The association fights neuromuscular diseases through research, public health education, and a broad program of direct services for U.S. residents affected by these disorders.

National AMBUCS Inc.
4285 Regency Court
High Point, NC 27265

336-852-0052
ambucs@ambucs.com
http://www.ambucs.com
Disability Served: various
This organization's mission is to create opportunities and
   independence for people with disabilities. Services
   include providing scholarships and giving away
   AmTrykes, therapeutic tricycles for children.

National Amputation Foundation
40 Church Street
Malverne, NY 11565
516-887-3600
amps76@aol.com
http://www.nationalamputation.org
Disability Served: physically disabled
The foundation provides amputees with legal counsel,
   vocational guidance and placement, social activities,
   psychological aid, and training on prosthetic devices.

National Association for Down Syndrome
PO Box 206
Wilmette, IL 60091
630-325-9112
info@ndss.org
http://www.nads.org
Disability Served: Down Syndrome
The association provides support, education, and
   information for children and adults with Down
   Syndrome who live in the Chicago area.

National Association for Parents of the Visually Impaired Inc.
PO Box 317
Watertown, MA 02272-0317
617-972-7441, 800-562-6265
napvi@perkins.org
http://www.napvi.org
Disability Served: vision
This organization helps parents find information and
   resources for their blind and visually impaired children.

National Ataxia Foundation
2600 Fernbrook Lane
Minneapolis, MN 55447
763-553-0020
http://www.ataxia.org
Disability Served: physically disabled
This organization provides education, service, and
   research programs to combat hereditary ataxias.

The foundation also publishes a quarterly newsletter,
Generations.

National Braille Association Inc.
3 Townline Circle
Rochester, NY 14623-2513
585-427-8260
nbaoffice@nationalbraille.org
http://www.nationalbraille.org
Disability Served: vision
This organization provides continuing education to
   those who prepare Braille, and provides Braille
   materials to persons who are visually impaired.

National Catholic AIDS Network
10 East Pearson Street
Chicago, IL 60611
312-915-7790
info@ncan.org
http://www.ncan.org
Disability Served: AIDS
This organization offers help and support for Catholics
   suffering from AIDS/HIV.

National Center for Learning Disabilities
381 Park Avenue South, Suite 1401
New York, NY 10016-8806
212-545-7510, ext. 233
mcarey@ncld.org
http://www.ncld.org
Disability Served: learning disabled
This national organization offers information and referral,
   advocacy services, education, and other services for
   persons with learning disabilities, their families, and
   professionals who work with the learning disabled.

National Chronic Pain Outreach Association
PO Box 274
Millboro, VA 24460
540-862-9437
http://www.chronicpain.org
Disability Served: chronic pain
The association provides support and services to
   those suffering from chronic pain. It also publishes
   a quarterly newsletter, *Lifeline,* which provides
   information on pain management methods and
   coping techniques.

National Council on Independent Living
1710 Rhode Island Avenue NW
Washington, DC 20036

703-525-3406, 703-525-4153 (TTY)
ncil@ncil.org
http://www.ncil.org
Disability Served: various
This organization provides information and referral,
advocacy, and resources for persons with disabilities
who live independently.

National Cued Speech Association
23970 Hermitage Road
Cleveland, OH 44122
800-459-3529 (Voice/TTY)
http://www.cuedspeech.org
Disability Served: hearing
The association offers training, support services, and
information regarding cued speech and hearing loss.

National Diabetes Information Clearinghouse
1 Information Way
Bethesda, MD 20892-3560
800-860-8747
ndic@info.niddk.nih.gov
http://diabetes.niddk.nih.gov
Disability Served: diabetes
This clearinghouse disseminates educational materials,
informational publications, and referrals to support
groups and diabetes organizations.

National Digestive Diseases Information
Clearinghouse
2 Information Way
Bethesda, MD 20892-3570
800-891-5389
nddic@info.niddk.nih.gov
http://digestive.niddk.nih.gov
Disability Served: various
This clearinghouse disseminates information on digestive
diseases and is affiliated with the National Institute of
Diabetes and Digestive and Kidney Diseases.

National Dissemination Center for Children
with Disabilities
PO Box 1492
Washington, DC 20013-1492
202-884-8200, 800-695-0285
http://www.nichcy.org
Disability Served: various
This clearinghouse provides information on disabilities
and disability-related issues regarding children.

Services include personal responses to questions,
referrals to state or national organizations,
publications, and technical assistance to families
and professionals.

National Down Syndrome Society
666 Broadway, 8th Floor
New York, NY 10012
212-460-9330, 800-221-4602
info@ndss.org
http://www.ndss.org
Disability Served: Down Syndrome
This organization works so that all people with Down
Syndrome are provided the opportunity to reach
their full potential through education, research,
advocacy, and information and referral.

National Federation of the Blind (NFB)
1800 Johnson Street
Baltimore, MD 21230-4914
410-659-9314
http://www.nfb.org
Disability Served: vision
This federation works to improve opportunities
for the blind, and understanding of blindness
by the general public. The NFB offers public
education, information and referrals, scholarships,
publications about blindness, adaptive equipment
for the blind, advocacy services, job opportunities,
and support.

National Federation of the Blind of California
175 East Olive Avenue, Suite 308
Burbank, CA 91502
818-558-6524
nfbcal@sbcglobal.net
http://www.nfbcal.org
Disability Served: vision
This membership organization for the blind offers
scholarships, referral services, and represents
California in the JOB network.

National Health Information Center
PO Box 1133
Washington, DC 20013-1133
301-468-1273
healthfinder@nhic.org
http://www.healthfinder.gov
Disability Served: various

The center matches consumer requests with appropriate health agencies and information services.

National Hemophilia Foundation
116 West 32nd Street, 11th Floor
New York, NY 10001
212-328-3700
handi@hemophilia.org
http://www.hemophilia.org
Disability Served: inherited bleeding disorders
The foundation is dedicated to finding cures for inherited bleeding disorders, and to the prevention and treatment of their complications through education, advocacy, and research.

National Hydrocephalus Foundation
12413 Centralia Road
Lakewood, CA 90715-1623
888-857-3434
nhf@earthlink.net
http://www.nhfonline.org
Disability Served: hydrocephalus
The foundation provides information on hydrocephaly through publications, support services, and educational materials.

National Institute of Arthritis and Musculoskeletal and Skin Diseases
Information Clearinghouse
National Institutes of Health
1 AMS Circle
Bethesda, MD 20892-3675
301-565-2966, 877-22-NIAMS
niamsinfo@mail.nih.gov
http://www.niams.nih.gov
Disability Served: various
The organization supports research into the causes, treatment, and prevention of arthritis and musculoskeletal and skin diseases, the training of basic and clinical scientists to carry out this research, and the dissemination of information on research progress in these diseases.

National Institute of Neurological Disorders and Stroke
PO Box 5801
Bethesda, MD 20824
301-496-5751, 800-352-9424, 301-468-5981 (TTY)
http://www.ninds.nih.gov
Disability Served: various

The institute conducts research and provides information, educational materials, and publications on brain and nervous system disorders to the public and to medical professionals.

National Lekotek Center
3204 West Armitage Avenue
Chicago, IL 60647
773-276-5164, 800-366-PLAY
lekotek@lekotek.org
http://www.lekotek.org
Disability Served: various
This organization provides play-centered programs to maximize development and facilitate enjoyment for children with disabilities, and their families, through a network of national sites. Toy lending libraries, computer programs, and direct services are available.

National Mental Health Association
2001 North Beauregard Street, 12th Floor
Alexandria, VA 22311
703-684-7722, 800-433-5959
http://www.nmha.org
Disability Served: mental health
The association provides mental health information and/or referrals through its 24-hour information center.

National Mental Health Consumer's Self-Help Clearinghouse
1211 Chestnut Street, Suite 1207
Philadelphia, PA 19107
800-553-4539
info@mhselfhelp.org
http://www.mhselfhelp.org
Disability Served: mental health
The clearinghouse provides information and support to encourage the organization of self-help groups across the nation.

National Multiple Sclerosis Society
733 Third Avenue
New York, NY 10017
800-344-4867
http://www.nationalmssociety.org
Disability Served: multiple sclerosis
The society provides education, information and referral, and supports research on multiple sclerosis.

National Network for the Learning Disabled
808 North 82nd Street, Suite F2
Scottsdale, AZ 85257
602-941-5112
Disability Served: learning disabled
This is a network of adults with learning disabilities
devoted to providing support, advice, and
information to others with learning disabilities.

National Organization for Rare Disorders (NORD)
55 Kenosia Avenue, PO Box 1968
Danbury, CT 06813-1968
203-744-0100, 800-999-6673, 203-797-9590 (TDD)
orphan@rarediseases.org
http://www.rarediseases.org
Disability Served: various
NORD is an clearinghouse for those seeking information
on rare 'orphan' disorders. NORD also offers
networking, referrals to support groups, and
advocacy services.

National Organization on Disability
910 16th Street, NW, Suite 600
Washington, DC 20006
202-293-5960
ability@nod.org
http://www.nod.org
Disability Served: various
This national disability network organization helps
people with disabilities participate in their
communities.

National Parkinson Foundation
1501 Northwest Ninth Avenue
Miami, FL 33136-1494
305-243-6666, 800-327-4545
contact@parkinson.org
http://www.parkinson.org
Disability Served: physically disabled
The foundation's mission is to find the cause and cure for
Parkinson's Disease, and other neurological disorders,
through research; to educate medical practitioners
on how to detect early warning signs of Parkinson's;
to educate patients and the general public; and to
provide diagnostic and therapeutic services.

National Rehabilitation Association
633 South Washington Street
Alexandria, VA 22314
703-836-0850, 703-836-0849 (TDD)

info@nationalrehab.org
http://www.nationalrehab.org/website
Disability Served: various
This organization promotes rehabilitation services for
persons with disabilities and provides information
to professionals and the general public.

**National Voluntary Organizations for Independent
Living for the Aging**
1730 Rhode Island Avenue, SW, Suite 1200
Washington, DC 20036
202-872-0888
http://www.n4a.org
Disability Served: elderly
This organization is dedicated to educating and assisting
organizations that work to maintain independent
lives for the elderly.

Neil Squire Foundation
2250 Boundary Road
Burnaby, BC V5M 3Z3
Canada
604-473-9363
info@neilsquire.ca
http://www.neilsquire.ca
Disability Served: physically disabled
This nonprofit organization provides programs and
services incorporating assistive technology for
persons with physical disabilities.

**Northern Virginia Resource Center for Deaf
and Hard of Hearing Persons**
3951 Pender Drive
Fairfax, VA 22030
703-352-9055, 703-352-9056 (TTY)
http://www.nvrc.org
Disability Served: hearing
This resource center provides information, education,
advocacy, and support services to persons with hearing
impairments, and to their families and caregivers.

Obsessive-Compulsive Foundation Inc.
676 State Street
New Haven, CT 06511
203-401-2070
info@ocfoundation.org
http://www.ocfoundation.org
Disability Served: mental health
The foundation offers free information and support
on obsessive-compulsive disorder (OCD). They

also support research into the causes and effective treatments of OCD and related disorders.

Okada Hearing Guide and Specialty Dogs
7509 East Saviors Path
Floral City, FL 34436
352-344-2212
http://www.okadadogs.com
Disability Served: mental health, physically disabled
This organization trains dogs to help persons with physical or mental disabilities. The majority of the dogs come from animal shelters.

Orchard Village
7670 Marmora Manor
Skokie, IL 60077
847-967-1800
http://www.orchardvillage.org
Disability Served: developmentally disabled
This nonprofit organization provides residential and vocational support for adults with developmental disabilities.

Outdoor Buddies
PO Box 37283
Denver, CO 80237
303-771-8216
outbud@juno.com
http://www.outbud.freeservers.com
Disability Served: physically disabled
This nonprofit organization provides outdoor opportunities for people with physical disabilities. Volunteer hunters and anglers help the disabled enjoy outdoor activities and sports in Colorado.

Paralyzed Veterans of America
801 18th Street, NW
Washington, DC 20006-3517
800-424-8200, 800-795-4327 (TTY)
info@pva.org
http://www.pva.org
Disability Served: physically disabled, spinal-cord injury
This organization serves veterans who are paralyzed due to spinal cord injury or disease.

Parent Information Center
PO Box 2405
Concord, NH 03301-2405

603-224-7005 (Voice/TDD), 800-232-7005
picinfo@parentinformationcenter.org
http://www.parentinformationcenter.org
Disability Served: various
The center is a nonprofit organization that provides information, support services, and training to parents of children with disabilities. The center serves the state of New Hampshire.

Parents Helping Parents
3041 Olcott Street
Santa Clara, CA 95054-3222
408-727-5775
info@php.com
http://www.php.com
Disability Served: various
This organization provides information and referral, support programs, peer counseling, siblings programs, and networking programs to families of children with disabilities or illness.

Parent Support Network of Rhode Island
400 Warwick
Warwick, RI 02888
800-483-8844
Disability Served: various
The network is designed to provide advocacy, education, and support to parents of children in Rhode Island with emotional and behavioral disorders.

Parents of Children with Down Syndrome
c/o The Arc of Montgomery County
PO Box 10416
Rockville, MD 20849
301-916-4985
information@podsmc.org
http://www.podsmc.org
Disability Served: Down Syndrome
This organization is a support group of parents who have children with Down Syndrome.

Pediatric Projects Inc.
PO Box 57155
Tarzana, CA 91357
818-705-3660
http://www.westsiderc.org/f/sg_osg.htm
Disability Served: various
This organization helps families of children with special needs.

Pioneer Center of McHenry County

4001 Dayton Street
McHenry, IL 60050
815-344-1230
http://www.pioneercenter.org
Disability Served: developmentally disabled, mental health, traumatic brain injury
This agency provides case management and residential and vocational services to adults with mental illness, developmental disabilities, or traumatic brain injuries. It also offers early intervention services to children with developmental disabilities.

Post-Polio Health International

4207 Lindell Boulevard, #110
St Louis, MO 63108-2915
314-534-0475
info@post-polio.org
http://www.post-polio.org
Disability Served: various
The institute provides information, newsletters, educational materials, and resources for people with disabilities, especially survivors of polio and users of home mechanical ventilation.

Presbyterian Health, Education and Welfare Association

100 Witherspoon Street, #4617
Louisville, KY 40202
502-569-5800, 888-728-7228, ext. 5800
ntroy@pcusa.org
http://www.pcusa.org/phewa/about.htm
Disability Served: various
The association provides support services as well as information and referral for persons with disabilities.

R. A. Bloch Cancer Foundation Inc.

4400 Main Street
Kansas City, MO 64111
800-433-0464
hotline@hrblock.com
http://www.blochcancer.org
Disability Served: cancer patients and survivors
This organization matches newly diagnosed cancer patients with survivors of the same type of cancer. It also offers the following free books: *Fighting Cancer* (also available in Spanish), *Cancer . . . There's Hope*, and *Guide for Cancer Supporters*.

Rainbow Alliance of the Deaf

309 Millside Drive
Columbus, OH 43230
president@rad.org
http://www.rad.org
Disability Served: hearing
This organization provides support services to persons with hearing impairments who are members of the gay and lesbian community.

Recording for the Blind and Dyslexic

20 Roszel Road
Princeton, NJ 08540
866-RFBD-585, 800-221-4792
http://www.rfbd.org
Disability Served: dyslexic, vision
This nonprofit organization provides recorded books for persons with visual impairments and dyslexia.

Reginald S. Lourie Center for Infants and Young Children

Therapeutic Nursery Program
12301 Academy Way
Rockville, MD 20852
301-984-4444
http://www.louriecenter.org/beta/lc/index.html
Disability Served: emotionally disabled adolescents
The therapeutic nursery program is a specialized preschool that addresses the needs of young children three to five years of age who have emotional and behavioral problems that may interfere with success in a regular preschool or day care setting.

Rehabilitation Opportunities

5100 Philadelphia Way, #A
Lanham, MD 20706
301-731-4242
generalinfo@roiworks.org
http://www.roiworks.org
Disability Served: developmentally disabled, physical disabled
This organization provides workshops, evaluation, and day and work adjustment programs for persons with developmental disabilities.

Rehabilitation Research and Training Center on Blindness and Low Vision

Mississippi State University
PO Drawer 6189

Mississippi State, MS 39762
662-325-2001, 662-325-8693 (TDD)
jemoore@colled.msstate.edu
http://www.blind.msstate.edu
Disability Served: vision
This center conducts research and training activities
that prevent or alleviate the vocational, personal,
and economic effects of blindness.

Resources for Rehabilitation
22 Bonad Road
Winchester, MA 01890
781-368-9094
info@rfr.org
http://www.rfr.org
Disability Served: various
This organization provides training and resources to
professionals and the public about the needs of
people with disabilities. Publications on various
disabilities and issues are offered.

Rhode Island Parent Information Network Inc. (RIPIN)
175 Main Street
Pawtucket, RI 02860
401-727-4144, 800-464-3399
heffernan@ripin.org
http://www.ripin.org
Disability Served: various
RIPIN is a training and information center for parents
of children with disabilities. It provides information,
support, guidance, training, and consultation
services.

Rock Creek Foundation
700 Roeder Road, 6th Floor
Silver Spring, MD 20910-4457
301-589-8303, 301-925-2735 (TTY/TTD)
http://ddamaryland.org/rockCreek.htm
Disability Served: chemical dependency, developmentally
disabled, mental health
The foundation provides a variety of services for adults
with development disabilities, chronic mental illness,
and substance abuse. It also operates a national
training program for professionals who serve people
with these disabilities.

Rocky Mountain ADA Technical Assistance Center
3630 Sinton Road, Suite 103
Colorado Springs, CO 80907-5072

719-444-0268, 800-949-4232
rmdbtac@mtc-inc.com
http://www.adainformation.org
Disability Served: various
This Americans with Disabilities Act information center
provides technical assistance, materials, training, and
referral for residents of the Rocky Mountain states.

Ronald McDonald House Charities
1 Kroc Drive
Oak Brook, IL 60523
630-623-7048
http://www.rmhc.org
Disability Served: various
This organization provides temporary housing for
families of children hospitalized in nearby facilities.
There are more than 150 Ronald McDonald houses
in nine countries. McDonald's owners, local
businesses, civic organizations, members of the
medical community, and other volunteers run each
house.

Rum River Special Education Cooperative
315 17th Lane, NE
Cambridge, MN 55008
763-689-3600
http://www.cambridge.k12.mn.us/~rumriversec
Disability Served: various
This program is operated by a Minnesota school district
and provides services, including school psychology,
occupational and physical therapy, and vision and
hearing testing, to disabled students within three
Minnesota counties.

San Diego Regional Center (SDRC)
4355 Ruffin Road, Suite 200
San Diego, CA 92123
858-576-2996
http://www.sdrc.org
Disability Served: developmentally disabled
The SDRC offers support and education for people
with developmental disabilities and their families.

Scottish Rite Center for Childhood Language Disorders
Children's Hospital
1630 Columbia Road, NW
Washington, DC 20009
202-939-4703

http://www.srmason-sj.org/council/temple/booklet/
cldp.htm
Disability Served: communication, hearing
The center provides evaluations, consultations,
treatment services, and more, for children with
hearing and language disorders.

The Seeing Eye
PO Box 375
Morristown, NJ 07963-0375
973-539-4425
info@seeingeye.org
http://www.seeingeye.org
Disability Served: vision
This organization breeds, raises, and trains dogs as
guides for blind people and instructs blind people
in the proper use and care of the dogs.

Sign Language Associates Inc.
11002 Veirs Mill Road, Suite 506
Silver Spring, MD 20910-3803
301-946-9710
http://www.signlanguage.com
Disability Served: hearing
This organization provides sign language interpreting
services to local and national clients. It also offers
on-demand remote interpreting services, emergency
response systems, and professional education
programs.

Simon Foundation for Continence
PO Box 815
Wilmette, IL 60091
847-864-3913, 800-237-4666
cbgartley@simonfoundation.org
http://www.simonfoundation.org
Disability Served: physically disabled
This organization provides information on incontinence.

Slingerland Institute
One Bellevue Center
411 108th Avenue NE, Suite 560
Bellevue, WA 98004
425-453-1190
mail@slingerland.org
http://www.slingerland.org
Disability Served: dyslexia
This organization provides teacher education in the
identification, diagnosis, and teaching of children
and adults with dyslexia.

Southeast Missouri Easter Seal Society
PO Box 366
Cape Girardeau, MO 63701
573-335-3377
Disability Served: various
The society provides an early learning center and an
early intervention program in southeast Missouri
for children at risk as well as those with a diagnosed
disability.

Special Interest on Accessible Computing
Association for Computing Machinery
1515 Broadway
New York, NY 10036
212-626-0500, 800-342-6626
http://www.acm.org/sigaccess
Disability Served: physically disabled
This organization provides information, resources,
and advocacy services for computer users who
are physically disabled.

Spina Bifida Association of America
4590 MacArthur Boulevard, NW, Suite 250
Washington, DC 20007-4226
202-944-3285, 800-621-3141
sbaa@sbaa.org
http://www.sbaa.org
Disability Served: spina bifida
The association provides information and referral,
counseling, support services, and more, for the
spina bifida population.

Stuttering Foundation of America
PO Box 11749
Memphis, TN 38111-0749
800-992-9392
info@stutteringhelp.org
http://www.stutteringhelp.org
Disability Served: communication
This foundation provides a toll-free hotline on stuttering,
as well as information, books, and brochures.
Workshops and conferences on stuttering are also
offered.

Taping for the Blind Inc.
3935 Essex Lane
Houston, TX 77027
713-622-2767
http://www.tapingfortheblind.org
Disability Served: vision

This organization offers custom recording, radio reading, and audio description services.

Technology for Life and Learning Center
10 Quakerbridge Plaza
Trenton, NJ 08625
609-588-3157, 609-584-4355 (TTY)
http://www.state.nj.us/humanservices/ooe/tllc.html
Disability Served: communication
The center provides a multidisciplinary assessment for augmentative communication devices and other assistive technologies. A loan program is also available.

Telecommunications for the Deaf Inc.
8630 Fenton Street, #604
Silver Spring, MD 20910
301-589-3786, 301-589-3006
info@tdi-online.org
http://www.tdi-online.org
Disability Served: hearing
This organization disseminates information on telecommunications issues and regulations regarding persons with hearing impairments.

Tourette Syndrome Association
42-40 Bell Boulevard
Bayside, NY 11361-2820
718-224-2999, 800-237-0717
ts@tsa-usa.org
http://tsa-usa.org
Disability Served: Tourette Syndrome
The association disseminates information and educational materials regarding Tourette Syndrome. It also hosts seminars, conferences, and support groups for its members.

Trace Research and Development Center
2107 Engineering Centers Building,
    1550 Engineering Drive
Madison, WI 53706
608-262-6966, 608-263-5408 (TTY)
info@trace.wisc.edu
http://trace.wisc.edu
Disability Served: various
The Trace Center focuses on making off-the-shelf technologies and systems more usable for everyone. The center's work is in great part funded through the National Institute on Disability and Rehabilitation Research, which is part of the U.S. Department of Education. Trace is designated as the Rehabilitation Engineering Research Center (RERC) on information technology access and is also a partner in the RERC on universal telecommunications access.

Travelin' Talk Network
travelin@travelintalk.net
http://www.travelintalk.net
Disability Served: various
This Web site is a global meeting place for the disabled and the non-disabled who are interested in learning more about travel.

United Cerebral Palsy Association
1660 L Street, NW, Suite 700
Washington, DC 20036
202-776-0406, 800-872-5827
http://www.ucp.org
Disability Served: cerebral palsy
This national organization provides a number of services for persons with cerebral palsy and their families, including information and referral, counseling, grant funding, advocacy services, and more.

United States Association for Blind Athletes
Brown Hall, 33 North Institute Street
Colorado Springs, CO 80903
719-630-0422
http://www.usaba.org
Disability Served: vision
This athletic association represents blind athletes.

United States International Council on Disability
1630 Connecticut Avenue, NW, Suite 201
Washington, DC 20009
202-462-1893
usicd@earthlink.net
http://www.usicd.org
Disability Served: various
This organization's goal is to create an international standard for rehabilitation programs for persons with disabilities.

The University of Montana Rural Institute: Center for Excellence in Disability Education, Research, and Service
52 Corbin Hall
Missoula, MT 59812-7056
406-243-5467
rural@ruralinstitute.umt.edu

http://www.ruralinstitute.umt.edu
Disability Served: various
This research and training center provides training in rural employment, economic development strategies, health and wellness for people with disabilities, and rural accessible transportation models.

Variety Club
1520 Locust Street, Suite 900
Philadelphia, PA 19102-4496
215-735-0803
http://www.varietyphila.org
Disability Served: various
The club provides advocacy and services, including assessment and computer training, for children with disabilities.

Vision World Wide Inc.
5707 Brockton Drive, Suite 302
Indianapolis, IN 46220-5481
317-254-1332
info@visionww.org
http://www.visionww.org
Disability Served: vision
This nonprofit organization provides information and referrals for the vision impaired through a worldwide telephone and Internet service; training; and publications. The organization also publishes an online journal, *Vision Enhancement.*

Volunteers for Medical Engineering Inc. (VME)
2301 Argonne Drive
Baltimore, MD 21218
410-243-7495
vme@toad.net
http://www.toad.net/~vme
Disability Served: various
VME is an organization of volunteers working to improve the independence of individuals with disabilities through uniquely engineered solutions. Services include custom devices, modifications, and computer loans.

VSA Arts
818 Connecticut Avenue, NW, Suite 600
Washington, DC 20006
202-628-2800, 800-933-8721
info@vsarts.org
http://www.vsarts.org
Disability Served: various
This organization promotes arts, education, and creative expression involving children and adults with disabilities.

West Coast Cued Speech Programs
348 Cernon Street, Suite D
Vacaville, CA 95688
707-448-4060
http://www.cuedspeech.org/sub/about/affiliates.asp
Disability Served: hearing
This organization provides information, resources, support services, and cued speech training to persons who are hearing impaired.

Wheelchair Sports, USA
1668 320th Way
Earlham, IA 50072
515-833-2450
wsusa@aol.com
http://www.wsusa.org
Disability Served: physically disabled
This is an association for wheelchair athletics.

Winners on Wheels
302 East Church Street
Lewisville, TX 75057
800-WOW-TALK
info@wowusa.com
http://www.wowusa.com
Disability Served: physically disabled
This organization seeks to empower children who are in wheelchairs through creative learning and expanded life experiences.

World Association of Persons with Disabilities (WAPD)
5016 Alan Lane
Oklahoma City, OK 73135
405-672-4440
http://www.wapd.org
Disability Served: various
This nonprofit organization provides information and support to people with disabilities. The WAPD's Web site serves as a clearinghouse for information about disabilities.

World Institute on Disability (WID)
510 16th Street, Suite 100
Oakland, CA 94612

510-763-4100
wid@wid.org
http://www.wid.org
Disability Served: *various*
The WID is a nonprofit research and public policy
center that promotes the civil rights and full societal
inclusion of people with disabilities. It focuses on
four areas: employment-development, health access,
inclusive technology design, and international
disability and development.

World Recreation Association of the Deaf Inc.
PO Box 3211
Quartz Hill, CA 93586
wradceo@aol.com
http://www.wrad.org
Disability Served: *hearing*
The association promotes recreational and cultural
activities for the hearing impaired.

WTFUSA
2351 Parkwood Road
Snellville, GA 30039
770-972-1298
bewing@bellsouth.net
Disability Served: *physically disabled*
WTFUSA is an association for wheelchair athletics.

TECHNOLOGY ACCESS ORGANIZATIONS

Technology access organizations—many of which are jointly sponsored by the Alliance for Technology Access and Microsoft—provide assistive technology information and support services to children and adults with disabilities.

ALABAMA

Birmingham Alliance for Technology Access Center
206 13th Street South
Birmingham, AL 35233
205-251-2223 (Voice/TTY)
bilc@bellsouth.net
http://www.birminghamilc.org
Disability Served: various

Technology Assistance for Special Consumers
915 Monroe Street, PO Box 443
Huntsville, AL 35804
205-532-5996
tasc@hiwaay.net
http://tasc.ataccess.org
Disability Served: various

ARIZONA

Technology Access Center of Tucson Inc.
4710 East 29th Street, PO Box 13178
Tucson, AZ 85732-3178
520-745-5588, ext. 412
tactaz@aol.com
http://www.ed.arizona.edu/tact
Disability Served: various

ARKANSAS

Technology Resource Center
c/o Arkansas Easter Seal Society
3920 Woodland Heights Road
Little Rock, AR 72212
501-227-3600
crctech@ar.seaterseals.com
http://www.iser.com/easterseal-AR.html
Disability Served: various

CALIFORNIA

Alliance for Technology Access
1304 Southpoint Boulevard, Suite 240
Petaluma, CA 94954
707-778-3011, 707-778-3015 (TTY)

ATAinfo@ATAccess.org
http://www.ATAccess.org
Disability Served: various

Center for Accessible Technology
2547 8th Street, #12A
Berkeley, CA 94710
510-841-3224, 510-841-5621 (TTY)
info@cforat.org
http://www.cforat.org
Disability Served: various

Computer Access Center
6234 West 87th Street
Los Angeles, CA 90045
310-388-1597
info@cac.org
http://www.cac.org
Disability Served: various

iTECH-Parents Helping Parents
3041 Olcott Street
Santa Clara, CA 95054-3222
408-727-5775
iTech@php.com
http://www.php.com
Disability Served: various

Kern Assistive Technology Center
3101 North Sillect Avenue, Suite 101
Bakersfield, CA 93308
661-852-3399, 661-852-3336 (TTY)
katc2003@sbcglobal.net
Disability Served: various

SACC Assistive Technology Center
Simi Valley Hospital, Rehabilitation North, PO Box 1325
Simi Valley, CA 93062
805-582-1881
Disability Served: various

Sacramento Center for Assistive Technology
4370 Mather School Road
Sacramento, CA 95655-0301
916-361-0553

scatca@aol.com
Disability Served: various

San Diego Assistive Technology Center
c/o United Cerebral Palsy Association
6153 Fairmount Avenue, Suite 150
San Diego, CA 92120
858-278-5420
sdatc@ucpsd.org
http://www.ucpsd.org
Disability Served: various

Special Technology Center
590 Castro Street
Mountain View, CA 94041
650-961-6789
Disability Served: various

Team of Advocates for Special Kids-Main Office
100 Cerritos Avenue
Anaheim, CA 92805
714-533-8275
taskca@yahoo.com
http://www.taskca.org
Disability Served: various

Team of Advocates for Special Kids-San Diego Branch Office
4550 Kearney Villa Road, #102
San Diego, CA 92123
858-874-2386
taskca@yahoo.com
http://www.taskca.org
Disability Served: various

DISTRICT OF COLUMBIA
District of Columbia Assistive Technology Program
810 First Street, NE, 9th Floor
Washington, DC 20002
202-589-0288, 202-589-1260 (TTY)
democenter@mindspring.com
http://www.atpdc.org
Disability Served: various

FLORIDA
Florida Alliance for Assistive Services and Technology
Building 400, 325 John Knox Road
Tallahassee, FL 32303

850-487-3278, 888-788-9216
faast@faast.org
http://www.faast.org
Disability Served: various

Lighthouse Central Florida Inc.
215 East New Hampshire Street
Orlando, FL 32804
407-898-2483
citeinfo@cite-fl.com
http://www.lighthousecentralflorida.org
Disability Served: various

GEORGIA
Tech-Able Inc.
1114 Brett Drive
Conyers, GA 30094
770-922-6768, 770-922-6768 (TTY)
techweb@techable.org
http://www.techable.org
Disability Served: various

HAWAII
Aloha Special Technology Access Center
710 Green Street
Honolulu, HI 96813
808-523-5547
astachi@yahoo.com
http://www.geocities.com/astachi
Disability Served: various

Assistive Technology Resource Centers of Hawaii
414 Kuwili Street, Suite 104
Honolulu, HI 96817
808-532-7110 (Voice/TTY)
atrc-info@atrc.org
http://www.atrc.org
Disability Served: various

IDAHO
United Cerebral Palsy of Idaho Inc.
5420 West Franklin Road, Suite A
Boise, ID 83705
208-377-8070, 888-289-3259
info@ucpidaho.org
http://www.ucp.org/ucp_local.cfm/66
Disability Served: various

ILLINOIS

Northern Illinois Center for Adaptive Technology
3615 Louisiana Road
Rockford, IL 61108-6195
815-229-2163
davegrass@earthlink.net
http://nicat.ataccess.org
Disability Served: various

Technical Aids and Assistance for the Disabled Center
1950 West Roosevelt Road
Chicago, IL 60608
312-421-3373, 800-346-2939
Disability Served: various

INDIANA

Assistive Technology Training and Information Center
1721 Washington Avenue
Vincennes, IN 47591
812-886-0575, 877-96-ATTIC
inattic1@aol.com
http://www.wvc.net/~attic
Disability Served: various

KANSAS

Missouri Assistive Technology Program
Coalition for Independence, 4911 State Avenue
Kansas City, KS 66102
913-321-5140, 913-321-5216 (TTY)
http://cfi-kc.org
Disability Served: various

Technology Resource Solutions for People
1710 West Schilling Road
Salina, KS 67402-1160
785-827-9383 (Voice/TDD)
occk@occk.com
http://www.occk.com
Disability Served: various

KENTUCKY

AbleTech Assistive Technology Resource Center
36 West Fifth Street
Covington, KY 41011
800-209-7112

abletech@unidial.com
Disability Served: various

Bluegrass Technology Center
961 Beasley Street, Suite 103A
Lexington, KY 40509
859-294-4343, 800-209-7767
office@bluegrass-tech.org
http://www.bluegrass-tech.org
Disability Served: various

Enabling Technologies of Kentuckiana
Administration Building, 851 South 4th Street, Room 011
Louisville, KY 40203
502-585-9911, 800-896-8941, ext. 2648
rstacy@spaulding.edu
Disability Served: various

Western Kentucky Assistive Technology Center
815 Triplett Street
Owensboro, KY 42303
270-689-1738
wkatcmurray@yahoo.com
http://wkatc.org
Disability Served: various

MAINE

Maine Assistive Technology Program
Maine Department of Labor
Portland Career Center, 150 State House Station
Augusta, ME 04333
207-624-5956
http://www.mainecareercenter.com
Disability Served: various

Technical Exploration Center
Evergreen Woods, 700 Mount Hope Avenue, Suite 302
Bangor, ME 04401
877-603-0030
lynn@tecmaine.org
Disability Served: various

MARYLAND

Learning Independence Through Computers Inc.
1001 Eastern Avenue, 3rd Floor
Baltimore, MD 21202
410-659-5462, 410-843-0219 (TTY)

info@linc.org
http://www.linc.org
Disability Served: various

MASSACHUSETTS
Massachusetts Special Technology Access Center
12 Mudge Way 1-6
Bedford, MA 01730
617-275-2446
Disability Served: various

MICHIGAN
Living and Learning Resource Centre
601 West Maple Street
Lansing, MI 48906
517-487-0883, 800-833-1996
Disability Served: various

Michigan's Assistive Technology Resource
1023 South US 27, Suite B31
St Johns, MI 48879-2423
989-224-0333, 989-224-0246 (TTY)
matr@match.org
http://www.cenmi.org/matr
Disability Served: various

MINNESOTA
Minnesota STAR Program
50 Sherburne Avenue, Room 309
St Paul, MN 55155
651-201-2640, 888-234-1267
star.program@state.mn.us
http://www.admin.state.mn.us/assistivetechnology
Disability Served: various

PACER Computer Resource Center
8161 Normandale Boulevard
Minneapolis, MN 55437
952-838-9000, 952-838-0190 (TTY)
pacer@pacer.org
http://www.pacer.org/stc
Disability Served: various

MISSOURI
Technology Access Center
12110 Clayton Road
Town and Country, MO 63131

314-989-8404, 314-989-8446 (TTY)
mostltac@aol.com
http://stlouis.missouri.org/501c/mostltac
Disability Served: various

MONTANA
Montana Technology Access Center
634 Eddy Avenue, CHS 009
Missoula, MT 59812
406-243-5467
http://montech.ruralinstitute.umt.edu
Disability Served: various

Parents, Let's Unite for Kids
526 North 32nd Street
Billings, MT 59101
406-255-0540, 800-222-7585
plukinfo@pluk.org
http://www.pluk.org
Disability Served: various

NEW HAMPSHIRE
Assistive Technology, Education and Community Health
67 Communications Drive
Laconia, NH 03246
603-528-3060, 800-932-5837
http://www.nhassistivetechnology.org
Disability Served: various

NEW JERSEY
Center for Enabling Technology
622 Route 10 West, Suite 22B
Whippany, NJ 07981
973-428-1455, 973-428-1450 (TTY)
cetnj@aol.com
Disability Served: various

TECHConnection
35 Haddon Avenue
Shrewsbury, NJ 07702
732-747-5310
info@techconnection.org
http://www.techconnection.org
Disability Served: various

NEW YORK

New York Assistive Technology Program-ENABLE
1603 Court Street
Syracuse, NY 13208
315-455-7591, 315-455-1794 (TTY)
info@enablecny.org
http://www.enablecny.org
Disability Served: various

Resource Center for Independent Living
401-409 Columbia Street, PO Box 210
Utica, NY 13503-0210
315-797-4642
tamara.marrioti@rcil.com
http://www.rcil.com
Disability Served: various

NORTH CAROLINA

Carolina Computer Access Center
401 East Ninth Street
Charlotte, NC 28202
704-342-3004
ccacnc@bellsouth.net
http://ccac.ataccess.org
Disability Served: various

North Carolina Assistive Technology Program
1110 Navaho Drive, Suite 101
Raleigh, NC 27609
919-850-2787
http://www.ncatp.org
Disability Served: various

NORTH DAKOTA

Pathfinder Parent Training and Information Center
1600 2nd Avenue, SW, Suite 19
Minot, ND 58701
701-837-7500, 800-245-5840
ndpath01@minot.ndak.net
http://www.pathfinder.minot.com
Disability Served: various

OHIO

Assistive Technology of Ohio
Building L, 445 East Dublin-Granville Road
Worthington, OH 43085

614-293-9134
atohio03@osu.edu
http://www.atohio.org
Disability Served: various

Technology Resource Center
1133 Edwin C. Moses Boulevard, #370
Dayton, OH 45408-2094
937-461-3305
k.leonard@goodwilldayton.org
http://www.trcd.org
Disability Served: various

OREGON

Access Technologies Inc.
3070 Lancaster Drive, NE
Salem, OR 97305
503-361-1201 (Voice/TTY)
http://www.accesstechnologiesinc.org
Disability Served: various

RHODE ISLAND

TechACCESS of Rhode Island
110 Jefferson Boulevard, Suite I
Warwick, RI 02888-3854
401-463-0202, 800-916-TECH
techaccess@techaccess-ri.org
http://techaccess-ri.org
Disability Served: various

SOUTH DAKOTA

Career Learning Center of the Black Hills
730 East Watertown Street
Rapid City, SD 57701
605-394-5120
http://www.clcbh.org
Disability Served: various

TENNESSEE

East Tennessee Technology Access Center
4918 North Broadway
Knoxville, TN 37918
865-219-0130 (Voice/TTY)
etstactn@aol.com
http://www.korrnet.org/ettac
Disability Served: various

Mid-South Access Center for Technology
University of Memphis, Patterson Hall, Room 119
Memphis, TN 38152
901-678-1489
act@memphis.edu
http://coe.memphis.edu/ACT/midsouthaccess.htm
Disability Served: various

Signal Center's Assistive Technology Center
.109 North Germantown Road
Chattanooga, TN 37411
423-698-8528
info@signal.chattanooga.net
http://www.signalcenters.org
Disability Served: various

Technology Access Center of Middle Tennessee
2222 Metrocenter Boulevard, Suite 126
Nashville, TN 37221
615-248-6733, 800-368-4651, 615-248-6733 (TTY)
techaccess@mindstate.com
http://tac.ataccess.org
Disability Served: various

**West Tennessee Special Technology Access
  Resource Center**
The STAR Center, 1119 Old Humboldt Road
Jackson, TN 38305
731-668-3888, 800-464-5619
information@starcenter.tn.org
http://www.starcenter.tn.org
Disability Served: various

UTAH
Computer Center for Citizens with Disabilities
1595 West 500 South
Salt Lake City, UT 84104
801-887-9533, 888-866-5550
cboogaar@utah.gov
http://www.usor.utah.gov/ucat/computers.htm
Disability Served: various

VIRGINIA
Tidewater Center for Technology Access
1413 Laskin Road
Virginia Beach, VA 23451
757-437-6542
tcta@aol.com

http://tcta.ataccess.org
Disability Served: various

WASHINGTON
Center for Technology and Disabilities Studies
University of Washington, Box 357920
Seattle, WA 98195-7920
206-685-4181 (Voice/TTY)
uwctds@u.washington.edu
http://uwctds.washington.edu
Disability Served: various

Microsoft Accessibility Resource Centers
One Microsoft Way
Redmond, WA 98052-6399
http://www.microsoft.com/enable/centers
Disability Served: various

WEST VIRGINIA
Eastern Panhandle Technology Access Center Inc.
300 South Lawrence Street, PO Box 987
Charles Town, WV 25414
304-725-6473
eptac@webcombo.net
http://eptac.ataccess.org
Disability Served: various

WISCONSIN
IndependenceFirst
600 West Virginia Street, 4th Floor
Milwaukee, WI 53204-1516
414-291-7520 (Voice/TTY)
http://www.independencefirst.org
Disability Served: various

VETERANS ORGANIZATIONS

This is a listing of Veterans Administration Medical Centers and regional offices.

ALABAMA

Veterans Administration Medical Center-Birmingham
700 South 19th Street
Birmingham, AL 35233
205-933-8101
http://www1.va.gov/directory/guide/facility.
    asp?ID=16&dnum=ALL&map=1
Disability Served: various

Veterans Administration Medical Center-Montgomery
215 Perry Hill Road
Montgomery, AL 36109
334-272-4670
http://www1.va.gov/directory/guide/facility.
    asp?ID=91&dnum=ALL&map=1
Disability Served: various

Veterans Administration Medical Center-Tuscaloosa
3701 Loop Road East
Tuscaloosa, AL 35404
205-554-2000
http://www1.va.gov/directory
Disability Served: various

Veterans Administration Medical Center-Tuskegee
2400 Hospital Road
Tuskegee, AL 36083-5001
334-727-0550
http://www1.va.gov/directory
Disability Served: various

ALASKA

**Veterans Administration Medical Center-and
    Regional Office**
2925 DeBarr Road
Anchorage, AK 99508
907-257-4700, 888-353-7574
http://www1.va.gov/directory
Disability Served: various

ARIZONA

Veterans Administration Medical Center-Phoenix
Carl T. Hayden VA Medical Center
650 East Indian School Road
Phoenix, AZ 85012-1892

602-277-5551
kristi.miller@med.va.gov
http://www.phoenix.med.va.gov
Disability Served: various

Veterans Administration Medical Center-Prescott
500 North Highway 89
Prescott, AZ 86313
520-445-4860
http://www1.va.gov/directory
Disability Served: various

Veterans Administration Medical Center-Tucson
3601 South Sixth Avenue
Tucson, AZ 85723
520-792-1450, 800-470-8262
http://www.va.gov/678savahcs
Disability Served: various

Veterans Administration Regional Office-Phoenix
3225 North Central Avenue
Phoenix, AZ 85012
800-827-1000
http://www1.va.gov/directory
Disability Served: various

ARKANSAS

Veterans Administration Medical Center-Fayetteville
1100 North College Avenue
Fayetteville, AR 72703
479-443-4301
http://www1.va.gov/directory
Disability Served: various

Veterans Administration Medical Center-Little Rock
John L. McClellan Memorial Veterans Hospital
4300 West 7th Street
Little Rock, AR 72205-5484
501-257-1000
http://www1.va.gov/directory
Disability Served: various

**Veterans Administration Regional Office-
    North Little Rock**
Building 65, 2200 Fort Roots Drive
North Little Rock, AR 72114-1756

800-827-1000
http://www1.va.gov/directory
Disability Served: various

CALIFORNIA

Veterans Administration Medical Center-Fresno
2615 East Clinton Avenue
Fresno, CA 93703
559-225-6100
http://www1.va.gov/directory
Disability Served: various

Veterans Administration Medical Center-Livermore
4951 Arroyo Road
Livermore, CA 94550
925-373-4700
http://www1.va.gov/directory
Disability Served: various

Veterans Administration Medical Center-Loma Linda
11201 Benton Street
Loma Linda, CA 92357
909-825-7084
http://www1.va.gov/directory
Disability Served: various

Veterans Administration Medical Center-Long Beach
5901 East Seventh Street
Long Beach, CA 90822
562-826-8000
http://www1.va.gov/directory
Disability Served: various

Veterans Administration Medical Center-Los Angeles
11301 Willshire Boulevard
Los Angeles, CA 90073
310-478-3711
http://www1.va.gov/directory
Disability Served: various

Veterans Administration Medical Center-Menlo Park
795 Willow Road
Menlo Park, CA 94025
650-493-5000
http://www1.va.gov/directory
Disability Served: various

Veterans Administration Medical Center-Palo Alto
3801 Miranda Avenue
Palo Alto, CA 94304-1290
650-493-5000
http://www.palo-alto.med.va.gov
Disability Served: various

Veterans Administration Medical Center-Sacramento
10535 Hospital Way
Sacramento, CA 95655
916-366-5366
http://www1.va.gov/directory
Disability Served: various

Veterans Administration Medical Center-San Diego
3350 La Jolla Village Drive
San Diego, CA 92161
858-552-8585, 800-331-8387, 858-552-7541 (TDD)
http://www.san-diego.med.va.gov/start.htm
Disability Served: various

Veterans Administration Medical Center-San Francisco
4150 Clement Street
San Francisco, CA 94121
415-221-4810
http://www.sf.med.va.gov
Disability Served: various

Veterans Administration Regional Office-Los Angeles
Federal Building
11000 Wilshire Boulevard
Los Angeles, CA 90024
800-827-1000
http://www1.va.gov/directory
Disability Served: various

Veterans Administration Regional Office-Oakland
1301 Clay Street, Room 1300 North
Oakland, CA 94612
800-827-1000
http://www1.va.gov/directory
Disability Served: various

Veterans Administration Regional Office-San Diego
8810 Rio San Diego Drive
San Diego, CA 92108
800-827-1000
http://www1.va.gov/directory
Disability Served: various

COLORADO

Veterans Administration Medical Center-Grand Junction
2121 North Avenue
Grand Junction, CO 81501
970-242-0731,866-206-6415
http://www1.va.gov/directory
Disability Served: various

Veterans Administration Regional Office-Denver (Lakewood)
155 Van Gordon Street, PO Box 25126
Lakewood, CO 80228
800-827-1000
http://www1.va.gov/directory
Disability Served: various

CONNECTICUT

Veterans Administration Medical Center-Newington
555 Willard Avenue
Newington, CT 06111
860-666-6951
http://www.visn1.med.va.gov/vact
Disability Served: various

Veterans Administration Medical Center-West Haven
950 Campbell Avenue
West Haven, CT 06516
203-932-5711
http://www.visn1.med.va.gov/vact
Disability Served: various

Veterans Administration Regional Office-Hartford
450 Main Street
Hartford, CT 06103
800-827-1000
http://www1.va.gov/directory
Disability Served: various

DELAWARE

Veterans Administration Regional Office-Wilmington
1601 Kirkwood Highway
Wilmington, DE 19805
302-994-2511, 800-827-1000
http://www1.va.gov/directory
Disability Served: various

DISTRICT OF COLUMBIA

Veterans Administration Medical Center-Washington, D.C.
50 Irving Street, NW
Washington, DC 20422
202-745-8000
http://www1.va.gov/washington
Disability Served: various

Veterans Administration Regional Office-Washington, D.C.
1722 I Street, NW
Washington, DC 20421
800-827-1000
http://www1.va.gov/directory
Disability Served: various

FLORIDA

Veterans Administration Medical Center-Bay Pines
10000 Bay Pines Boulevard, North
Bay Pines, FL 33744
727-398-6661
http://www.visn8.med.va.gov/baypines
Disability Served: various

Veterans Administration Medical Center-Gainesville
Malcom Randall VA Medical Center
1601 Southwest Archer Road
Gainesville, FL 32608-1197
352-376-1611, 800-324-8387
http://www.visn8.med.va.gov/nfsg
Disability Served: various

Veterans Administration Medical Center-Lake City
619 South Marion Avenue
Lake City, FL 32025-5808
386-755-3016, 800-308-8387
http://www.visn8.med.va.gov/nfsg/facilities/
  LakeCity.asp
Disability Served: various

Veterans Administration Medical Center-Miami
1201 Northwest 16th Street
Miami, FL 33125
305-575-7000
http://www.visn8.med.va.gov/miami
Disability Served: various

Veterans Administration Medical Center-Tampa
James A. Haley VA Medical Center
13000 Bruce B. Downs Boulevard
Tampa, FL 33612
813-972-2000
http://www.visn8.med.va.gov/Tampa
Disability Served: various

Veterans Administration Medical Center-West Palm Beach
7305 North Military Trail
West Palm Beach, FL 33410-6400
561-882-8262
http://www.visn8.med.va.gov/westpalm
Disability Served: various

Veterans Administration Regional Office-St Petersburg
9500 Bay Pines Boulevard
St Petersburg, FL 33708
800-827-1000
http://www.vba.va.gov/ro/south/spete
Disability Served: various

GEORGIA
Veterans Administration Medical Center-Augusta
One Freedom Way
Augusta, GA 30904-6285
706-733-0188
http://www1.va.gov/directory
Disability Served: various

Veterans Administration Medical Center-Decatur
1670 Clairmont Road
Decatur, GA 30033
404-321-6111
Bart.Lewis@med.va.gov
http://www1.va.gov/atlanta
Disability Served: various

Veterans Administration Medical Center-Dublin
Carl Vinson VA Medical Center
1826 Veteran's Boulevard
Dublin, GA 31021
912-272-1210
http://www1.va.gov/directory
Disability Served: various

Veterans Administration Regional Office-Atlanta
1700 Clairmont Road
Decatur, GA 30033

800-827-1000
http://www.vba.va.gov/ro/atlanta/rlc/index.htm
Disability Served: various

HAWAII
Veterans Administration Medical Center-Honolulu
459 Patterson Road
Honolulu, HI 96819-1522
808-433-0600
http://www.va.gov/hawaii
Disability Served: various

Veterans Administration Regional Office-Honolulu
459 Patterson Road, E-Wing
Honolulu, HI 96819-1522
808-566-1000
http://www.va.gov/hawaii
Disability Served: various

IDAHO
Veterans Administration Medical Center-Boise
500 West Fort Street
Boise, ID 83702
208-422-1000
http://www1.va.gov/directory
Disability Served: various

Veterans Administration Regional Office-Boise
805 West Franklin Street
Boise, ID 83702
208-334-1245
http://www1.va.gov/directory
Disability Served: various

ILLINOIS
Veterans Administration Medical Center-Chicago Westside
Jesse Brown VA Medical Center
820 South Damen Avenue
Chicago, IL 60612
312-569-8387
http://www.visn12.med.va.gov/chicago
Disability Served: various

Veterans Administration Medical Center-Danville
1900 East Main Street
Danville, IL 61832-5198

217-442-8200
http://www1.va.gov/directory
Disability Served: various

Veterans Administration Medical Center-Hines
Edward Hines Jr. VA Hospital
Fifth & Roosevelt Road, PO Box 5000
Hines, IL 60141
708-202-8387
http://www.visn12.med.va.gov/hines
Disability Served: various

Veterans Administration Medical Center-Marion, IL
2401 West Main Street
Marion, IL 62959
618-997-5311
http://www1.va.gov/directory
Disability Served: various

Veterans Administration Medical Center-North Chicago
3001 Green Bay Road
North Chicago, IL 60064
847-688-1900
http://www1.va.gov/directory
Disability Served: various

Veterans Administration Regional Office-Chicago
2122 West Taylor Street
Chicago, IL 60612
800-827-1000
http://www1.va.gov/directory
Disability Served: various

INDIANA
Veterans Administration Medical Center-Fort Wayne
2121 Lake Avenue
Ft Wayne, IN 46805
260-426-5431
http://www1.va.gov/directory
Disability Served: various

Veterans Administration Medical Center-Indianapolis
Richard L. Roudebush VA Medical Center
1481 West Tenth Street
Indianapolis, IN 46202
317-554-0000
http://www1.va.gov/directory
Disability Served: various

Veterans Administration Regional Office-Indianapolis
575 North Pennsylvania Street
Indianapolis, IN 46204
800-827-1000
http://www1.va.gov/directory
Disability Served: various

IOWA
Veterans Administration Medical Center-Des Moines
3600 30th Street
Des Moines, IA 50310-5774
515-699-5999
http://www1.va.gov/directory
Disability Served: various

Veterans Administration Medical Center-Iowa City
601 Highway 6 West
Iowa City, IA 52246-2208
319-338-0581, 800-637-0128
http://www.iowa-city.med.va.gov
Disability Served: various

Veterans Administration Medical Center-Knoxville
1515 West Pleasant Street
Knoxville, IA 50138
515-842-3101
http://www1.va.gov/directory
Disability Served: various

Veterans Administration Regional Office-Des Moines
210 Walnut Street
Des Moines, IA 50309
800-827-1000
http://www1.va.gov/directory
Disability Served: various

KANSAS
Veterans Administration Medical Center-Leavenworth
Dwight D. Eisenhower VA Medical Center
4101 South 4th Street
Leavenworth, KS 66048-5055
913-682-2000
http://www1.va.gov/directory
Disability Served: various

Veterans Administration Medical Center-Topeka
Colmery-O'Neil VA Medical Center
2200 Southwest Gage Boulevard

Topeka, KS 66622
785-350-3111
http://www1.va.gov/directory
Disability Served: various

Veterans Administration Regional Office-Wichita

Robert J. Dole Department of Veterans Affairs Medical
    and Regional Office Center
5500 East Kellogg
Wichita, KS 67218
316-685-2221, 800-827-1000
http://www1.va.gov/directory
Disability Served: various

KENTUCKY
Veterans Administration Medical Center-Lexington

1101 Veterans Drive
Lexington, KY 40502-2236
859-233-4511
http://www1.va.gov/directory
Disability Served: various

Veterans Administration Medical Center-Louisville

800 Zorn Avenue
Louisville, KY 40206
502-287-4000, 800-376-8387
http://www.va.gov/603Louisville
Disability Served: various

Veterans Administration Regional Office-Louisville

545 South Third Street
Louisville, KY 40202
502-584-2231, 800-827-1000
http://www1.va.gov/directory
Disability Served: various

LOUISIANA
Veterans Administration Medical Center-Alexandria

PO Box 69004
Alexandria, LA 71306-9004
318-473-0010, 800-375-8387
barbara.watkins@med.va.gov
http://www.alexandria.med.va.gov
Disability Served: various

Veterans Administration Medical Center-Baton Rouge

7968 Essen Park Lane
Baton Rouge, LA 70808

504-568-0811
http://www1.va.gov/directory
Disability Served: various

Veterans Administration Medical Center-Shreveport

Overton Brooks VA Medical Center
510 East Stoner Avenue
Shreveport, LA 71101-4295
318-221-8411
http://www1.va.gov/directory
Disability Served: various

Veterans Administration Regional Office-New Orleans

701 Loyola Avenue
New Orleans, LA 70113
504-589-7191, 800-827-1000
neworleans.query@vba.va.gov
http://www.vba.va.gov/ro/new-orleans/index.htm
Disability Served: various

MAINE
Veterans Administration Medical Center-Augusta

1 VA Center
Augusta, ME 04330-6795
207-623-8411, 800-827-1000, 800-829-4833 (TDD)
Togus.query@vba.va.gov
http://www.vba.va.gov/ro/east/togus/index.htm
Disability Served: various

Veterans Administration Regional Office-Togus

1 VA Center
Augusta, ME 04330
207-623-8000, 877-421-8263
http://www.visn1.med.va.gov/togus
Disability Served: various

MARYLAND
Veterans Administration Medical Center-Baltimore

Baltimore Veterans Affairs Medical Center
10 North Greene Street
Baltimore, MD 21201
410-605-7000
http://www.vamhcs.med.va.gov
Disability Served: various

Veterans Administration Medical Center-Perry Point

Perry Point VA Medical Center
Perry Point, MD 21902

410-642-2411
http://www.vamhcs.med.va.gov
Disability Served: various

Veterans Administration Regional Office-Baltimore
31 Hopkins Plaza Federal Building
Baltimore, MD 21201
800-827-1000
http://www1.va.gov/directory
Disability Served: various

MASSACHUSETTS
Veterans Administration Medical Center-Bedford
Edith Nourse Rogers Memorial Veterans Hospital
200 Springs Road
Bedford, MA 01730
781-687-2000
http://www.visn1.med.va.gov/bedford
Disability Served: various

Veterans Administration Medical Center-Brockton
940 Belmont Street
Brockton, MA 02301
508-583-4500
http://www.visn1.med.va.gov/boston/brock.htm
Disability Served: various

Veterans Administration Medical Center-Jamaica Plain
150 South Huntington Avenue
Jamaica Plain, MA 02130
617-232-9500
http://www.visn1.med.va.gov/boston/jplain.htm
Disability Served: various

Veterans Administration Medical Center-Leeds
421 North Main Street
Leeds, MA 01053-9764
413-584-4040, 800-892-1522
http://www.visn1.med.va.gov/northampton
Disability Served: various

Veterans Administration Medical Center-West Roxbury
1400 VFW Parkway
West Roxbury, MA 02132
617-323-7700
http://www.visn1.med.va.gov/boston/wrox.htm
Disability Served: various

Veterans Administration Regional Office-Boston
JFK Federal Building, Government Center
Boston, MA 02203
617-227-4600, 800-827-1000
http://www1.va.gov/directory
Disability Served: various

MICHIGAN
Veterans Administration Medical Center-Ann Arbor
2215 Fuller Road
Ann Arbor, MI 48105
734-769-7100
http://www1.va.gov/directory
Disability Served: various

Veterans Administration Medical Center-Battle Creek
5500 Armstrong Road
Battle Creek, MI 49015
269-966-5600
http://www1.va.gov/directory
Disability Served: various

Veterans Administration Medical Center-Detroit
John D. Dingell VA Medical Center
4646 John Road
Detroit, MI 48201
313-576-1000
http://www1.va.gov/directory
Disability Served: various

Veterans Administration Medical Center-Iron Mountain
325 East H Street
Iron Mountain, MI 49801
906-774-3300
http://www.visn12.med.va.gov/ironmountain
Disability Served: various

Veterans Administration Medical Center-Saginaw
Aleda E. Lutz VA Medical Center
1500 Weiss Street
Saginaw, MI 48602
989-497-2500
http://www1.va.gov/directory
Disability Served: various

Veterans Administration Regional Office-Detroit
Patrick V. McNamara Federal Building
477 Michigan Avenue

Detroit, MI 48226
313-226-4183
vsdemill@vba.va.gov
http://www1.va.gov/directory
Disability Served: various

MINNESOTA
Veterans Administration Medical Center-Minneapolis
One Veterans Drive
Minneapolis, MN 55417
612-725-2000
http://www1.va.gov/directory
Disability Served: various

Veterans Administration Medical Center-St. Cloud
4801 Veterans Drive
St Cloud, MN 56303
320-252-1670
http://www1.va.gov/directory/guide
Disability Served: various

Veterans Administration Regional Office-St Paul
1 Federal Drive, Fort Snelling
St Paul, MN 55111-4050
800-827-1000
VBCINQ@VBA.VA.GOV
http://www1.va.gov/directory/guide
Disability Served: various

MISSISSIPPI
Veterans Administration Medical Center-Biloxi
400 Veterans Avenue
Biloxi, MS 39531
228-523-5000
http://www.va.gov/biloxi
Disability Served: various

Veterans Administration Medical Center-Jackson
G.V. (Sonny) Montgomery VA Medical Center
1500 East Woodrow Wilson Drive
Jackson, MS 39216
601-362-4471
http://www1.va.gov/directory
Disability Served: various

Veterans Administration Regional Office-Jackson
1600 East Woodrow Wilson Avenue
Jackson, MS 39269

601-364-7000, 800-827-1000
IRM9@VBA.VA.GOV
http://www.vba.va.gov/ro/south/jacks/jackson.htm
Disability Served: various

MISSOURI
Veterans Administration Medical Center-Columbia
Harry S. Truman Memorial
800 Hospital Drive
Columbia, MO 65201-5297
573-814-6000
http://www1.va.gov/directory
Disability Served: various

Veterans Administration Medical Center-Kansas City
4801 Linwood Boulevard
Kansas City, MO 64128
816-861-4700
http://www1.va.gov/directory
Disability Served: various

Veterans Administration Medical Center-Poplar Bluff
John J. Pershing VA Medical Center
1500 North Westwood Boulevard
Poplar Bluff, MO 63901
783-686-4151, 888-557-8262
http://www.visn15.med.va.gov/facilities/pb/popbluff.htm
Disability Served: various

Veterans Administration Medical Center-St. Louis
John Cochran Division
915 North Grand Avenue
St Louis, MO 63106-1621
314-652-4100
http://www1.va.gov/stlouis
Disability Served: various

Veterans Administration Regional Office-St Louis
Federal Building
400 South 18th Street
St Louis, MO 63103
800-827-1000
http://www1.va.gov/directory
Disability Served: various

MONTANA
Veterans Administration Medical Center-Fort Harrison
1892 Williams Street
Ft Harrison, MT 59636

406-442-6410
http://www1.va.gov/directory
Disability Served: various

Veterans Administration Regional Office-Fort Harrison
Williams Street off Highway 12 West
Fort Harrison, MT 59636
800-827-1000
http://www1.va.gov/directory
Disability Served: various

NEBRASKA

Veterans Administration Medical Center-Grand Island
2201 North Broadwell Avenue
Grand Island, NE 68803-2196
308-382-3660
http://www1.va.gov/directory
Disability Served: various

Veterans Administration Medical Center-Lincoln
600 South 70th Street
Lincoln, NE 68510
402-489-3802
 http://www1.va.gov/directory
Disability Served: various

Veterans Administration Medical Center-Omaha
4101 Woolworth Avenue
Omaha, NE 68105
402-346-8800
http://www1.va.gov/directory
Disability Served: various

Veterans Administration Regional Office-Lincoln
5631 South 48th Street
Lincoln, NE 68516
402-420-4275, 800-827-1000
http://www1.va.gov/directory
Disability Served: various

NEVADA

Veterans Administration Medical Center-Las Vegas
901 Rancho Lane
Las Vegas, NV 89106
702-636-3000

http://www.las-vegas.med.va.gov
Disability Served: various

Veterans Administration Medical Center-Reno
1000 Locust Street
Reno, NV 89520
775-786-7200
http://www1.va.gov/directory
Disability Served: various

Veterans Administration Regional Office-Reno
1201 Terminal Way
Reno, NV 89520
800-827-1000
http://www1.va.gov/directory
Disability Served: various

NEW HAMPSHIRE

Veterans Administration Medical Center-Manchester
718 Smyth Road
Manchester, NH 03104
603-624-4366, 800-892-8384
http://www.visn1.med.va.gov/manchester
Disability Served: various

Veterans Administration Regional Office-Manchester
Norris Cotton Federal Building
275 Chestnut Street
Manchester, NH 03101
800-827-1000
http://www1.va.gov/directory/guide/state.
    asp?STATE=NH&dnum=ALL
Disability Served: various

NEW JERSEY

Veterans Administration Medical Center-East Orange
385 Tremont Avenue
East Orange, NJ 07018
973-676-1000
http://www1.va.gov/visns/visn03
Disability Served: various

Veterans Administration Medical Center-Lyons
151 Knollcroft Road
Lyons, NJ 07939
908-647-0180

http://www1.va.gov/visns/visn03/lyonsinfo.asp
Disability Served: various

Veterans Administration Regional Office-Newark
20 Washington Place
Newark, NJ 07102
800-827-1000
http://www1.va.gov/directory
Disability Served: various

NEW MEXICO
Veterans Administration Medical Center-Albuquerque
1501 San Pedro Drive, SE
Albuquerque, NM 87108-5153
505-265-1711
http://www1.va.gov/directory
Disability Served: various

Veterans Administration Regional Office-Albuquerque
Dennis Chavez Federal Building
500 Gold Avenue, SW
Albuquerque, NM 87102
800-827-1000
http://www1.va.gov/directory
Disability Served: various

NEW YORK
Veterans Administration Medical Center-Albany
Samuel S. Stratton VA Medical Center
113 Holland Avenue
Albany, NY 12208
518-626-5000
http://www1.va.gov/visns/visn02/albany.html
Disability Served: various

Veterans Administration Medical Center-Batavia
222 Richmond Avenue
Batavia, NY 14020
716-343-7500
http://www1.va.gov/visns/visn02/batavia.html
Disability Served: various

Veterans Administration Medical Center-Bath
76 Veterans Avenue
Bath, NY 14810
607-664-4000

http://www1.va.gov/visns/visn02/bath.html
Disability Served: various

Veterans Administration Medical Center-Bronx
130 West Kingsbridge Road
Bronx, NY 10468
718-584-9000
http://www1.va.gov/visns/visn03/bronxinfo.asp
Disability Served: various

Veterans Administration Medical Center-Brooklyn
800 Poly Place
Brooklyn, NY 11209
718-836-6600
http://www1.va.gov/visns/visn03/brooklyninfo.asp
Disability Served: various

Veterans Administration Medical Center-Buffalo
3495 Bailey Avenue
Buffalo, NY 14215
716-834-9200
http://www1.va.gov/directory
Disability Served: various

Veterans Administration Medical Center-Canandaigua
400 Fort Hill Avenue
Canandaigua, NY 14424
585-394-2000
http://www1.va.gov/visns/visn02/canandaigua.html
Disability Served: various

Veterans Administration Medical Center-Castle Point
Route 9D
Castle Point, NY 12511
845-831-2000
http://www1.va.gov/visns/visn03/castinfo.asp
Disability Served: various

Veterans Administration Medical Center-Montrose
Franklin Delano Roosevelt Campus
2094 Albany Post Road, Route 9A, PO Box 100
Montrose, NY 10548
914-737-4400
http://www1.va.gov/visns/visn03/mtrsinfo.asp
Disability Served: various

Veterans Administration Medical Center-New York
423 East 23rd Street
New York, NY 10010

212-686-7500
http://www1.va.gov/visns/visn03/nyinfo.asp
Disability Served: various

Veterans Administration Medical Center-Northport
79 Middleville Road
Northport, NY 11768
631-261-4400
http://www1.va.gov/visns/visn03/nrptinfo.asp
Disability Served: various

Veterans Administration Medical Center-Syracuse
800 Irving Avenue
Syracuse, NY 13210
315-425-4400
http://www1.va.gov/visns/visn02
Disability Served: various

Veterans Administration Regional Office-Buffalo
130 South Elmwood Avenue
Buffalo, NY 14202
800-827-1000
 http://www.vba.va.gov/ro/buffalo/default.htm
Disability Served: various

Veterans Administration Regional Office-New York
245 West Houston Street
New York, NY 10014
212-807-7229, 800-827-1000
http://www1.va.gov/directory
Disability Served: various

NORTH CAROLINA
Veterans Administration Medical Center-Asheville
1100 Tunnel Road
Asheville, NC 28805
828-298-7911, 800-932-6408
http://www1.va.gov/midatlantic/facilities/asheville.htm
Disability Served: various

Veterans Administration Medical Center-Durham
508 Fulton Street
Durham, NC 27705
919-286-0411, 888-878-6890
http://www1.va.gov/midatlantic/facilities/durham.htm
Disability Served: various

Veterans Administration Medical Center-Fayetteville, NC
2300 Ramsey Street
Fayetteville, NC 28301

910-488-2120, 800-771-6106
http://www1.va.gov/midatlantic/facilities/fayetteville.
  htm
Disability Served: various

Veterans Administration Medical Center-Salisbury
W.G. (Bill) Hefner VA Medical Center
1601 Brenner Avenue
Salisbury, NC 28144
704-683-9000, 800-469-8262
http://www1.va.gov/midatlantic/facilities/salisbury.
  htm
Disability Served: various

Veterans Administration Regional Office-Winston-Salem
Federal Building
251 North Main Street
Winston-Salem, NC 27155
800 827 1000
http://www1.va.gov/directory
Disability Served: various

NORTH DAKOTA
Veterans Administration Medical Center-Fargo
2101 Elm Street
Fargo, ND 58102
701-232-3241
http://www1.va.gov/directory
Disability Served: various

Veterans Administration Regional Office-Fargo
2101 Elm Street
Fargo, ND 58102
701-451-4600
 http://www1.va.gov/directory
Disability Served: various

OHIO
Veterans Administration Medical Center-Brecksville
Louis Stokes VA Medical Center
10000 Brecksville Road
Brecksville, OH 44141
440-526-3030
http://www.cleveland.med.va.gov/facilities/
  brecksville.htm
Disability Served: various

Veterans Administration Medical Center-Chillicothe
17273 State Route 104
Chillicothe, OH 45601
740-773-1141
http://www.chillicothe.med.va.gov
Disability Served: various

Veterans Administration Medical Center-Cincinnati
3200 Vine Street
Cincinnati, OH 45220
513-861-3100
http://www1.va.gov/directory
Disability Served: various

Veterans Administration Medical Center-Cleveland
Louis Stokes VA Medical Center
10701 East Boulevard
Cleveland, OH 44106
216-791-3800
http://www.cleveland.med.va.gov
Disability Served: various

Veterans Administration Medical Center-Dayton
4100 West Third Street
Dayton, OH 45428
937-268-6511
daytonprweb@med.va.gov
http://www.dayton.med.va.gov
Disability Served: various

Veterans Administration Regional Office-Cleveland
Anthony J. Celebrezze Federal Building
1240 East Ninth Street
Cleveland, OH 44199
800-827-1000
http://www1.va.gov/directory
Disability Served: various

OKLAHOMA
Veterans Administration Medical Center-Muskogee
1011 Honor Heights Drive
Muskogee, OK 74401
918-683-3261
http://www1.va.gov/directory
Disability Served: various

Veterans Administration Medical Center-Oklahoma City
921 Northeast 13th Street
Oklahoma City, OK 73104

405-270-0501
http://www1.va.gov/directory
Disability Served: various

Veterans Administration Regional Office-Muskogee
Federal Building
125 South Main Street
Muskogee, OK 74401
800-827-1000
http://www.vba.va.gov/ro/muskogee
Disability Served: various

OREGON
Veterans Administration Medical Center-Portland
3710 Southwest U.S. Veterans Hospital Road
Portland, OR 97239
503-220-8262
http://www1.va.gov/directory
Disability Served: various

Veterans Administration Medical Center-Roseburg
913 Northwest Garden Valley Boulevard
Roseburg, OR 97470-6513
541-440-1000
http://www1.va.gov/directory
Disability Served: various

Veterans Administration Regional Office-Portland
Federal Building
1220 Southwest Third Avenue
Portland, OR 97204
800-827-1000
http://www1.va.gov/directory
Disability Served: various

PENNSYLVANIA
Veterans Administration Medical Center-Altoona
James E. Van Zandt VA Medical Center
2907 Pleasant Valley Boulevard
Altoona, PA 16602-4377
814-943-8164
http://www1.va.gov/directory
Disability Served: various

Veterans Administration Medical Center-Butler
325 New Castle Road
Butler, PA 16001-2480
724-287-4781, 800-362-8262

http://www.butler.med.va.gov/butlerva
Disability Served: various

Veterans Administration Medical Center-Coatesville
1400 Black Horse Hill Road
Coatesville, PA 19320-2096
610-384-7711, 800-290-6172
Coatesville.Query@med.va.gov
http://www.coatesville.med.va.gov
Disability Served: various

Veterans Administration Medical Center-Erie
135 East 38th Street
Erie, PA 16504
814-868-8661
http://www1.va.gov/directory
Disability Served: various

Veterans Administration Medical Center-Lebanon
1700 South Lincoln Avenue
Lebanon, PA 17042
717-272-6621, 800-409-8771
zzask.va@lebanon.med.va.gov
http://www.starsandstripes.med.va.gov/visn4/page.
   cfm?pg=34
Disability Served: various

Veterans Administration Medical Center-Pittsburgh
H. John Heinz III Progressive Care Center
University Drive
Pittsburgh, PA 15240
866-482-7488
http://www.va.gov/pittsburgh/heinz.htm
Disability Served: various

Veterans Administration Medical Center-Pittsburgh
7180 Highland Drive
Pittsburgh, PA 15206
866-4VAPITT, 800- 647-6220
http://www.va.gov/pittsburgh/highland.htm
Disability Served: various

Veterans Administration Medical Center-Wilkes-Barre
1111 East End Boulevard
Wilkes-Barre, PA 18711
570-824-3521, 877-928-2621
http://www1.va.gov/vamcwb
Disability Served: various

Veterans Administration Regional Office-Philadelphia
5000 Wissahickon Avenue
Philadelphia, PA 19101
800-827-1000
http://www1.va.gov/directory
Disability Served: various

Veterans Administration Regional Office-Pittsburgh
1000 Liberty Avenue
Pittsburgh, PA 15222
800-827-1000
http://www1.va.gov/directory
Disability Served: various

RHODE ISLAND
Veterans Administration Medical Center-Providence
830 Chalkstone Avenue
Providence, RI 02908-4799
401-273-7100
http://www.visn1.med.va.gov/providence
Disability Served: various

Veterans Administration Regional Office-Providence
380 Westminster Mall
Providence, RI 02903
800 827 1000
http://www1.va.gov/directory
Disability Served: various

SOUTH CAROLINA
Veterans Administration Medical Center-Charleston
Ralph H. Johnson VA Medical Center
109 Bee Street
Charleston, SC 29401-5799
843-577-5011
http://www1.va.gov/directory
Disability Served: various

Veterans Administration Medical Center-Columbia
William Jennings Bryan Dorn VA Medical Center
6439 Garners Ferry Road
Columbia, SC 29209-1639
803-776-4000
http://www1.va.gov/directory
Disability Served: various

Veterans Administration Regional Office-Columbia
1801 Assembly Street
Columbia, SC 29201
800-827-1000
http://www1.va.gov/directory
Disability Served: various

SOUTH DAKOTA
**Veterans Administration Medical Center-
Fort Meade**
113 Comanche Road
Ft Meade, SD 57741
605-347-2511
http://www1.va.gov/directory
Disability Served: various

**Veterans Administration Medical Center-
Hot Springs**
500 North Fifth Street
Hot Springs, SD 57747
605-745-2000
http://www1.va.gov/directory
Disability Served: various

**Veterans Administration Medical Center-
Sioux Falls**
2501 West 22nd Street, PO Box 5046
Sioux Falls, SD 57117-5046
605-336-3230
http://www1.va.gov/directory
Disability Served: various

**Veterans Administration Regional Office-
Sioux Falls**
2501 West 22nd Street, PO Box 5046
Sioux Falls, SD 57117
800-827-1000
http://www1.va.gov/directory
Disability Served: various

TENNESSEE
Veterans Administration Medical Center-Memphis
1030 Jefferson Avenue
Memphis, TN 38104
901-523-8990
http://www1.va.gov/directory
Disability Served: various

**Veterans Administration Medical Center-
Mountain Home**
James H. Quillen VA Medical Center
PO Box 4000
Mountain Home, TN 37684
423-926-1171
http://www1.va.gov/directory
Disability Served: various

Veterans Administration Medical Center-Murfreesboro
3400 Lebanon Pike
Murfreesboro, TN 37129
615-867-6000
http://www1.va.gov/directory
Disability Served: various

Veterans Administration Medical Center-Nashville
1310 24th Avenue South
Nashville, TN 37212-2637
615-327-4751
http://www1.va.gov/directory
Disability Served: various

Veterans Administration Regional Office-Nashville
110 Ninth Avenue South
Nashville, TN 37203
800-827-1000
http://www1.va.gov/directory
Disability Served: various

TEXAS
Veterans Administration Medical Center-Amarillo
6010 Amarillo Boulevard West
Amarillo, TX 79106
806-355-9703
http://www1.va.gov/directory
Disability Served: various

Veterans Administration Medical Center-Big Spring
300 Veterans Boulevard
Big Spring, TX 79720
432-263-7361
http://www1.va.gov/directory
Disability Served: various

Veterans Administration Medical Center-Bonham
Sam Rayburn Memorial Veterans Center
1201 East Ninth Street

Bonham, TX 75418
903-583-2111, 800-792-3271
ntx_internet_information@med.va.gov
http://www.north-texas.med.va.gov
Disability Served: various

Veterans Administration Medical Center-Dallas
4500 South Lancaster Road
Dallas, TX 75216
214-742-8387
(800) 849-3597
ntx_internet_information@med.va.gov
http://www.north-texas.med.va.gov/dallasgeninfo.htm
Disability Served: various

Veterans Administration Medical Center-El Paso
5001 North Piedras Street
El Paso, TX 79930-4211
915-564-6100
http://www1.va.gov/directory
Disability Served: various

Veterans Administration Medical Center-Houston
Michael E. DeBakey VA Medical Center
2002 Holcombe Boulevard
Houston, TX 77030-4298
713-791-1414, 800-553-2278
vhahougeneralquestions@med.va.gov
http://www.houston.med.va.gov
Disability Served: various

Veterans Administration Medical Center-Kerrville
3600 Memorial Boulevard
Kerrville, TX 78028
830-896-2020
http://www.vasthcs.med.va.gov/kd.htm
Disability Served: various

Veterans Administration Medical Center-Marlin
1016 Ward Street
Marlin, TX 76661
254-883-3511
http://www.central-texas.med.va.gov/main
Disability Served: various

Veterans Administration Medical Center-San Antonio
7400 Merton Minter Boulevard
San Antonio, TX 78229
210-617-5300

http://www.vasthcs.med.va.gov
Disability Served: various

Veterans Administration Medical Center-Temple
Olin E Teague Veterans' Center
1901 Veterans Memorial Drive
Temple, TX 76504-7451
254-778-4811
http://www.central-texas.med.va.gov/main
Disability Served: various

Veterans Administration Regional Office-Houston
6900 Almeda Road
Houston, TX 77030
800-827-1000
http://www1.va.gov/directory
Disability Served: various

Veterans Administration Regional Office-Waco
701 Clay Avenue
Waco, TX 76799
800-827-1000
http://www1.va.gov/directory
Disability Served: various

UTAH
Veterans Administration Medical Center-Salt Lake City
500 Foothill Drive
Salt Lake City, UT 84148
801-582-1565, 800-613-4012
http://www1.va.gov/directory
Disability Served: various

Veterans Administration Regional Office-Salt Lake City
550 Foothill Drive
Salt Lake City, UT 84158
801-326-2375
http://www1.va.gov/directory
Disability Served: various

VERMONT
Veterans Administration Medical Center-White River Junction
215 North Main Street
White River Junction, VT 05009

802-295-9363, 866-OUR-VETS
http://www.visn1.med.va.gov/wrj/wrjweb1.html
Disability Served: various

Veterans Administration Regional Office-
**   White River Junction**
North Hartland Road
White River Junction, VT 05009
800 827 1000
http://www1.va.gov/directory
Disability Served: various

VIRGINIA

Veterans Administration Medical Center-Hampton
100 Emancipation Drive
Hampton, VA 23667
757-722-9961, 888-869-6060
http://www1.va.gov/midatlantic/facilities/hampton.htm
Disability Served: various

Veterans Administration Medical Center-Richmond
Hunter Holmes McGuire VA Medical Center
1201 Broad Rock Boulevard
Richmond, VA 23249
804-675-5000, 800-784-8381
http://www1.va.gov/midatlantic/facilities/richmond.
    htm
Disability Served: various

Veterans Administration Medical Center-Salem
1970 Roanoke Boulevard
Salem, VA 24153
540-982-2463, 888-982-2463
http://www1.va.gov/midatlantic/facilities/salem.htm
Disability Served: various

Veterans Administration Regional Office-Roanoke
210 Franklin Road, SW
Roanoke, VA 24011
800-827-1000
http://www1.va.gov/directory
Disability Served: various

WASHINGTON

Veterans Administration Medical Center-Spokane
4815 North Assembly Street
Spokane, WA 99205-6197

509-434-7000
http://www1.va.gov/directory
Disability Served: various

Veterans Administration Medical Center-Tacoma
Building 81
9600 Veterans Drive,
Tacoma, WA 98493
800-329-8387
http://www1.va.gov/PSprim_care/page.cfm?pg=4
Disability Served: various

Veterans Administration Medical Center-Walla Walla
Jonathan M. Wainwright Memorial VA Medical Center
77 Wainwright Drive
Walla Walla, WA 99362
509-525-5200
http://www1.va.gov/directory
Disability Served: various

Veterans Administration Regional Office-Seattle
Federal Building
915 Second Avenue
Seattle, WA 98174
800-827-1000
http://www1.va.gov/directory
Disability Served: various

WEST VIRGINIA

Veterans Administration Medical Center-Beckley
200 Veterans Avenue
Beckley, WV 25801
304-255-2121, 877-902-5142
http://www1.va.gov/midatlantic/facilities/beckley.htm
Disability Served: various

Veterans Administration Medical Center-Clarksburg
Louis A. Johnson VA Medical Center
One Medical Center Drive
Clarksburg, WV 26301
304-623-3461
http://www1.va.gov/directory
Disability Served: various

Veterans Administration Medical Center-Huntington
1540 Spring Valley Drive
Huntington, WV 25704
304-429-6741

http://www1.va.gov/directory
Disability Served: various

Veterans Administration Medical Center-Martinsburg
510 Butler Avenue
Martinsburg, WV 25410
304-263-0811
http://www1.va.gov/directory
Disability Served: various

Veterans Administration Regional Office-Huntington
640 Fourth Avenue
Huntington, WV 25701
800-827-1000
http://www1.va.gov/directory
Disability Served: various

WISCONSIN
Veterans Administration Medical Center-Madison
William S. Middleton Memorial Veterans Hospital
2500 Overlook Terrace
Madison, WI 53705-2286
608-256-1901
http://www.visn12.med.va.gov/madison
Disability Served: various

Veterans Administration Medical Center-Milwaukee
Clement J. Zablocki Veterans Affairs Medical Center
5000 West National Avenue
Milwaukee, WI 53295-1000
414-384-2000
http://www.visn12.med.va.gov/milwaukee
Disability Served: various

Veterans Administration Medical Center-Tomah
500 East Veterans Street
Tomah, WI 54660
608-372-3971
john.renda@med.va.gov
http://www1.va.gov/TomahVAMC
Disability Served: various

Veterans Administration Regional Office-Milwaukee
5400 West National Avenue
Milwaukee, WI 53214
800-827-1000
http://www1.va.gov/directory
Disability Served: various

WYOMING
Veterans Administration Medical Center-Cheyenne
2360 East Pershing Boulevard
Cheyenne, WY 82001
307-778-7550
http://www1.va.gov/directory
Disability Served: various

Veterans Administration Medical Center-Sheridan
1898 Fort Road
Sheridan, WY 82801
307-672-3473
http://www1.va.gov/directory
Disability Served: various

Veterans Administration Regional Office-Cheyenne
2360 East Pershing Boulevard
Cheyenne, WY 82001
800-827-1000
http://www1.va.gov/directory
Disability Served: various

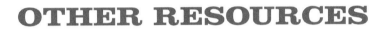

OTHER RESOURCES

ARTS PROGRAMS

These organizations offer opportunities for people with disabilities to become involved in music, performing arts, or visual arts for the purposes of self-expression, for therapeutic benefits, or to increase public awareness and tolerance.

VARIOUS

Alan Short Center
c/o DDSO Inc.
928 East Rose Street
Stockton, CA 95202-1849
209-948-5759
alanshortcenter@sbcglobal.net
http://www.ddso.org
Disability Served: developmentally disabled
The center offers creative art programs, drama classes, support groups, and vocational programs for adults with developmental disabilities.

Growth Thru Art
7 North 31st Street
Billings, MT 59101
406-247-4785
growththruart@imt.net
http://www.imt.net/~dist7hrdc/growth.htm
Disability Served: various
Growth Thru Art offers arts programs in the performing arts and visual arts for individuals with disabilities.

Hope University
800 South Lemon Street
Anaheim, CA 92805
714-778-4440
info@hope-arts.org
http://www.hopeu.com
Disability Served: developmentally disabled
Hope University is a fine-arts facility for adults with developmental disabilities. Students receive full-time arts education, including visual arts, music, dance, drama, and storytelling.

Interact Center for the Visual And Performing Arts
212 Third Avenue North, Suite 140
Minneapolis, MN 55401
612-339-5145
info@interactcenter.com
http://www.interactcenter.com
Disability Served: various
Interact is a nonprofit center for artists with disabilities. Actors, musicians, visual artists, and writers are able to develop skills, perform, and exhibit their work.

International Cent er on Deafness and the Arts
614 Anthony Trail
Northbrook, IL 60062
847-509-8260, 847-509-8257 (TTY)
icoda@aol.com
http://www.icodaarts.org
Disability Served: hearing
This organization provides educational resources and professional arts opportunities that instill principles, cultivate character, and nurture talent in children who are deaf and hard of hearing and assist their development in becoming successful adults. Productions are produced simultaneously in American Sign Language and voice.

Little City Foundation Center for the Arts
1760 West Algonquin Road
Palatine, IL 60067-4799
847-358-5510
jwaters@littlecity.org
http://www.littlecity.org
Disability Served: developmentally disabled
The center hosts visual and media arts programs, including painting, sculpture, and printmaking, for both children and adults with developmental disabilities. Its media arts program produces a cable access show, supports individual video projects, and collaborates with local performance companies.

Marnie Paul Arts Center
9508 Jollyville Road, Suite 101
Austin, TX 78753
512-342-0490
mpac@marniepaul.org
http://www.marniepaul.org
Disability Served: various
The center provides expression through art, music, and dance, and arts therapies to young adults with disabilities, ages 18 to 25.

National Arts and Disability Center (NADC)
UCLA University Affiliated Program
300 UCLA Medical Plaza, Suite 3330
Los Angeles, CA 90095-6967
310-794-1141, 310-267-2356 (TTY)

oraynor@mednet.ucla.edu

http://nadc.ucla.edu

Disability Served: various

The NADC is the national information dissemination, technical assistance, and referral center specializing in the field of arts and disability. The NADC is dedicated to promoting the full inclusion of children and adults with disabilities into the visual-, performing-, media-, and literary-arts communities.

National Endowment for the Arts (NEA)

Office for AccessAbility

1100 Pennsylvania Avenue, NW

Washington, DC 20506

202-682-5532, 202-682-5496 (TTY)

http://www.arts.gov

Disability Served: various

The Office for AccessAbility is the advocacy-technical-assistance arm of the NEA for people with disabilities, older adults, veterans, and people living in institutions.

VSA Arts

818 Connecticut Avenue, NW, Suite 600

Washington, DC 20006

202-628-2800, 800-933-8721, 202-737-0645 (TDD)

info@vsarts.org

http://www.vsarts.org

Disability Served: various

With an affiliate network that now spans the United States and 83 other countries worldwide, VSA Arts offers opportunities for people with disabilities of all ages to engage in the arts as a means of creative self-expression, positive change, and personal and professional growth.

MUSIC

Coalition for Disabled Musicians Inc.

PO Box 1002M

Bay Shore, NY 11706

631-586-0366

cdmnews@aol.com

http://www.disabled-musicians.org

Disability Served: various

Coalition for Disabled Musicians introduces disabled musicians to each other, gives access to handicapped-accessible rehearsal and recording studios, and creates adaptive techniques for pain, endurance, and other limitations. It holds live performances, produces recordings, and holds music workshops and seminars. It promotes public awareness of the disabled community.

Special Music by Special People

Welles Park

2333 West Sunnyside Avenue

Chicago, IL 60625

312-742-PLAY

http://www.specialmusic.org

Disability Served: developmentally disabled

Special Music by Special People is a Chicago Park District music program for people with developmental disabilities. Participants in the program use music performances, song writing, and music writing as creative and social outlets.

Vancouver Adapted Music Society

770 Pacific Boulevard South, Plaza of Nations, Box 27, Suite A-304

Vancouver, BC V6B 5E7

Canada

604-688-6464, ext. 107

vams@disabilityfoundation.org

http://www.reachdisability.org/vams/about.htm

Disability Served: various

The society has a roster of volunteers and musicians with disabilities who are available for performances. These musicians play benefit concerts to rehabilitate disabled people through involvement in musical activities, to raise awareness of the musical capabilities of people with disabilities, and to promote quality music.

VISUAL ARTS

Accessible Arts Inc.

1100 State Avenue

Kansas City, KS 66102-4411

913-281-1133 (Voice/TYY)

accarts@accessiblearts.org

http://www.accessiblearts.org

Disability Served: various

This is a not-for-profit organization dedicated to providing equal access to the arts for children and youth with physical, emotional, and psychological disabilities. Training workshops, art demonstrations, an art resource center, and various educational materials are used to introduce children to the arts.

Arts for All Inc.
2520 North Oracle Road
Tucson, AZ 85705
520-622-4100
adminassist@artsforallinc.org
http://www.artsforallinc.org
Disability Served: various
Arts for All's mission is to provide accessible education, training, and experiences in the arts for children, particularly those with special needs.

Cedars Textile Arts Center
PO Box 947
Ross, CA 94957
415-453-4240
info@cedarsofmarin.org
http://www.thecedarsofmarin.org
Disability Served: various
Cedars Textile Arts Center offers a creative art educational program for individuals with disabilities. Program components include hand weaving, gardening, animal husbandry, adaptive homemaking/home living skills, arts and crafts, functional academics, and job preparation skills.

Creative Growth Art Center
355 24th Street
Oakland, CA 94612
510- 836-2340
info@creativegrowth.org
http://www.creativegrowth.org
Disability Served: various
Creative Growth Art Center serves physically, mentally, and developmentally disabled adult artists, providing a stimulating environment for artistic instruction, gallery promotion, and personal expression.

Creative Spirit Art Centre
PO Box, 16 Postal Station "P"
Toronto, ON M5S 2S6
Canada
416-588-8801
http://www.creativespirit.on.ca
Disability Served: various
This center provides art education and studio space to individuals with disabilities who cannot access art classes,

Creativity Explored of San Francisco
3245 16th Street
San Francisco, CA 94103
415-863-2108
info@creativityexplored.org
http://www.creativityexplored.org
Disability Served: various
Creativity Explored provides adults with disabilities the opportunity to express themselves through the creation of art.

Exceptional Children's Foundation Art Center
3750 West Martin Luther King Jr. Boulevard
Los Angeles, CA 90008
323-290-6030
http://www.ecfartcenter.com
Disability Served: developmentally disabled
The center offers professional arts training, studio facilities, and educational programs, to adults with developmental disabilities.

First Street Gallery Art Center
250 West First Street, Suite 120
Claremont, CA 91711
909-626-5455
http://www.1ststreetgallery.org
Disability Served: various
Professional artists provide instruction to people with disabilities in drawing, painting, ceramics, and printmaking.

Gateway Crafts/Vinfen
62 Harvard Street
Brookline, MA 02445
617-734-1577
gateway@shore.net
http://www.vinfen.org
Disability Served: various
This organization provides creative, alternative, vocational opportunities and programs for adults with developmental and other disabilities.

Handicapped Artist Painting Productions and You
c/o Saint Martin in the Field
140 Southeast 28th Avenue
Pompano Beach, FL 33062
954-742-7791
happy@asclepius.com
http://www.asclepius.com/happy/index.htm
Disability Served: various
This nonprofit organization provides artists with disabilities with a medium for self-expression through art.

National Institute of Arts and Disabilities (NIAD)
551 23rd Street
Richmond, CA 94804
510-620-0290
admin@niadart.org
http://www.niadart.org
Disability Served: various
The NIAD's mission is to provide an art environment for
people with developmental and other disabilities
that promotes creative expression, independence,
dignity and community integration. It serves up
to 50 adults each day with training in painting,
printmaking, sculpture, ceramics, textiles, decorative
arts, and more. Client artwork is actively promoted
through an exhibitions program.

Passion Works
21 South Campbell Street
Athens, OH 45701
740-592-6659, ext. 252
patty@passionworks.org
http://www.passionworks.org
Disability Served: developmentally disabled
This studio offers art opportunities for people with
developmental disabilities, artists, and other
community members.

Short Center South
1250 Sutterville Road
Sacramento, CA 95822
916-737-2397
http://www.shortcentersouth.org
Disability Served: various
The Short Center South offers art classes for individuals
with disabilities.

Sister Kenny Institute
800 East 28th Street
Minneapolis, MN 55407
612-863-4466
http://www.allina.com/ahs/ski.nsf
Disability Served: various
The institute sponsors a contest for the best art pieces by
artists with disabilities and the top nine contestants
win a monetary prize.

Southside Art Center
8583 Elder Creek Road, Suite 200
Sacramento, CA 95828

916-387-8080
info@southsideartcenter.com
http://www.southsideartcenter.com
Disability Served: developmentally disabled
The Southside Art Center offers choices for individuals
with developmental disabilities, including creative
art programs, computer skills training, and vocational
opportunities.

THEATRE

Amaryllis Theater Company
100 South Broad Street
Philadelphia, PA 19110
215-564-2431, 215-564-2481 (TTY)
info@amaryllistheatre.org
http://www.amaryllistheatre.org
Disability Served: various
Amaryllis Theater Company is a professional theater
dedicated to the principles of inclusion and the
celebration of difference.

**Changing Perceptions: Theater by the Blind and
Physically Disabled**
11271 Ventura Boulevard, Suite 455
Studio City, CA 591604
323-660-4607
Disability Served: physically disabled, vision
Theater by the Blind and Physically Disabled provides
the disabled community with free dramatic arts
education. Its drama classes empower 50 to 60
visually or physically disabled students between
the ages of 25 and 85. Four weekly classes, in basic
acting, improvisation, theatre games, movement,
voice, emotional strengthening, and tuning are
offered year round and free of charge.

Cleveland Signstage Theatre
8500 Euclid Avenue
Cleveland, OH 44106
216-229-2838, 216-229-0431 (TTY)
deaftheatre@signstage.org
http://www.signstage.org
Disability Served: hearing
Deaf and hearing cast members perform simultaneously
in spoken English and American Sign Language in
pursuit of their mission to "produce extraordinary
theater that brings deaf and hearing people
together."

Deaf West Theatre

5112 Lankershim Boulevard
North Hollywood, CA 91601
818-762-2998, 818-508-8389 (TDD)
info@deafwest.org
http://www.deafwest.org
Disability Served: hearing
DWT presents professional main stage productions in American Sign Language with simultaneous voice translation, thereby bridging the gap between deaf and hearing worlds. Activities of DWT include three productions annually, including one targeted for young audiences. Deaf West's Conservatory program provides professional training for deaf and hard of hearing individuals (ages 18+) in theater arts. DWT conducts educational outreach drama workshops that serve deaf and hard of hearing children (K-12) in inner-city schools, and a Saturday morning storytelling workshop during the summer that is open to deaf and hearing children and their parents.

Firehouse Theater Company

PO Box 69913
West Hollywood, CA 90069-0913
310-659-6744
oppenheimz@aol.com
http://www.firehousetheatercompany.org
Disability Served: various
The Firehouse Theatre Company both produces and assists in creating innovative, inclusive, theatrical, musical, and visual arts events. It works as an advocate for artists and audiences with physical or sensory disabilities.

National Theater of the Deaf

139 North Main Street
West Hartford, CT 06107
860-300-5179, 860-724-5179 (TTY)
info@ntd.org
http://www.ntd.org
Disability Served: hearing
National Theater of the Deaf has a national and international reputation as the world's premiere deaf theatre company.

Paradigm Players

2001 North Adams, Suite 919
Arlington, VA 22201
703-807-0785
http://dcmdva-arts.org/sourceth/paradigm.htm
Disability Served: various
Paradigm Theater provides opportunities for individuals with and without disabilities to participate in community theatre. It serves the Greater Washington, D.C., area.

Performing Arts Studio West

438 South Market Street
Inglewood, CA 90301
310-674-1346
pastudiowest@earthlink.net
http://www.pastudiowest.com
Disability Served: developmentally disabled
Performing Arts Studio West provides an environment where adults with developmental disabilities can enhance self-esteem, social skills, and vocational skills through participation in a performing arts curriculum, professionally staged productions, and vocational training. Entertainment industry professionals teach all classes. This setting brings together actors, singers, musicians, and technical personnel—with and without disabilities—and combines their talents to produce quality, original entertainment.

PHAMALy

PO Box 44216
Denver, CO 80201-4216
303-575-0005
phamaly@worldnet.att.net
http://www.phamaly-colorado.org
Disability Served: physically disabled
PHAMALy is a theatre group and touring company that enables physically challenged performers to showcase their talents and abilities and to make the performing arts more accessible to everyone. PHAMALy is dedicated to producing traditional theater in nontraditional ways.

Short Center Repertory

265 Second Avenue
Sacramento, CA 95818
916-857-0636, 916-737-2709 (TDD)
shortrep@sbcglobal.net
Disability Served: developmentally disabled
This touring company of adult actors with developmental disabilities tours classical and modern plays throughout the West Coast. It uses

fully integrated American Sign Language in all productions.

Theatre by the Blind
306 West 18th Street, Suite 3A
New York, NY 10011
212-243-4337
gar@nyc.rr.com
http://www.tbtb.org
Disability Served: vision
This integrated company of blind, visually impaired, and sighted artists is dedicated to finding, developing, and exhibiting blind theatrical talent.

Theatre in Motion
LFanelli@Theatreinmotion.com
http://www.theatreinmotion.com
Disability Served: various
Theatre in Motion is a participatory, educational theatre company that uses nontraditional casting that includes people with and without disabilities.

Theater Unlimited
The Janet Pomeroy Center
207 Skyline Boulevard
San Francisco, CA 94132
415-665-4100
info@janetpomeroy.org
http://www.janetpomeroy.org
Disability Served: various
Theater Unlimited is a program of The Janet Pomeroy Center, a nonprofit organization that provides recreational, educational, and vocational rehabilitation, and respite care for people with disabilities. Theatre Unlimited is an ensemble company dedicated to providing theatre training and performance opportunities for actors and dancers with and without disabilities.

Triumvirate Pi Theatre Company
PO Box 1452
Culver City, CA 90232
310-836-2961
triumviratepi@earthlink.net
http://www.tri-pi.org
Disability Served: various
Triumvirate Pi Theatre Company is a nonprofit playwrights collective and producing organization. It seeks to bring together artists and audiences from California's diverse communities. Its goal is to create live theatre that encourages understanding and breaks down perceived barriers of race, gender, and disability.

Unlimited Potential Theater Company
VSA Arts of New Jersey
703 Jersey Avenue
New Brunswick, NJ 08901
732-745-3885, 732-745-5935, 732-745-3913 (TTY)
info@vsanj.org
http://www.vsanj.org
Disability Served: various
This theater company integrates the talents of actors, age 16 and over, with and without disabilities. Performances are fully accessible for both audience and cast members.

CAMPS

These resources will help you find short-term camps and recreational programs for children and adults with disabilities.

GUIDES AND LISTS

American Camp Association
5000 State Road 67 North
Martinsville, IN 46151-7902
765-342-8456
http://www.acacamps.org
Disability Served: various

Camps for Children with Diabetes
http://www.childrenwithdiabetes.com/camps
Disability Served: diabetes

Camps for Children with Spina Bifida
4590 MacArthur Boulevard, NW, Suite 250
Washington, DC 20007-4226
202-944-3285, 800-621-3141
sbaa@sbaa.org
http://www.sbaa.org
Disability Served: spina bifida

The Candlelighters—Childhood Cancer Foundation Camp List for Children with Cancer
PO Box 498
Kensington, MD 20895-0498
301-962-3520; 800-366-2223
info@candlelighters.org
http://www.candlelighters.org/supportcamps.stm
Disability Served: various

Learning Disabilities Association of America— Directory of Summer Camps for Children with Learning Disabilities
4156 Library Road
Pittsburgh, PA 15234
412-341-1515, 412-341-8077
http://www.ldaamerica.org
Disability Served: learning disabled

Porter Sargent Publishers Inc.—*Guide to Summer Camps and Summer Schools*
400 Bedford Street
Manchester, NH 03101
800-342-7470
info@portersargent.com
http://www.portersargent.com
Disability Served: various

Resources for Children with Special Needs Inc.— *Camps 2005: A Directory of Camps and Summer Programs for Children and Youth with Disabilities and Special Needs in the Metro New York Area*
116 East 16th Street, 5th Floor
New York, NY 10003
212-677-4650
info@resourcesnyc.org
http://www.resourcesnyc.org
Disability Served: various

CAMPS BY GEOGRAPHIC REGION

CALIFORNIA

Camp Rubber Soul
PO Box 942
Mendocino, CA 95460
smiller@mcn.org
http://www.camprubbersoul.org
Disability Served: various
This recreational camp offers one-week overnight sessions for children with varying degrees of disabilities. A one-to-one counselor ratio gives a unique, fulfilling, and rewarding experience.

Junior Blind of America
5300 Angeles Vista Boulevard
Los Angeles, CA 90043
323-295-4555, 800-352-2290
info@fjb.org
http://www.fjb.org
Disability Served: vision
This organization offers extensive camp and recreation programs for young people of all ages who are blind or visually impaired.

COLORADO

Learning Camp
PO Box 1146
Vail, CO 81658
970-926-2706
information@learningcamp.com
http://www.learningcamp.com
Disability Served: learning disabled

The mission of the Learning Camp is to provide a loving and nurturing adventure experience where children with learning disabilities can practice basic reading, writing, and math, and build self-esteem and independence.

DISTRICT OF COLUMBIA
Summer Camps for Children Who Are Deaf or Hard of Hearing
Gallaudet University
Laurent Clerc National Deaf Education Center
800 Florida Avenue, NE
Washington, DC 20002
202-651-5000 (Voice/TTY)
http://clerccenter.gallaudet.edu/InfoToGo/142.html
Disability Served: hearing

FLORIDA
Sertoma Camp Endeavor Inc.
PO Box 910
Dundee, FL 33838-0910
863-439-1300
directordeluca@aol.com
http://sertomacampendeavor.com
Disability Served: hearing
The mission of this camp is to provide an education program for deaf and hard of hearing youth that promotes social/personal growth, environmental awareness, independence, and citizenship.

GEORGIA
Georgia's Lions Camp for the Blind
5626 Laura Walker Road
Waycross, GA 31503
912-283-4320, 888-297-1775
glcblind@accessatc.net
http://www.glcb.org
Disability Served: vision
The Georgia Lions' Camp for the Blind Inc. provides personal growth experiences for children, teens, and adults with visual impairments through the use of recreation, education, socialization, and rehabilitation in an outdoor setting.

ILLINOIS
Easter Seals Camping and Recreation List
Easter Seals-National Office
230 West Monroe Street, Suite 1800
Chicago, IL 60606
312-726-6200, 800-221-6827, 312-726-4258 (TTY)
info@easterseals.com
http://www.easterseals.com/site/PageServer?page name=ntl_directory_camprec
Disability Served: various

IOWA
Camp Courageous of Iowa
12007 190th Street, PO Box 418
Monticello, IA 52310-0418
319-465-5916
info@campcourageous.org
http://www.campcourageous.org
Disability Served: various
Camp Courageous of Iowa is a year-round respite and recreational facility for individuals of all ages with disabilities.

LOUISIANA
Louisiana Lions Camp
PO Box 171
Leesville, LA 71496
337-239-0782, 800-348-6567
http://www.lionscamp.org
Disability Served: various
This summer camp is for physically challenged, mentally challenged, and diabetic youth of Louisiana.

MARYLAND
Lions Camp Merrick/Glyndon
3650 Rick Hamilton Place
Nanjemoy, MD 20662
301-870-5858
administrator@lionscampmerrick.org
http://www.lionscampmerrick.org
Disability Served: diabetes, hearing, vision
Lions Camp Merrick provides weeklong residential camping experiences for children who are deaf, blind, or have diabetes, ages 6 through 16. Additionally the camp provides many shorter weekend retreats and daylong sessions for related activities, including scouting and 4-H.

MICHIGAN
Great Lakes Burn Camp
1709 North West Avenue, Suite 138
Jackson, MI 49202

800-989-2571
glbcsr@aol.com
http://www.greatlakesburncamp.com/index.htm
Disability Served: burns
Great Lakes Burn Camp is open to burn-injured children
ages 6 through 17.

NEW YORK

Camp Huntington
56 Bruceville Road
High Falls, NY 12440
845-687-7840
camphtgtn@aol.com
http://www.camphuntington.com
Disability Served: attention deficit order, autism,
developmentally disabled, learning disabled
Camp Huntington's recreation program is specifically
designed for children and teenagers with learning
disabilities, ADD/ADHD, and neurological impairments.
Campers participate in a variety of daily activities
which are much like those offered at a camp for the
nondisabled.

Camp Jened
Adams Road, PO Box 483
Rock Hill, NY 12775
845-434-2220
http://www.campjened.org
Disability Served: various
This camp provides a vacation for adults who have
a wide range of physical and developmental
disabilities, such as cerebral palsy, Down Syndrome,
autism and behavior disorders.

Camp Northwood
132 State Route 365
Remsen, NY 13438-5700
315-831-3621
campinfo@nwood.com
http://www.nwood.com
Disability Served: learning disabled
Camp Northwood provides programming to socially
immature, isolated, nonaggressive children, ranging
in age from 8 to 18 that experience difficulties in
social and academic settings due to a variety of
learning challenges.

Herbert G. Birch Family Camp
Herbert G. Birch Services
275 Seventh Avenue, 19th Floor
New York, NY 10001
212-741-6522
hgbgerrym@aol.com
http://www.hgbirch.org
Disability Served: AIDS
This weeklong retreat provides a sanctuary for children
and families living with AIDS.

NEW JERSEY

Camp Oakhurst
111 Monmouth Road
Oakhurst, NJ 07755
732-531-0215
Oakhurst06@aol.com
http://www.campchannel.com/campoakhurst
Disability Served: physically disabled
Camp Oakhurst serves children and adults with physical
disabilities. There is a summer camp, a year round
respite, and vacation programs. Scholarships are
available.

NORTH CAROLINA

SOAR
PO Box 388
Balsam, NC 28707-0388
828-456-3435
jonathan@soarnc.org
http://www.soarnc.org
Disability Served: learning disabled
Students participating in SOAR's summer camps,
weekend, winter break, and semester courses take
part in adventure experiences, such as camping,
rock climbing, whitewater rafting, scuba diving, sea
kayaking, and horseback riding.

Stone Mountain School
126 Camp Elliott Road
Black Mountain, NC 28711
828-669-8639
info@stonemountainschool.com
http://www.stonemountainschool.org
Disability Served: attention deficit disorder, behavioral
disorders, emotionally disabled adolescents, learning
disabled
This camp serves boys ages 10 through 17 who have
learning disabilities, attention deficit disorder,
hyperactivity, emotional problems, or behavioral
problems.

OHIO

Camp Nuhop
404 Hillcrest Drive
Ashland, OH 44805
419-938-7151
http://www.campnuhop.org
Disability Served: attention deficit disorder, behavioral disorders, learning disabled
This summer residential program is for any youngster from age 6 to 16 with a learning disability, behavior disorder, or attention deficit disorder. Among its camp choices are an exploration camp and a wilderness camp.

PENNSYLVANIA

Camp Lee Mar
Summer Address: 450 Route 590
Lackawaxen, PA 18435
570-685-7188
Winter Address: 805 Redgate Road
Dresher, PA 19025
215-658-1708
gtour400@aol.com
http://www.leemar.com
Disability Served: various
Camp Lee Mar is a private residential special needs camp for children and young adults with mild to moderate learning and developmental challenges, including but not limited to the following: mental retardation, developmental disabilities, Down Syndrome, autism, learning disabilities, Williams Syndrome, Asperger Syndrome, ADD, Prader Willi, and ADHD.

TENNESSEE

Tennessee Camp for Diabetic Children
2622 Lee Pike
Soddy, TN 37379
bgabriel_tcdc@yahoo.com
http://www.tcdc.net
Disability Served: diabetes
The Tennessee Camp for Diabetic Children is located on Lake Chickamauga in Soddy, Tennessee, just north of Chattanooga. The camp is committed to teaching children with diabetes how to live a normal and active life.

VIRGINIA

Camp Optimism Foundation
703 South 23rd Street
Arlington, VA 22202
703-486-2257
CampOptimism@juno.com
http://novaplaza.com/campoptimism
Disability Served: various
This residential summer camp is for children with mental or physical disabilities. There is a fee for this camp, however no child will ever be denied admission to the camp due to an inability to pay, subject to available funds.

WEST VIRGINIA

Space Camp for Interested Visually Impaired Students
West Virginia School for the Blind
PO Box 1034
Romney, WV 26757
304-822-4883
scivis@atlanticbb.net
http://www.tsbvi.edu/space
Disability Served: vision
This is a weeklong camp that takes place at the U.S. Space and Rocket Center in Huntsville, Alabama.

CANADA

Camp Winston
9005 Leslie Street, Unit 203
Richmond Hill, ON L4B 1G7
Canada
905-707-3427
mail@campwinston.com
http://www.campwinston.com
Disability Served: various
Camp Winston operates a residential recreational summer program for campers with complex neurological disorders. It also provides behavior management and skills workshops and weekend retreats.

CONFERENCES

The following conferences focus on disability-related topics and issues.

Alexander Graham Bell Association for Deaf Annual Conference
PO Box 235
Irvington, NY 10533
914-591-4565
agbell@agbellny.org
http://www.agbellny.org
Disability Served: hearing
The association hosts an annual conference that offers information on the latest developments regarding hearing impairments. The conference is held in June.

American Academy for Cerebral Palsy and Developmental Medicine Conference
6300 North River Road, Suite 727
Rosemont, IL 60018-4226
847-698 1635
http://www.aacpdm.org/index?service=page/Home
Disability Served: cerebral palsy
An annual conference featuring educational seminars regarding developments in cerebral palsy takes place each October.

American Association of Spinal Cord Injury Psychologists and Social Workers Conference
75-20 Astoria Boulevard
Jackson Heights, NY 11370-1177
718-803-3782
aascipsw@unitedspinal.org
http://www.aascipsw.org
Disability Served: spinal-cord injury
The association's annual conference explores clinical, scientific, and technological advances in the field of spinal cord injury.

American Association on Mental Retardation Conference
444 North Capitol Street, NW, Suite 846
Washington, DC 20001-1512
202-387-1968, 800-424-3688
http://www.aamr.org
Disability Served: developmentally disabled
The conference offers seminars, workshops, and social activities. It is held annually in the last week of May.

American Council of the Blind Annual Convention
1155 15th Street, NW, Suite 1004
Washington, DC 20001
202-467-5081, 800-424-8666
info@acb.org
http://www.acb.org
Disability Served: vision
This convention is geared toward persons who are blind or visually impaired and offers information booths and workshops. It is held annually in early summer.

American Diabetes Association Annual Meeting and Scientific Sessions
1701 North Beauregard Street
Alexandria, VA 22311
800-DIABETES
http://www.diabetes.org
Disability Served: diabetes
The association's annual conference is a trade show that focuses on equipment, technology, and supplies used in the treatment of diabetes. The conference is geared toward medical professionals.

American Physical Therapy Association
1111 North Fairfax Street
Alexandria, VA 22314-1488
703-684-2782, 800-999-APTA, 703-683-6748 (TDD)
http://www.apta.org
Disability Served: various
This professional association promotes National Physical Therapy Week every October. It is designed to inform the public about healthy living and offers fitness clinics, exercise activities, seminars, and more.

American Rehabilitation Counseling Association Conference
c/o American Counseling Association
5999 Stevenson Avenue
Alexandria, VA 22304
http://www.arcaweb.org/.html
Disability Served: various
The association hosts a conference for its members every March or April. Seminars, workshops, and presentations on research studies and developments in rehabilitation counseling are offered.

American Speech-Language-Hearing Association Annual Convention
10801 Rockville Pike
Rockville, MD 20852-3279
800-498-2071, 301-897-5700 (TTY)
http://www.asha.org
Disability Served: communication
This national conference focuses on products and services related to speech pathology, audiology, and speech and hearing science. The conference takes place in November.

Approaches to Developmental and Learning Disorders in Infants and Children Conference
Interdisciplinary Council on Developmental and Learning Disorders
4938 Hampden Lane, Suite 800
Bethesda, MD 20814
301-656-2667
http://www.icdl.com
Disability Served: developmentally disabled, learning disabled
This regional conference is designed for educators, administrators, and professionals who work with the developmentally and learning disabled. The conference is held in November.

Association for Persons in Supported Employment Conference
1627 Monument Avenue
Richmond, VA 23220
804-278-9187
apse@apse.org
http://www.apse.org
Disability Served: various
This nonprofit organization hosts the world's largest annual conference on supported employment. The conference is held in July. Registration materials are available in January.

Center for School Mental Health Analysis and Action National Conference on Advancing School-Based Mental Health Services
University of Maryland-Baltimore
Department of Psychiatry
737 West Lombard Street, 4th Floor
Baltimore, MD 21201
410-706-0980, 888-706-0980
http://csmha.umaryland.edu
Disability Served: mental health

This conference takes place each fall and focuses on mental health issues in schools.

Children and Adults With Attention-Deficit/Hyperactivity Disorder Annual International Conference
8181 Professional Place, Suite 150
Landover, MD 20785
301-306-7070
http://www.chadd.org
Disability Served: attention deficit disorder
This conference is geared toward professionals working with attention deficit disorder. The conference is held each October.

Closing The Gap Annual Conference
526 Main Street, PO Box 68
Henderson, MN 56044
507-248-3294
ckneip@closingthegap.com
http://www.closingthegap.com
Disability Served: various
Closing the Gap, an organization that researches microcomputer technology in special education and rehabilitation, sponsors an annual conference in October.

Commonwealth Institute for Child and Family Studies Conference
PO Box 980489
Richmond, VA 23298-0489
804-828-4393
vmarinelli@vcu.edu
http://www.cicfs.vcu.edu
Disability Served: behavioral disorders, developmentally disabled, emotionally disabled adolescents
This university research institute disseminates information on children and adolescents with emotional and behavioral disorders. Its annual conference is held each October.

Council for Exceptional Children Conference
1110 North Glebe Road, Suite 300
Arlington, VA 22201-5704
703-620-3660, 888-CEC-SPED, 866-915-5000 (TTY)
http://www.cec.sped.org
Disability Served: various
The council hosts an annual conference in April for educators and administrators in the field of special education.

Discovery Low Vision Conference

Deicke Center for Visual Rehabilitation
219 East Cole Avenue
Wheaton, IL 60187
630-690-7115
dlevine@deicke.org
http://www.deicke.org
Disability Served: vision
This statewide conference focuses on low-vision issues
and related products.

Federation of Families for Children's Mental Health Annual Conference

1101 King Street, Suite 420
Alexandria, VA 22314
703-684-7710
ffcmhc@ffcmh.org
http://www.ffcmh.org
Disability Served: mental health
This regional conference takes place in November and
is geared toward mental health professionals.

Geneva Centre for Autism Symposium

112 Merton Street
Toronto, ON M4S 1H2
Canada
416-322-7877, 866-Geneva-9
info@autism.net
http://www.autism.net
Disability Served: autism
The centre provides a biennial Symposium on autism-
related issues.

Institute for Inclusive Education Annual Conference

1460 Craig Road
St Louis, MO 63146
314-872-8282, 800-835-8282
http://csd.org/csdrpdc
Disability Served: various
This regional conference targets school professionals
and focuses on inclusive education. The conference
is held in October.

International Conference on Learning Disabilities

Council for Learning Disabilities
PO Box 4014
Leesburg, VA 20177
571-258-1010
http://www.cldinternational.org
Disability Served: learning disabled

This international conference focuses on developments
in the field of learning disability and is geared toward
educators and other professionals.

International Conference on Parents with Disabilities and their Families

Through the Looking Glass
2198 Sixth Street, Suite 100
Berkeley, CA 94710-2204
800-644-2666, 800-804-1616 (TTY)
TLG@lookingglass.org
http://www.lookingglass.org
Disability Served: various
This conference focuses on research findings, theories,
and practical strategies regarding parenting with a
disability.

International Dyslexia Association Annual Conference

Chester Building, 8600 LaSalle Road, Suite 382
Baltimore, MD 21286-2044
410-296-0232
http://www.interdys.org
Disability Served: dyslexic
This conference focuses on dyslexia and is designed
for school professionals and educators.

Learning Disabilities Association of America- Annual International Conference

4156 Library Road
Pittsburgh, PA 15234-1349
412-341-1515
http://www.ldanatl.org
Disability Served: learning disabled
This international conference focuses on the latest developments in learning disabilities and is geared toward
professionals. The conference is held each March.

Lowe Syndrome Association Conference

18919 Voss Road
Dallas, TX 75287-2766
612-869-5693
info@lowesyndrome.org
http://www.lowesyndrome.org
Disability Served: various
The association fosters communication among families,
provides information, and sponsors research. A
newsletter and other printed materials are available.
Conferences are held every two years.

MedTrade Conferences
SEMCO Productions
1145 Sanctuary Parkway, Suite 355
Alpharetta, GA 30004
770-569-1540
http://www.medtrade.com
Disability Served: various
This trade show features the latest in health care
products and services and is geared toward
medical professionals.

Midwest Symposium on Therapeutic Recreation
344 Hearnes Center
Columbia, MO 65211
573-882-9558
Disability Served: various
This conference, held each April, focuses on therapeutic
recreation and adapted physical activities.

**National Alliance for the Mentally Ill Annual
Conference**
Colonial Place Three, 2107 Wilson Boulevard, Suite 300
Arlington, VA 22201-3042
800-950-NAMI
ann@nami.org
http://www.nami.org
Disability Served: mental health
This organization hosts an annual conference each
summer to discuss recent developments, legislation,
advocacy issues, and more regarding mental health.

**National Council for Community Behavioral
Healthcare Conference**
12300 Twinbrook Parkway, Suite 320
Rockville, MD 20852
301-984-6200
nolam@nccbh.org
http://www.nccbh.org
Disability Served: mental health
This conference takes place every spring and offers
booths and exhibits of products and services.

National Council on the Aging Conference
Conference Department
300 D Street, SW, Suite 801
Washington, DC 20024
202-479-1200, 202-479-6674 (TDD)
info@ncoa.org
http://www.ncoa.org

Disability Served: elderly
This conference is held every spring and is designed for
administrators and professionals who are interested
in continuing education and improvement of their
skills.

National Down Syndrome Society Conference
666 Broadway, Suite 810
New York, NY 10012-2317
212-460-9330, 800-221-4602
info@ndss.org
http://www.ndss.org
Disability Served: Down Syndrome
This international conference brings together research
specialists, professionals, and others to discuss
findings regarding Down Syndrome. It is held in
October.

National Hemophilia Foundation Annual Meeting
116 West 32nd Street, 11th Floor
New York, NY 10001
212-328-3700
handi@hemophilia.org
http://www.hemophilia.org
Disability Served: inherited bleeding disorders
This national conference is designed for medical
professionals and others concerned with
hemophilia. The conference is held in October
or November.

National Managed Health Care Congress
212-661-3500 ext. 3013
MAntonelli@IIRUSA.com
http://www.nmhcc.com
Disability Served: various
This conference is a gathering of managed care
professionals and representatives.

**National Organization on Rare Disorders Annual
Patient Family Conference**
55 Kenosia Avenue, PO Box 1968
Danbury, CT 06813-1968
203-744-0100, 800-999-6673, 203-797-9590 (TDD)
orphan@rarediseases.org
http://www.rarediseases.org
Disability Served: various
This national conference focuses on research findings,
developments, and current trends concerning rare
disorders. The conference takes place in the fall.

Partnerships: Linkages for Success
National Association for the Dually Diagnosed
132 Fair Street
Kingston, NY 12401
845-331-4336, 800-331-5362
info@thenadd.org
http://www.thenadd.org
Disability Served: developmentally disabled, mental health, mental retardation
This national conference, held in October, focuses on issues of mental health, mental retardation, developmental disabilities, and mental illness.

Registry for Interpreters for the Deaf Annual Conference
333 Commerce Street
Alexandria, VA 22314
703-838-0030, 703-838-0459 (TTY)
http://www.rid.org
Disability Served: hearing
This annual conference, held each August, focuses on hearing issues and is open to the general public.

Rehabilitation Engineering and Assistive Technology Society of North America (RESNA) Annual Conference
1700 North Moore Street, Suite 1540
Arlington, VA 22209-1903
703-524-6686
info@resna.org
http://www.resna.org
Disability Served: various
RESNA hosts an annual conference each June. Rehabilitation and assistive-technology professionals gather to, network, and discuss and learn about the latest developments in rehabilitation and assistive technologies.

Southeast Augmentative Communication Conference
2430 11th Avenue, North
Birmingham, AL 35234
205-251-0165
http://www2.edc.org/NCIP/library/ec/Seac.htm
Disability Served: communication
This regional conference focuses on augmentative communication developments. Held each October, the conference is appropriate for professionals.

Students Actively Involved in Leadership (S.A.I.L.) Conference
Landmark College
River Road South
Putney, VT 05346
802-387-6700
http://www.landmark.edu
Disability Served: attention deficit disorder, dyslexic, learning disabled
This conference at Landmark College offers leadership training opportunities for students.

TASH (The Association for Persons with Severe Handicaps)
29 West Susquehanna Avenue, Suite 210
Baltimore, MD 21204
410-828-8274
http://tash.org
Disability Served: various
The annual TASH conference provides a forum for individuals with disabilities, families, researchers, educators, scholars, and others to create dialogue around creating action for social and systems reform.

MULTIMEDIA AND FILM

The following companies offer multimedia products for people with disabilities, their educators, parents, care-givers, and the public. Also listed are companies that offer video services, such as captioning and descriptive narration.

Alexander Graham Bell Association for the Deaf and Hard of Hearing
3417 Volta Place, NW
Washington, DC 20007
866-337-5220, 202-337-5221 (TTY)
publications@agbell.org
http://www.agbell.org
Disability Served: hearing
This organization provides educational materials, including a video that shows rehabilitation therapists working with students who have had a cochlear implant and a video that details hearing development in the first three years of life.

ASL Access
4217 Adrienne Drive
Alexandria, VA 22309
ASLAccess@aol.com
http://www.aslaccess.org
Disability Served: hearing
This nonprofit organization provides American Sign Language video resources to libraries.

Aylmer Press
PO Box 2302
Madison, WI 53701
888-SIGNIT2
steve@signit2.com
http://www.signit2.com
Disability Served: hearing
This company offers videos that teach kids sign language.

CCMaker
822 Guilford Avenue, #148
Baltimore, MD 21202
800-527-0551
wGallant@CCmaker.com
http://www.ccmaker.com
Disability Served: hearing
This company adds closed-captioning to videos produced by its customers.

Deaf Connection Inc.
330 Hawthorne Lane
Vero Beach, FL 32962

info@signlanguagemadesimple.com
http://www.signlanguagemadesimple.com
Disability Served: hearing
This company offers videos that allows users to learn 1,500 American Sign Language signs, the Manual Alphabet, and numbers.

DeBee Communications
3900 Monet Court South
Pittsburgh, PA 15101-3221
412-492-8214 (TTY)
customer@debee.com
http://www.debee.com
Disability Served: hearing
This company offers educational videos for the hearing impaired.

Educators Publishing Service
PO Box 9031
Cambridge, MA 02139-9031
800-435-7728
customer_service@epsbooks.com
http://www.epsbooks.com
Disability Served: learning disabled
This company offers the Dyslexia Training Program, by the Texas Scottish Rite Hospital, designed to teach reading and writing through the use of videotapes and accompanying texts.

Fanlight Productions
4196 Washington Street
Boston, MA 02131
617-469-4999, 800-937-4113
info@fanlight.com
http://www.fanlight.com
Disability Served: various
This company distributes educational videotapes on disabilities, mental health, gerontology, and general health care.

Harris Communications
15155 Technology Drive
Eden Prairie, MN 55344
952-906-1180, 952-906-1198 (TTY), 800-825-6758, 800-825-9187 (TTY)

info@harriscomm.com
http://www.harriscomm.com
Disability Served: hearing
This company has videotapes and books on sign
language instruction, deaf culture, and other
topics related to hearing disabilities.

Health Tapes Inc.
13225 Capital Street
Oak Park, MI 48237-3106
248-662-5100
Disability Served: cancer, Parkinson's disease
This company produces exercise videotapes for persons
with Parkinson's disease and for persons who have
had breast cancer surgery.

Heartsong Communications
PO Box 2455
Glenview, IL 60025
800-484-8041, ext. 0800
hrtsngComm@aol.com
http://members.aol.com/gaiasign
Disability Served: hearing
This company manufactures children's sign language
and music videotapes by Gaia.

HOPE Inc.
1856 North 1200 East
North Logan, UT 84341
435-245-2888
hope@hopepubl.com
http://www.hopepubl.com
Disability Served: various
This company offers books and videos for people with
a variety of disabilities.

Interax Training
170 Cedar Lane
Portland, TN 37148
800-242-5583
contact@signcourse.com
http://www.signcourse.com
Disability Served: hearing
This company offers the Interax Video Sign Language
Course, a video series about the signs and introductory
concepts of American Sign Language.

Magic Lamp Production
1838 Washington Way
Venice, CA 90291-4704

800-367-9661
videopage@earthlink.net
http://www.aslvideos.com
Disability Served: hearing
This company offers nearly 150 videos about American
Sign Language.

Research Press
Department 25W, PO Box 9177
Champaign, IL 61826
217-352-3273, 800-519-2707
rp@researchpress.com
http://www.researchpress.com
Disability Served: various
This company provides teachers with educational
materials, including videos and workbooks.

Sign Media Inc.
4020 Blackburn Lane
Burtonsville, MD 20866-1167
301-421-0268, 800-475-4756
http://www.signmedia.com
Disability Served: hearing
This company offers videotapes and text material on
American Sign Language and American Deaf Culture.

SignQuest Publishers
4409 Old Colony Drive
Flint, MI 48507
sqp@massoud.org
http://www.massoud.org/sqp
Disability Served: hearing
This company offers books and videos that help people
to learn American Sign Language.

Sign2Me/Northlight Communications
11395 5th Avenue, NE, Suite B
Seattle, WA 98125
206-361-0307 (Voice/TTY), 877-744-6263
http://www.sign2me.com
Disability Served: hearing
This company offers resources that help hearing parents
and their hearing children communicate through
American Sign Language.

PUBLICATIONS

Following are titles of books, magazines, newsletters, and other publications on a wide variety of disability-related topics that may be of interest to people with disabilities and their caregivers, educators, librarians, medical professionals, counselors, and others.

Ability Magazine
1001 West 17th Street
Costa Mesa, CA 92627
949-854-8700
subscriptions@abilitymagazine.com
http://www.abilitymagazine.com
Disability Served: various
This magazine offers employment news and classified ads for persons with disabilities.

About Down Syndrome
National Down Syndrome Society
666 Broadway
New York, NY 10012
800-221-4602
info@ndss.org
http://www.ndss.org/content.cfm?fuseaction=InfoRes.
SrchResMat
Disability Served: Down Syndrome
This free brochure discusses Down Syndrome.

About Heart Transplants: Our Guide for Transplant Patients, Their Families and Donor Families
American Heart Association
7272 Greenville Avenue
Dallas, TX 75231
800-242-8721
http://www.americanheart.org/presenter.
jhtml?identifier=3001740
Disability Served: physically disabled
This free booklet serves as a resource for patients and family members who are facing heart transplantation.

About Your Bypass Surgery: Our Guide to Understanding Coronary Artery Bypass Graft Surgery
American Heart Association
7272 Greenville Avenue
Dallas, TX 75231
800-242-8721
http://www.americanheart.org/presenter.
jhtml?identifier=3001740
Disability Served: physically disabled
This free brochure provides a complete overview of coronary artery bypass graft surgery.

Abstracts in Social Gerontology
National Council on the Aging
300 D Street, SW, Suite 801
Washington, DC 20024
202-479-1200
info@ncoa.org
http://www.ncoa.org/content.cfm?sectionID=30
Disability Served: elderly
This quarterly journal features the latest information in the field of gerontology.

Accessibility Services
United Spinal Association
75-20 Astoria Boulevard
Jackson Heights, NY 11370
718-803-3782, 800-444-0120
publications@unitedspinal.org
http://www.unitedspinal.org/pages.php?catid=7
Disability Served: spinal-cord injury
This free brochure outlines the services provided by the United Spinal Association.

Accessible Air Travel
United Spinal Association
75-20 Astoria Boulevard
Jackson Heights, NY 11370
718-803-3782, 800-444-0120
publications@unitedspinal.org
http://www.unitedspinal.org/pages.php?catid=7
Disability Served: physically disabled
This free booklet provides people who use wheelchairs and other mobility aids with all the information they need to have a safe and enjoyable flight.

Accessible Transit and The Law
Paralyzed Veterans of America
801 Eighteenth Street, NW
Washington, DC 20006-3517
301-932-7834, 888-860-7244
info@pva.org
http://www.pva.org/cgi-bin/pvastore/products.cgi?id=2
Disability Served: various
This free publication details the types of transportation facilities (except air transport) covered by the Americans with Disabilities Act.

Access Info
Access to Independence
2345 Atwood Avenue
Madison, WI 53704
608-242-8484
http://www.accesstoind.org
Disability Served: various
This quarterly newsletter provides news to disabled
people living in Dane, Columbia, Green, and Dodge
counties in Wisconsin.

Accessing Treatment Information-PDQ
R.A. Bloch Cancer Foundation Inc.
4400 Main Street
Kansas City, MO 64111
816-932-8453, 800-433-0464
http://www.blochcancer.org
Disability Served: cancer patients and survivors
This free, online publication helps patients find the latest
state-of-the-art treatment as well as experimental
protocols.

Achieving Physical and Communication Accessibility
Adaptive Environments
374 Congress Street, Suite 301
Boston, MA 02120
617-695-1225
info@adaptiveenvironments.org
http://www.adaptenv.org/index.php?option=Resource&
topicid=25
Disability Served: physically disabled
This book provides businesses with information and tips
about access issues relating to different disabilities
and suggests a variety of accommodations that
provide cost-effective ways to make services
accessible.

**Activities of Daily Living: Practical Pointers for
Parkinson Disease**
National Parkinson Foundation
1501 Northwest Ninth Avenue/Bob Hope Road
Miami, FL 33136-1454
305-243-6666, 800-327-4545
contact@parkinson.org
http://www.parkinson.org/site/pp.asp?c=9dJFJLPwB&b
=71407
Disability Served: Parkinson's Disease
This free booklet includes chapters on bathing, grooming,
toileting, dressing, rest and sleeping, eating, getting
around, and recreation and exercise.

**Adaptations and Accommodations for Students
with Disabilities**
National Dissemination Center for Children with Disabilities
PO Box 1492
Washington, DC 20013
800-695-0285
nichcy@aed.org
http://nichcy.org/publist.asp
Disability Served: various
This free resource guide includes 37 resources for
adapting classrooms and curricula so that the unique
needs of students with disabilities can be met.

Adapted Physical Activity Quarterly
Human Kinetics Publishers Inc.
PO Box 5076
Champaign, IL 61826
217-351-5076, 800-747-4457
http://www.humankinetics.com/APAQ/journalAbout.cfm
Disability Served: various
This quarterly professional journal reports on research
findings, current opinions, and legislative issues
regarding adapted physical activity.

Adult Attention Deficit Disorder (ADD)
National Mental Health Association
2001 North Beauregard Street, 12th Floor
Alexandria, VA 22311
703-684-7722, 800-969-6642
http://www.nmha.org/infoctr/factsheets
Disability Served: attention deficit disorder
This free fact sheet offers information under the
following subject areas on adult attention deficit
disorder (ADD): causes, diagnosis, ADD with or
without hyperactivity, characteristics of adults
with ADD, tips, and additional resources.

Adults with Dyslexia in the Workplace
International Dyslexia Association
Chester Building, 8600 LaSalle Road, Suite 382
Baltimore, MD 21286-2044
410-296-0232
http://www.interdys.org
Disability Served: dyslexic
This online brochure covers important issues for dyslexic
job seekers.

Advocacy Resource List
National Down Syndrome Society
666 Broadway

New York, NY 10012
800-221-4602
info@ndss.org
http://www.ndss.org/content.cfm?fuseaction=InfoRes.
    SrchResMat
Disability Served: Down Syndrome
This free publication offers an annotated bibliography
    of useful organizations and materials on advocacy for
    people with Down Syndrome.

The Advocate
Autism Society of America
7910 Woodmont Avenue, Suite 300
Bethesda, MD 20814-3067
301-657-0881, 800-328-8476
http://www.autism-society.org/site/PageServer?page
    name=AdvocateMagazine
Disability Served: autism
This quarterly magazine for members of the Autism
    Society of America offers the latest information on
    research, legislation, and tips on living with autism.

Advocating for Your Pre-School Child
National Center for Learning Disabilities
381 Park Avenue South, Suite 1401
New York, NY 10016
212-545-7510
http://www.ld.org/LDInfoZone/InfoZone_FactSheet
    Index.cfm
Disability Served: learning disabled
This free fact sheet provides an introductory guide to
    help parents and guardians get help and services,
    if they believe their young child has a learning
    disability.

Advocating for Your School-Aged Child
National Center for Learning Disabilities
381 Park Avenue South, Suite 1401
New York, NY 10016
212-545-7510
http://www.ld.org/LDInfoZone/InfoZone_FactSheet
    Index.cfm
Disability Served: learning disabled
This free fact sheet offers an introductory guide to help
    parents and guardians get help and services if they
    believe their school-aged child has a learning disability.

After Your Heart Attack: Our Guide to Help You Recover
American Heart Association
7272 Greenville Avenue

Dallas, TX 75231
800-242-8721
http://www.americanheart.org/presenter.
    jhtml?identifier=3001740
Disability Served: physically disabled
This free brochure provides useful information for
    patients as they recover from a heart attack.

Aging News Alert
CD Publications
8204 Fenton Street
Silver Spring, MD 20910
301-588-6380, 800-666-6380
info@cdpublications.com
http://www.cdpublications.com/pubs/agingnews.php
Disability Served: elderly
This weekly report features legislative updates on aging
    issues.

AIDS Alert
American Health Consultants Inc.
PO Box 740056
Atlanta, GA 30374
404-262-7436
http://www.ahcpub.com
Disability Served: AIDS
This monthly publication discusses AIDS issues.

**The Air Carrier Access Act: Common Questions and
    Answers about Air Travel for Wheelchair Users**
Paralyzed Veterans of America
801 Eighteenth Street, NW
Washington, DC 20006-3517
301-932-7834, 888-860-7244
info@pva.org
http://www.pva.org/cgi-bin/pvastore/products.cgi?id=2
Disability Served: various
This free pamphlet responds to the most frequently
    asked questions concerning the implications of the
    Air Carrier Access Act.

**American Lung Association's Family Guide to Asthma
    and Allergies**
American Lung Association
61 Broadway
New York, NY 10006
212-315-8700, 800-LUNG
http://www.lungusa.org/site/pp.asp?c=dvLUK9O0
    E&b=22903
Disability Served: asthma

This book answers questions about asthma and allergies and explains how to manage asthma and allergies to lead an active, healthy life.

All Kinds of Minds

Educators Publishing Service Inc.
PO Box 9031
Cambridge, MA 02139-9031
800-435-7728
customer_service@epsbooks.com
http://www.epsbooks.com
Disability Served: learning disabled
This book provides fictional profiles of students and their learning disorders.

All You Need to Know About Back Pain

Arthritis Foundation
PO Box 7669
Atlanta, GA 30357
800-568-4045
http://www.arthritis.org/AFstore/CategoryHome.
asp?idCat=3
Disability Served: back injury, chronic pain
This book will help arthritis sufferers discover how to make the most of their medical treatment and therapies, make exercise routines less painful, build a stronger spine, learn to relax and relieve stress-related pain, and get a good night's sleep.

Alternative Therapies Resource List

National Down Syndrome Society
666 Broadway
New York, NY 10012
800-221-4602
info@ndss.org
http://www.ndss.org/content.cfm?fuseaction=InfoRes.
SrchResMat
Disability Served: Down Syndrome
This free publication offers an annotated bibliography of useful organizations and materials on alternative therapies for people with Down Syndrome.

Alzheimer's Disease

National Mental Health Association
2001 North Beauregard Street, 12th Floor
Alexandria, VA 22311
703-684-7722, 800-969-6642
http://www.nmha.org/infoctr/factsheets
Disability Served: dementia
This free fact sheet provides the following information

on Alzheimer's: symptoms, diagnosis, research for possible risk factors, treatment, and additional resources.

Alzheimer's Disease Resource List

National Down Syndrome Society
666 Broadway
New York, NY 10012
800-221-4602
info@ndss.org
http://www.ndss.org/content.cfm?fuseaction=InfoRes.
SrchResMat
Disability Served: dementia, Down Syndrome
This free publication offers an annotated bibliography of useful organizations and materials on Alzheimer's disease and Down Syndrome.

Alzheimer's: Searching for a Cure

Federal Citizen Information Center
1800 F Street, NW
Washington, DC 20405
888-878-3256
firstgov1@mail.fedinfo.gov
http://www.pueblo.gsa.gov/results.
tpl?id1=16&startat=1&--woSECTIONSdatarq=16&--
SECTIONSword=ww
Disability Served: dementia
This free brochure provides information on how Alzheimer's is diagnosed, its symptoms, current drug treatments, and lifestyle advice to help prolong mental health.

American Annals of the Deaf

Gallaudet University Press
800 Florida Avenue, NE
Washington, DC 20002
202-651-5488 (Voice/TTY)
valencia.simmons@gallaudet.edu
http://gupress.gallaudet.edu
Disability Served: hearing
Published quarterly, this well-known journal covers a variety of issues related to deafness and the education of deaf persons.

American Art Therapy Association Journal

American Art Therapy Association Inc.
1202 Allanson Road
Mundelein, IL 60060
847-949-6064
http://www.arttherapy.org

Disability Served: various
This quarterly journal provides information on art therapy and its application in the education, training, and development of disabled people.

American Association of Retired Persons Bulletin
American Association of Retired Persons
601 East Street, NW
Washington, DC 20049
888-687-2277
http://www.aarp.org/bulletin/prescription
Disability Served: various
This free, online news bulletin contains newsworthy events of interest to senior citizens. Common topics include issues with Medicaid and prescription drugs.

American Association of Retired Persons Health Guide
American Association of Retired Persons
601 East Street, NW
Washington, DC 20049
888-687-2277
http://www.aarp.org/health/healthguide
Disability Served: various
This free, online health guide offers reliable, easy-to-use information about health conditions and treatments. It includes information on medications; medical tests; self-help groups; Medicare rights, benefits and options at the federal and state level; and the importance of quality in healthcare.

American Association of Retired Persons: The Magazine
American Association of Retired Persons
601 East Street, NW
Washington, DC 20049
888-687-2277
http://www.aarpmagazine.org
Disability Served: various
This magazine discusses issues and topics of interest to retired persons in the United States.

American Cancer Society's Complete Guide to Prostate Cancer
American Cancer Society
1599 Clifton Road, PO Box 49528
Atlanta, GA 30359-0528
800-ACS-2346
http://www.cancer.org/docroot/PUB/PUB_
    1.asp?sitearea=PUB
Disability Served: cancer patients and survivors

This guidebook for men and their loved ones delivers the facts about prostate cancer—the latest advances in prevention, early detection, and treatment; the range of treatment options available and their advantages, expected outcomes, potential side effects; and how to cope with emotional stresses and potential physical side effects.

American Cancer Society's Consumer Guide to Cancer Drugs
American Cancer Society
1599 Clifton Road, PO Box 49528
Atlanta, GA 30359-0528
800-ACS-2346
http://www.cancer.org/docroot/PUB/PUB_
    1.asp?sitearea=PUB
Disability Served: cancer patients and survivors
This reference book provides the basic information that patients and their families need during cancer treatment in easy-to-understand language. Included are side effects and precautions for over 200 cancer-related medicines, explanations of the latest cancer drugs, how drugs are administered and taken, and a comprehensive glossary of cancer treatment terms.

American Cancer Society's Guide to Pain Control
American Cancer Society
1599 Clifton Road, PO Box 49528
Atlanta, GA 30359-0528
800-ACS-2346
http://www.cancer.org/docroot/PUB/PUB_
    1.asp?sitearea=PUB
Disability Served: cancer patients and survivors, chronic pain
This book helps people with cancer work with their health care teams to create effective pain-relief plans.

American Deafness and Rehabilitation Association Update
American Deafness and Rehabilitation Association
PO Box 480
Myersville, MD 21773
http://www.adara.org/pages/publications.shtml
Disability Served: hearing
This quarterly journal provides information on activities and news regarding the association.

American Diabetes Association Complete Guide to Diabetes
American Diabetes Association
1701 North Beauregard Street

Alexandria, VA 22311
800-342-2383
AskADA@diabetes.org
http://www.diabetes.org
Disability Served: diabetes
This sourcebook provides information on how to
    live an active, healthy life with diabetes. Self-care
    techniques, the latest medical breakthroughs,
    information about insulin, and dealing with
    workplace issues are just some of the topics covered.

American Foundation for the Blind Directory of
    Services for Blind and Visually Impaired Persons
    in the United States and Canada
American Foundation for the Blind
11 Penn Plaza, Suite 300
New York, NY 10001
212-502-7600, 800-232-5463
afbinfo@afb.net
http://www.afb.org
Disability Served: vision
This comprehensive resource book provides organizational
    profiles that include full contact information, including
    Web site addresses and key personnel, as well as useful
    descriptions of services offered that will help you
    identify the appropriate agency for your needs.

American Hearing Research Foundation Newsletter
American Hearing Research Foundation
8 South Michigan Avenue, Suite 814
Chicago, IL 60603-4539
312-726-9670
lkoch@american-hearing.org
http://www.american-hearing.org/name/about.html
Disability Served: hearing
This newsletter provides news on recent research studies
    and education programs related to hearing.

American Heart Association 365 Ways to Get Out
    the Fat: A Tip a Day to Trim the Fat Away
American Heart Association
7272 Greenville Avenue
Dallas, TX 75231
800-242-8721
http://www.americanheart.org/presenter.
    jhtml?identifier=3001740
Disability Served: physically disabled
This pocket guide is filled with tips on shopping,
    cooking, snacking, and preparing and customizing
    favorite foods.

American Journal of Orthopsychiatry
American Orthopsychiatric Association
Arizona State University
Department of Psychology
Box 1104
Tempe, AZ 85287-1104
480-727-7518
http://www.amerortho.org
Disability Served: mental health
This quarterly journal discusses mental health issues.

American Journal of Physical Medicine
    and Rehabilitation
Lippincott Williams and Wilkins
530 Walnut Street
Philadelphia, PA 19106-3621
215-521-8300
orders@lww.com
http://www.lww.com/product/?0894-9115
Disability Served: various
This journal focuses on the practice, research, and
    educational aspects of physical medicine and
    rehabilitation.

American Journal of Psychiatry
American Psychiatric Association
1000 Wilson Boulevard, Suite 1825
Arlington, VA 22209-3901
703-907-7300
apa@psych.org
http://www.psych.org
Disability Served: mental health
This monthly professional journal publishes scholarly
    articles on psychiatry.

American Journal of Public Health
American Public Health Association Inc.
800 I Street, NW
Washington, DC 20001-3710
202-777-APHA
http://www.apha.org/journal
Disability Served: various
This monthly journal provides scholarly articles on
    public health topics.

American Journal on Mental Retardation
American Association on Mental Retardation
444 North Capitol Street, NW, Suite 846
Washington, DC 20001-1512
800-424-3688

http://aamr.allenpress.com/aamronline/
?request=index-html
Disability Served: mental retardation
This journal provides scholarly articles on topics related
to mental retardation.

American Sign Language Handshape Flash Cards
Gallaudet University Press
800 Florida Avenue, NE
Washington, DC 20002
202-651-5488 (Voice/TTY)
valencia.simmons@gallaudet.edu
http://gupress.gallaudet.edu
Disability Served: hearing
These flash cards are designed to help students learn
American Sign Language.

American Sign Language-to-English Interpretation: Say It Like They Mean It
Registry of the Interpreters for the Deaf
333 Commerce Street
Alexandria, VA 22314
703-838-0030, 703-838-0459 (TTY)
info@rid.org
http://www.rid.org/pubs.html
Disability Served: hearing
This book looks at difficulties and issues that can arise
as interpreters work between ASL and English, with
exercises at the end of every chapter.

Americans with Disabilities Act Reference Packet
Disability Rights Education and Defense Fund
2212 Sixth Street
Berkeley, CA 94710
510-644-2555 (Voice/TTY)
dredf@dredf.org
http://www.dredf.org/publications.html
Disability Served: various
This guide analyzes all aspects of the Americans
with Disabilities Act.

Am I at Risk for Gestational Diabetes?
National Institute of Child Health and Human
Development
PO Box 2006
Rockville, MD 20847
800-370-2943
NICHDInformationResourceCenter@mail.nih.gov
http://www.nichd.nih.gov/publications/pubs.cfm
Disability Served: diabetes

This free brochure for pregnant women explains
gestational diabetes and lists the risk factors for
this condition.

Annals of Otology, Rhinology and Larynology
Annals Publishing Company
4507 Laclede Avenue
St Louis, MO 63108
314-367-4987
Manager@Annals.com
http://www.annals.com
Disability Served: various
This monthly publication provides articles on head
and neck injury,

Answering Your Questions about Epilepsy
Epilepsy Foundation
4351 Garden City Drive
Landover, MD 20785-7223
800-332-1000
http://www.epilepsyfoundation.org
Disability Served: epilepsy
This booklet contains basic information about epilepsy:
what it is, why people have it, what they can do to treat
it, and how they can take better care of themselves.

Answers for Employers
Stuttering Foundation of America
3100 Walnut Grove Road, Suite 603, PO Box 11749
Memphis, TN 38111-0749
901-452-7342, 800-992-9392
info@stutteringhelp.org
http://www.stutteringhelp.org/Default.aspx?tabid=131
Disability Served: communication
This free, downloadable brochure answers some
common questions about stuttering, and provides
additional resources for people who stutter, and their
colleagues in the workplace.

Antidepressant Medication and Children: Tips for Parents
National Mental Health Association
2001 North Beauregard Street, 12th Floor
Alexandria, VA 22311
703-684-7722, 800-969-6642
http://www.nmha.org/infoctr/factsheets
Disability Served: mental health
This free fact sheet helps parents better understand and
make decisions about the use of SSRI antidepressant
medication for their children.

Aphasia: What Is It?

The Speech Bin
1965 25th Avenue
Vero Beach, FL 32960
800-477-3324
info@speechbin.com
http://www.speechbin.com
Disability Served: communication, stroke
This set of brochures provides information on aphasic
language disorders that are caused by strokes. These
brochures are appropriate for families and caregivers
of persons with these disorders.

Archives of Neurology

American Medical Association
PO Box 10946
Chicago, IL 60610-0946
312-670-7827, 800-262-2350
ama-subs@ama-assn.org
http://pubs.ama-assn.org
Disability Served: various
This monthly publication provides scholarly articles
neurology-related topics.

Are You at Risk of Heart Attack or Stroke?

American Heart Association
7272 Greenville Avenue
Dallas, TX 75231
800-242-8721
http://www.americanheart.org/presenter.
jhtml?identifier=3001740
Disability Served: various
This free brochure can be used to educate those who
do not know the risk factors for heart disease and
stroke and to encourage them to see their healthcare
provider.

Art for Me Too!

Ablenet
2808 Fairview Avenue
Roseville, MN 55113-1308
800-322-0956
customerservice@ablenetinc.com
http://www.ablenetinc.com
Disability Served: physically disabled
This resource book helps support all students in art
activities using assistive technology. The functional
projects are based on proven and successful
education techniques.

Art Projects for the Mentally Retarded Child

Charles C. Thomas, Publisher
2600 South First Street
Springfield, IL 62704
800-258-8980
books@ccthomas.com
http://www.ccthomas.com
Disability Served: mental retardation
This text is designed to present art therapy projects to
the special education instructor.

Arthritis

American Occupational Therapy Association Inc.
4720 Montgomery Lane, PO Box 31220
Bethesda, MD 20824-1220
301-652-2682, 800-377-8555
http://www.aota.org/featured/area6/links/link02.asp
Disability Served: physically disabled
This free tip sheet provides information on the
modifications occupational therapists might
suggest to help people with arthritis work and live
independently while avoiding stress to the joints.

Arthritis and Rheumatic Diseases

Federal Citizen Information Center
1800 F Street, NW
Washington, DC 20405
888-878-3256
firstgov1@mail.fedinfo.gov
http://www.pueblo.gsa.gov/results.
tpl?id1=16&startat=1&--woSECTIONS
datarq=16&--SECTIONSword=ww
Disability Served: physically disabled
This free booklet provides basic facts about these
conditions, including examples of rheumatic
diseases, symptoms, causes, diagnosis, and
treatments.

Arthritis Drugs and More: An A to Z Guide

Arthritis Foundation
PO Box 7669
Atlanta, GA 30357
800-568-4045
http://www.arthritis.org/AFstore/CategoryHome.
asp?idCat=3
Disability Served: physically disabled
This book explores more than 260 prescription and over-
the-counter medications, including new COX-2 drugs,
pain-fighting analgesics, powerful new biologic
drugs, and more.

Arthritis: Timely Treatments for an Ageless Disease
Federal Citizen Information Center
1800 F Street, NW
Washington, DC 20405
888-878-3256
firstgov1@mail.fedinfo.gov
http://www.pueblo.gsa.gov/results.
    tpl?id1=16&startat=1&--woSECTIONS
    datarq=16&--SECTIONSword=ww
Disability Served: physically disabled
This free guide explains the types of arthritis, new
    treatments available, unproven remedies to guard
    against, and more.

Arthritis Today
Arthritis Foundation
PO Box 581
Mt. Morris, IL 61054-0581
800-283-7800
http://www.arthritis.org/AFstore/SubCatHome.
    asp?idCat=8&idSubCat=130
Disability Served: physically disabled
This magazine offers the latest information on research
    and new treatments and tips from experts and
    readers to help those with arthritis lead easier and
    more rewarding lives.

***Assessing Children for the Presence of a Disability:
    A Resource List You Can Use***
National Dissemination Center for Children with
    Disabilities
PO Box 1492
Washington, DC 20013
800-695-0285
nichcy@aed.org
http://nichcy.org/publist.asp
Disability Served: various
This free resource list will help schools as they plan
    assessments of individual students and instruction
    appropriate to the needs of students in special
    education.

***Assessing Learners with Special Needs:
    An Applied Approach***
Allyn & Bacon
75 Arlington Street, Suite 300
Boston, MA 02116
800-852-8024
http://www.ablongman.com
Disability Served: various

This book provides information for teachers in public
    schools who work with students who have mild to
    moderate disabling conditions.

Assistive Technologies: Principles and Practice
RESNA Press
1700 Moore Street, Suite 1540
Arlington, VA 22209-1903
703-524-6686, 703-524-6639 (TTY)
info@resna.org
http://www.resna.org/ProfResources/Publications/
    Publications2.php
Disability Served: various
This sourcebook offers information on assistive
    technology, including how and where to find it, how
    to evaluate it, the benefits of assistive technology,
    and more.

Assistive Technology Journal
AT Network/California Assistive Technology Systems
1029 J Street, Suite 120
Sacramento, CA 95814-2495
916-325-1690, 916-325-1695 (TTY)
http://www.atnet.org/news/index.html
Disability Served: various
This magazine, which is published twice a month,
    provides news and resources about assistive
    technology. It is available free online.

Asthma and Children Fact Sheet
American Lung Association
61 Broadway
New York, NY 10006
212-315-8700, 800-LUNG
http://www.lungusa.org/site/apps/s/content.asp?c=dvL
    UK9O0E&b=34706&ct=67462
Disability Served: asthma
This Web page provides facts and statistics on asthma in
    children.

Asthma in Adults Fact Sheet
American Lung Association
61 Broadway
New York, NY 10006
212-315-8700, 800-LUNG
http://www.lungusa.org/site/apps/s/content.asp?c=dvL
    UK9O0E&b=34706&ct=67470
Disability Served: asthma
This Web page provides facts and statistics on asthma in
    adults.

Asthma Magazine
American Lung Association
61 Broadway
New York, NY 10006
http://www.lungusa.org/site/pp.asp?c=dvLUK9O0E&b=
22903
Disability Served: asthma
This bimonthly publication is for people with asthma
who are interested in learning more about their
condition and how to manage it.

As You Get Older: Information for Teens
Cleft Palate Foundation
1504 East Franklin Street, Suite 102
Chapel Hill, NC 27514-2820
919-933-9044, 800-24CLEFT
info@cleftline.org
http://www.cleftline.org/publications
Disability Served: physically disabled
This free brochure discusses medical treatment, surgery,
braces, speech, and ear/nose/throat concerns, as well
as social relationships for teens born with clefts.

Ataxia Fact Sheet
National Ataxia Foundation
2600 Fernbrook Lane, Suite 119
Minneapolis, MN 55447
naf@ataxia.org
http://www.ataxia.org
Disability Served: physically disabled
This free brochure describes ataxia as a symptom (lack of
coordination) and its association with other medical
problems. It also discusses the hereditary types.

*Attention Deficit Disorder and the College Student:
A Guide for High School and College Students
with Attention Deficit Disorder*
Magination Press
750 First Street, NE
Washington, DC 20002-4242
800-374-2721
magination@apa.org
http://www.maginationpress.com
Disability Served: attention deficit disorder
This book provides advice for students with attention
deficit disorder who plan to attend college.

Attention Deficit Hyperactivity Disorder
American Occupational Therapy Association Inc.
4720 Montgomery Lane, PO Box 31220

Bethesda, MD 20824-1220
301-652-3682, 800-377-8555
http://www.aota.org/featured/area6/links/link02.asp
Disability Served: attention deficit disorder
This free tip sheet offers information to parents on
attention deficit hyperactivity disorder and how to
cope with the issues that arise from it. It also provides
an overview of how occupational therapists can help
a child with the disorder.

Attention Deficit/Hyperactivity Disorder
National Center for Learning Disabilities
381 Park Avenue South, Suite 1401
New York, NY 10016
212-545-7510
http://www.ld.org/LDInfoZone/InfoZone_
FactSheetIndex.cfm
Disability Served: attention deficit disorder
This free fact sheet provides a basic overview of this
disorder.

Attention Deficit/Hyperactivity Disorder
National Dissemination Center for Children
with Disabilities
PO Box 1492
Washington, DC 20013
800-695-0285
nichcy@aed.org
http://nichcy.org/publist.asp
Disability Served: attention deficit disorder
This free briefing paper is designed to help parents,
teachers, and others interested in Attention-Deficit/
Hyperactivity Disorder know what to look for, what to
do, and how to get help.

Attention Deficit/Hyperactivity Disorder
National Mental Health Association
2001 North Beauregard Street, 12th Floor
Alexandria, VA 22311
703-684-7722, 800-969-6642
http://www.nmha.org/infoctr/factsheets
Disability Served: attention deficit disorder
This free fact sheet offers information under the
following subject categories on attention-deficit/
hyperactivity disorder (ADHD): signs and symptoms,
affects on school and social life, other disorders
commonly occurring with ADHD, causes, treatments,
and additional resources for parents.

Attention-Deficit/Hyperactivity Disorder: What Every Parent Wants to Know

Paul H. Brookes Publishing Company Inc.
PO Box 10624
Baltimore, MD 21285-0624
800-638-3775
custserv@brookespublishing.com
http://www.pbrookes.com
Disability Served: attention deficit disorder
This useful text covers Attention-Deficit/Hyperactivity Disorder symptoms and diagnosis, medical interventions, instructional strategies, effective communication strategies, and other topics.

Augmentative and Alternative Communication

International Society of Augmentative and Alternative Communication
49 The Donway West, Suite 308
Toronto, ON M3C 3M9
Canada
416-385-0351
https://www1.securesiteserver.co.uk/isaaconline/en/publications/buy/aac.php
Disability Served: communication
This professional journal of the International Society of Augmentative and Alternative Communication reports on speech and language impairments.

Autism

American Occupational Therapy Association Inc.
4720 Montgomery Lane, PO Box 31220
Bethesda, MD 20824-1220
301-652-2682, 800-377-8555
http://www.aota.org/featured/area6/links/link02.asp
Disability Served: autism
This free tip sheet offers information to parents on what autism is and how to cope with specific situations. It also provides an overview of how occupational therapists can help an autistic child.

Autism

National Mental Health Association
2001 North Beauregard Street, 12th Floor
Alexandria, VA 22311
703-684-7722, 800-969-6642
http://www.nmha.org/infoctr/factsheets
Disability Served: autism
This free fact sheet offers information under the following subject categories on autism: definition, signs, causes, treatments, effects on the entire family, and additional resources for parents.

Autism and Genes

National Institute of Child Health and Human Development
PO Box 2006
Rockville, MD 20847
800-370-2943
NICHDInformationResourceCenter@mail.nih.gov
http://www.nichd.nih.gov/publications/pubs.cfm
Disability Served: autism
This free fact sheet for parents and families provides data related to autism spectrum disorders, genes, and Institute-supported research on the topic.

Autism and Pervasive Developmental Disorders Resources

National Dissemination Center for Children with Disabilities
PO Box 1492
Washington, DC 20013
800-695-0285
nichcy@aed.org
http://nichcy.org/publist.asp
Disability Served: autism
This resource list is designed to connect readers to some of the latest resources on these disorders.

Autism-Asperger's Digest

Future Horizons
721 West Abram Street
Arlington, TX 76013
800-489-0727
info@futurehorizons-autism.com
http://www.autismdigest.com
Disability Served: Asperger Syndrome, autism
This is a bimonthly digest that features articles and book reviews about autism-related topics.

The Autism Encyclopedia

Paul H. Brookes Publishing Company Inc.
PO Box 10624
Baltimore, MD 21285-0624
800-638-3775
custserv@brookespublishing.com
http://www.pbrookes.com
Disability Served: autism
This is an A-to-Z reference on autism that includes 500 entries.

Autism Fact Sheet

National Institute of Neurological Disorders and Stroke
PO Box 5801

Bethesda, MD 20824
301-496-5751, 800-352-9424
http://www.ninds.nih.gov/disorders/autism/autism.
htm#Publications
Disability Served: autism
This free fact sheet provides information on diagnosis
and treatment of autism.

Autism Overview: What We Know
National Institute of Child Health and Human
Development
PO Box 2006
Rockville, MD 20847
800-370-2943
NICHDInformationResourceCenter@mail.nih.gov
http://www.nichd.nih.gov/publications/pubs.cfm
Disability Served: autism
This free fact sheet for parents and families provides
data related to autism spectrum disorders and
institute-supported research on the topic.

Autism/Pervasive Developmental Disorders
National Dissemination Center for Children with
Disabilities
PO Box 1492
Washington, DC 20013
800-695-0285
nichcy@aed.org
http://nichcy.org/publist.asp
Disability Served: autism
This free fact sheet defines autism and related disorders
and provides information on the incidence,
characteristics, and educational implications of the
disorders, as well as lists additional resources and
associated organizations.

Autism Spectrum Disorders from A to Z
Future Horizons
721 West Abram Street
Arlington, TX 76013
800-489-0727
info@futurehorizons-autism.com
http://www.futurehorizons-autism.com/search_result.asp
Disability Served: autism
This publication covers symptoms, definitions, assessments, and diagnoses of autism spectrum disorders.

Awareness
National Association for Parents of Children with
Visual Impairments
PO Box 317

Watertown, MA 02471
admin@spedex.com
http://www.spedex.com/napvi/order.html
Disability Served: vision
This quarterly newsletter—free to members—is filled
with legislative updates, articles, notices regarding
conferences, ideas for activities, association regional
news and announcements, vendor advertisements,
thoughtful commentary, and letters to the editor.

Babies with Down Syndrome
Woodbine House
6510 Bells Mill Road
Bethesda, MD 20817
800-843-7323
http://www.woodbinehouse.com/Down-
Syndrome.29.0.0.2.htm
Disability Served: Down Syndrome
This guide for new parents covers all aspects of care
for babies and young children with Down Syndrome.
It includes daily care, family life, intervention,
education, and legal and medical issues.

Baby Talk: Helping Your Hearing-Impaired Baby Listen and Talk
Alexander Graham Bell Association of the Deaf
3417 Volta Place, NW
Washington, DC 20007
866-337-5220, 202-337-5221 (TTY)
publications@agbell.org
http://www.agbell.org
Disability Served: hearing
This is an instruction manual for parents of children,
from newborns to age four.

Back Injury Prevention Guide
LRP Publications
747 Dresher Road, Suite 500, PO Box 980
Horsham, PA 19044-0980
215-784-0860, 800-341-7874
http://www.shoplrp.com/product/p-31030.html
Disability Served: back injury
This pamphlet describes the common mistakes that
cause back injuries and shows people how to perform
their jobs pain- and injury-free. Includes details on
how to spot potential hazards and illustrations of
proper lifting and material-handling techniques.

Basic Home Care for ALS Patients
Amyotrophic Lateral Sclerosis Association
27001 Agoura Road, Suite 150

Calabasas Hills, CA 91301-5104
818-880-9007
info@alsa-national.org
http://www.alsa.org/resources/brochures.cfm?CFID=104
8742&CFTOKEN=97497558
Disability Served: physically disabled
This free, downloadable brochure provides basic
information about home care for people affected by
Amytrophic Lateral Sclerosis.

Be an Active Member of Your Health Care Team
Federal Citizen Information Center
1800 F Street, NW
Washington, DC 20405
888-878-3256
firstgov1@mail.fedinfo.gov
http://www.pueblo.gsa.gov/results.
tpl?id1=16&startat=1&--woSECTIONSdatarq=
16&--SECTIONSword=ww
Disability Served: various
This free brochure offers consumer protection tips and
describes how to get the most benefits from prescription and over-the-counter drugs. It includes a list of
questions to ask the doctor, nurse, or pharmacist.

Beautiful Universal Design: A Visual Guide
Adaptive Environments
374 Congress Street, Suite 301
Boston, MA 02120
617-695-1225
info@adaptiveenvironments.org
http://www.adaptenv.org/index.php?option=Resource
&topicid=25
Disability Served: physically disabled
This book discusses universal design and cultural
facilities.

Becoming a Parent
Multiple Sclerosis Society of Canada
175 Bloor Street East, Suite 700, North Tower
Toronto, ON M4W 3R8
Canada
416-922-6065, 800-268-7582
info@mssociety.ca
http://www.mssociety.ca/en/information/references.
htm
Disability Served: multiple sclerosis
This free, downloadable article addresses the question
of whether or not to become a parent if you are
a woman who has multiple sclerosis. The article

summarizes some of the latest research on this issue
and presents a positive point of view.

Behavioral Disorders
Council for Exceptional Children
1110 North Glebe Road, Suite 300
Arlington, VA 22201-5704
888-CEC-SPED, 866-915-5000 (TTY)
service@cec.sped.org
http://www.cec.sped.org
Disability Served: behavioral disorders
This quarterly journal discusses childhood behavioral
disorders, including assessment, educational
programs, and more.

Behavioral Evaluation of Hearing in Infants and Young Children
Alexander Graham Bell Association of the Deaf
3417 Volta Place, NW
Washington, DC 20007
866-337-5220, 202-337-5221 (TTY)
publications@agbell.org
http://www.agbell.org
Disability Served: hearing
This describes methods for conducting audiology
assessments in clinical settings.

Behavior Modification
SAGE Publications
2455 Teller Road
Thousand Oaks, CA 91320
805-499-9774, 800-818-7243
info@sagepub.com
http://www.sagepub.com
Disability Served: various
This quarterly publication is designed for therapists and
rehabilitation professionals and provides behavior
modification techniques.

Being Your Own Advocate
National Center for Learning Disabilities
381 Park Avenue South, Suite 1401
New York, NY 10016
212-545-7510
http://www.ld.org/LDInfoZone/InfoZone_
FactSheetIndex.cfm
Disability Served: learning disabled
This free fact sheet helps teens and adults with learning
disabilities become familiar with the rights and
responsibilities they have in school, college, and the
workplace.

The Bell

National Mental Health Association (NMHA)
2001 North Beauregard Street, 12th Floor
Alexandria, VA 22311
703-684-7722, 800-969-6642
thebell@nmha.org
http://www.nmha.org/newsroom/bell/index.cfm
Disability Served: mental health
This newsletter for NMHA members, affiliates, and
others helps people to stay informed about leading
issues and NMHA's advocacy efforts, and be aware of
educational and advocacy activities.

Be Smart about Your Heart. Control the ABC's of Diabetes: A1C, Blood Pressure, and Cholesterol

National Diabetes Information Clearinghouse
5 Information Way
Bethesda, MD 20892-3568
800-860-8747
catalog@niddk.nih.gov
http://catalog.niddk.nih.gov/AlphaList.cfm?CH=NDIC
Disability Served: diabetes
This brochure explains the link between diabetes and
heart disease and encourages people with diabetes
to take action to control the ABCs of diabetes: A1C,
blood pressure, and cholesterol. Single copies are
free.

The Best of Diabetes Self-Management

R.A. Rapaport Publishing Inc.
PO Box 11066
Des Moines, IA 50336-1066
800-664-9269
https://www.diabetesselfmanagement.com/eds/books.cfm
Disability Served: diabetes
This 460-page comprehensive desktop reference
provides effective ways of successfully managing all
aspects of diabetes.

Best Practices in Physical Activity

National Council on the Aging
300 D Street, SW, Suite 801
Washington, DC 20024
202-479-1200
info@ncoa.org
http://www.ncoa.org/content.cfm?sectionID=30
Disability Served: elderly
This free, downloadable document provides an overview
of the critical elements of programming necessary for
effective promotion of good health, physical activity,
and chronic disease self-management.

The Best Year of My Life: Book 1: Getting Diabetes

Juvenile Diabetes Foundation
120 Wall Street
New York, NY 10005-4001
800-533-2873
info@jdrf.org
http://www.jdrf.org/index.cfm?page_id=100250
Disability Served: diabetes
This inspirational story, written in the voice of a newly
diagnosed seven-year-old girl, helps families deal
with the emotional issues that accompany diabetes.

Better Communication and Hearing Aids: Guide to Hearing Aid Use

Alexander Graham Bell Association of the Deaf
3417 Volta Place, NW
Washington, DC 20007
866-337-5220, 202-337-5221 (TTY)
publications@agbell.org
http://www.agbell.org
Disability Served: hearing
This is a practical, how-to workbook that teaches people
how to get the most out of their hearing aids.

Beyond Traditional Cancer Care

American Cancer Society
1599 Clifton Road, PO Box 49528
Atlanta, GA 30359-0528
800-ACS-2346
http://www.cancer.org/docroot/PUB/PUB_1.asp?sitearea=PUB
Disability Served: cancer patients and survivors
This free, online guide to complementary and alternative
therapies provides the facts and philosophies behind
more than 100 such therapies.

Bipolar Disorder in Children

National Mental Health Association
2001 North Beauregard Street, 12th Floor
Alexandria, VA 22311
703-684-7722, 800-969-6642
http://www.nmha.org/infoctr/factsheets
Disability Served: mental health
This free fact sheet offers information under the
following subject categories: signs and symptoms,
what parents should do, and additional resources for
parents.

Blind Educator
National Federation of the Blind
1800 Johnson Street
Baltimore, MD 21230
410-659-9314
nfbstore@nfb.org
http://www.nfb.org/publications.html
Disability Served: vision
This newsletter is written by blind educators for
educators who are blind.

Blind Spots: The Communicative Performance of
Visual Impairment in Relationships and Social
Interaction
Charles C. Thomas, Publisher
2600 South First Street
Springfield, IL 62704
800-258-8980
books@ccthomas.com
http://www.ccthomas.com
Disability Served: vision
This text provides the results of a detailed survey of the
visually impaired to gauge how their disability affects
relationships and social interaction.

Board Games for Play and Say: School and Home
Board Games for Students with Speech and
Language Impairments
Pro-Ed Inc.
8700 Shoal Creek Boulevard
Austin, TX 78757-6897
800-897-3202
http://www.proedinc.com
Disability Served: communication
This set of educational games is designed to teach
speech sounds.

Braille Book Review
National Library Service for the Blind and Physically
Handicapped
1291 Taylor Street, NW
Washington, DC 20011
202-707-5100, 202-707-0744 (TDD)
nls@loc.gov
http://www.loc.gov/nls
Disability Served: vision
This publication provides information and reviews on
Braille books and other publications available at
cooperating libraries.

Braille Forum
American Council of the Blind
1155 15th Street, NW, Suite 1004
Washington, DC 20005
202-467-5081, 800-424-8666
http://www.acb.org
Disability Served: vision
This monthly publication provides news on council
activities and programs.

Braille Monitor
National Federation of the Blind
1800 Johnson Street
Baltimore, MD 21230
410-659-9314
nfbstore@nfb.org
http://www.nfb.org/publications.html
Disability Served: vision
This monthly newsletter covers the events and activities
of the National Federation of the Blind and addresses
many issues and concerns of the blind.

Brain Basics: Preventing Stroke
National Institute of Neurological Disorders and Stroke
PO Box 5801
Bethesda, MD 20824
301-496-5751, 800-352-9424
http://www.ninds.nih.gov/disorders/stroke/stroke.
htm#Publications
Disability Served: stroke
This free brochure provides information on stroke
prevention, including stroke risk factors and warning
signs.

Brain Injury
Brain Injury Association of America
8201 Greensboro Drive, Suite 611
McLean, VA 22102
703-761-0750, 800-444-6443
familyhelpline@biausa.org
http://www.biausa.org/Pages/facts_and_stats.html
Disability Served: traumatic brain injury
This free, downloadable fact sheet offers an overview
of brain injury, including its costs and consequences.

Brain Injury through the Years
Brain Injury Association of America
8201 Greensboro Drive, Suite 611
McLean, VA 22102
703-761-0750, 800-444-6443

familyhelpline@biausa.org
http://www.biausa.org/Pages/brochures.html#brain
Disability Served: traumatic brain injury
These free, downloadable brochures provide information about brain injury at different life stage. Brochures include *The ABC Years, The Teenage Years,* and *The Golden Years.*

Breast Cancer and Mammograms
Federal Citizen Information Center
1800 F Street, NW
Washington, DC 20405
888-878-3256
firstgov1@mail.fedinfo.gov
http://www.pueblo.gsa.gov/results.tpl?id1=16&startat=1
    &--woSECTIONSdatarq=16&--SECTIONSword=ww
Disability Served: cancer patients and survivors
This free brochure describes who is at risk for breast cancer, what you can do, and how a mammogram can help.

A Breast Cancer Journey
American Cancer Society
1599 Clifton Road, PO Box 49528
Atlanta, GA 30359-0528
800-ACS-2346
http://www.cancer.org/docroot/PUB/PUB_
    1.asp?sitearea=PUB
Disability Served: cancer patients and survivors
This book offers current information about diagnosis, treatment options, and beyond with input from readers, survivors, and experts.

Breathe Easy: Respiratory Care for Children with Muscular Dystrophy
Muscular Dystrophy Association
3300 East Sunrise Drive
Tucson, AZ 85718
800-572-1717
publications@mdausa.org
http://www.mdausa.org/publications
Disability Served: physically disabled
This free handbook provides information regarding the pulmonary aspects of muscular dystrophy and other neuromuscular diseases.

Breathe Easy: Young People's Guide to Asthma
Magination Press
750 First Street, NE
Washington, DC 20002-4242

800-374-2721
magination@apa.org
http://www.maginationpress.com
Disability Served: asthma
This book for children provides an overview of asthma, triggers, medications, and treatment options.

Bridging the Gap: A National Directory of Services for Women and Girls with Disabilities
Educational Equity Center at the Academy for Educational Development
100 Fifth Avenue, 8th Floor
New York, NY 10011
212-243-1110
information@edequity.org
http://www.edequity.org/programs_disability.php
Disability Served: various
This directory contains more than 200 listings of agencies and organizations that provide a wide variety of services or programs for women and girls with disabilities. A state-by-state listing makes it easy to find what is available in your area.

Building Bridges: A Manual on Including People with Disabilities
Mobility International USA/National Clearinghouse on Disability and Exchange
PO Box 10767
Eugene, OR 97440
541-343-1284 (Voice/TTY)
http://www.miusa.org/publications
Disability Served: various
This features suggestions and creative ideas for recruiting, including, and accommodating people with disabilities in international programs.

But You Look So Good!
National Multiple Sclerosis Society
733 Third Avenue
New York, NY 10017
800-344-4867
http://www.nationalmssociety.org/Newly%20
    Diagnosed.asp
Disability Served: multiple sclerosis
This free brochure provides information on invisible multiple sclerosis symptoms.

Buying Drugs Online
Federal Citizen Information Center
1800 F Street, NW
Washington, DC 20405

888-878-3256
firstgov1@mail.fedinfo.gov
http://www.pueblo.gsa.gov/results.
    tpl?id1=16&startat=1&--woSECTIONSdatarq=
    16&--SECTIONSword=ww
Disability Served: various
This free brochure describes the advantages of being
    able to buy prescription drugs online. It explains
    how online sales work, how to check for professional
    certification, and the warning signs of fraudulent
    Web sites.

Buying Prescription Medicines Online: A Consumer Safety Guide
Federal Citizen Information Center
1800 F Street, NW
Washington, DC 20405
888-878-3256
firstgov1@mail.fedinfo.gov
http://www.pueblo.gsa.gov/results.
    tpl?id1=16&startat=1&--woSECTIONSdatarq=
    16&--SECTIONSword=ww
Disability Served: various
This free brochure offers a helpful list of dos and don'ts
    when shopping for medications over the Internet.

Canadian Directory of Organizations for People with an Intellectual Disability
L'Institut Roeher Institute
York University, 4700 Keele Street
Toronto, ON M3J 1P3
Canada
416-661-9611, 800-856-2207
info@roeher.ca
http://www.roeher.ca
Disability Served: mentally disabled
This is a directory of Canadian organizations for people
    with mental disabilities, published in English and
    French as one text.

Cancer . . . There's Hope
R.A. Bloch Cancer Foundation Inc.
4400 Main Street
Kansas City, MO 64111
816-932-8453, 800-433-0464
http://www.blochcancer.org
Disability Served: cancer patients and survivors
This free, online inspirational book discusses lung cancer
    and cancer in general from a survivor's point of view.

Cancer: What Causes It, What Doesn't
American Cancer Society
1599 Clifton Road, PO Box 49528
Atlanta, GA 30359-0528
800-ACS-2346
http://www.cancer.org/docroot/PUB/PUB_
    1.asp?sitearea=PUB
Disability Served: cancer patients and survivors
This book provides the facts you need to judge which
    cancer risks you should be concerned about and
    which you can dismiss.

Career Development for Exceptional Individuals
Council for Exceptional Children
1110 North Glebe Road, Suite 300
Arlington, VA 22201-5704
service@cec.sped.org
http://www.cec.sped.org
Disability Served: various
This is a semiannual publication for educators who are
    transitioning exceptional individuals to the world of
    work.

Caregiving
Amytrophic Lateral Sclerosis Association
27001 Agoura Road, Suite 150
Calabasas Hills, CA 91301-5104
818-880-9007
info@alsa-national.org
http://www.alsa.org/resources/brochures.cfm?CFID=
    1048742&CFTOKEN=97497558
Disability Served: physically disabled
This free, downloadable brochure helps patients
    and families find effective ways to cope with the
    symptoms of the disease while coming to terms with
    the need for receiving help from others.

Caring for Your Child with Hemophilia
National Hemophilia Foundation
116 West 32nd Street, 11th Floor
New York, NY 10001
212-328-3700, 800-42-HANDI
handi@hemophilia.org
http://www.hemophilia.org/resources/handi_pubs.htm
Disability Served: inherited bleeding disorders
This publication provides parents of children newly
    diagnosed with hemophilia answers to their basic
    questions, including those regarding inheritance and
    current treatments, as well as sports and insurance
    issues. Single copies are free to members.

Caring for Your Parents: The Complete AARP Guide
American Association of Retired Persons (AARP)
601 East Street, NW
Washington, DC 20049
888-687-2277
http://www.aarp.org/fun/books_movies/books/caring_
for_your_parents_the_complete_aarp_guide.html
Disability Served: elderly
This guidebook offers a practical road map through the
complex emotional process of helping aging parents
live their lives to the fullest.

**Catalog of Accommodations for Students with TS,
ADHD, OCD**
Tourette Syndrome Association
42-40 Bell Boulevard
Bayside, NY 11361
718-224-2999
http://tsa-usa.org/Merchant2/merchant.mvc?Screen=
CTGY&Store_Code=TOS&Category_Code=E
*Disability Served: attention deficit disorder, Tourette
Syndrome*
This publication—written in response to requests from
dedicated teachers—suggests effective accommoda-
tions designed to promote learning and acceptance.

Cerebral Palsy
National Dissemination Center for Children with
Disabilities
PO Box 1492
Washington, DC 20013
800-695-0285
nichcy@aed.org
http://nichcy.org/publist.asp
Disability Served: cerebral palsy
This free fact sheet defines the disease and provides
information on its signs, symptoms, and
characteristics. It also provides tips for parents,
teachers, and schools, additional resources, and
associated organizations.

Cerebral Palsy
Pro-Ed Inc.
8700 Shoal Creek Boulevard
Austin, TX 78757-6897
800-897-3202
http://www.proedinc.com
Disability Served: cerebral palsy, communication
This text covers speech disorders associated with
cerebral palsy.

Cerebral Palsy: Hope through Research
National Institute of Neurological Disorders and Stroke
PO Box 5801
Bethesda, MD 20824
301-496-5751, 800-352-9424
http://www.ninds.nih.gov/disorders/cerebral_palsy/
cerebral_palsy.htm#Publications
Disability Served: cerebral palsy
This information booklet provides information about
the causes, risk factors, diagnosis, and treatments
available for cerebral palsy.

Charcot-Marie-Tooth Brochure
Charcot-Marie-Tooth Association
2700 Chestnut Street
Chester, PA 19013-4867
800-606-2682
info@charcot-marie-tooth.org
https://secure.charcot-marie-tooth.org/publications.php
Disability Served: Charcot-Marie-Tooth Disease
This brochure provides a quick overview of Charcot-
Marie-Tooth Disease.

**Charcot-Marie-Tooth Disorders: A Guide about
Genetics for Patients**
Charcot-Marie-Tooth Association
2700 Chestnut Street
Chester, PA 19013-4867
800-606-2682
info@charcot-marie-tooth.org
https://secure.charcot-marie-tooth.org/publications.php
Disability Served: Charcot-Marie-Tooth Disease
This booklet outlines the basics of genetic inheritance
and Charcot-Marie-Tooth Disease.

Charcot-Marie-Tooth FACTS IV
Charcot-Marie-Tooth Association
2700 Chestnut Street
Chester, PA 19013-4867
800-606-2682
info@charcot-marie-tooth.org
https://secure.charcot-marie-tooth.org/publications.php
Disability Served: Charcot-Marie-Tooth Disease
This resource book offers a wealth of information for
Charcot-Marie-Tooth patients.

Charcot-Marie-Tooth FACTS V
Charcot-Marie-Tooth Association
2700 Chestnut Street
Chester, PA 19013-4867

800-606-2682
info@charcot-marie-tooth.org
https://secure.charcot-marie-tooth.org/publications.php
Disability Served: Charcot-Marie-Tooth Disease
This publication is a sourcebook for information on
orthotics, pain, emotional issues, physical and
occupational therapy, Social Security Disability,
and more.

Child Care for Children with Complex Medical Needs
A.J. Pappanikou Center for Developmental Disabilities
University of Connecticut
263 Farmington Avenue, MC 6222
Farmington, CT 06030
http://www.uconnucedd.org
Disability Served: various
This free, online brochure provides information on
the care of children who have chronic physical,
developmental, behavioral, or emotional conditions.

Childhood Glaucoma
National Association for Parents of Children
with Visual Impairments
PO Box 317
Watertown, MA 02471
admin@spedex.com
http://www.spedex.com/napvi/order.html
Disability Served: vision
This free booklet covers all aspects of childhood
glaucoma including genetics, diagnosis, sibling
relationships, and more.

**The Child with a Bleeding Disorder: Guidelines
for Finding Childcare**
National Hemophilia Foundation
116 West 32nd Street, 11th Floor
New York, NY 10001
212-328-3700, 800-42-HANDI
handi@hemophilia.org
http://www.hemophilia.org/resources/handi_pubs.htm
Disability Served: inherited bleeding disorders
This brochure provides a helpful guide for parents
of children with bleeding disorders as they make
choices about in-home care, cooperative childcare,
center-based childcare, and choosing a daycare
center. Single copies are free to members.

Children Die, Too
Centering Corporation
7230 Maple Street

Omaha, NE 68134
402-533-1200
https://www.centeringcorp.com
Disability Served: various
This book for parents, and other children in the family,
talks about feelings, dealing with guilt, facing
sadness, and moving on when a child dies.

Children with Disabilities
Paul H. Brookes Publishing Company
PO Box 10624
Baltimore, MD 21285-0624
410-337-9580, 800-638-3775
custserv@brookespublishing.com
http://www.pbrookes.com
Disability Served: various
This comprehensive book provides information
on disabilities, including sections on specific
disabilities, genetics, behavior management,
and much more.

Children with Spina Bifida
Woodbine House
6510 Bells Mill Road
Bethesda, MD 20817
800-843-7323
http://www.woodbinehouse.com/Physical-Disabilities.1
9.0.0.2.htm
Disability Served: spina bifida
This comprehensive guide for parents of children with
spina bifida provides information, guidance, and
support to help meet a child's needs from birth
through childhood.

Children with Tourette Syndrome
Woodbine House
6510 Bells Mill Road
Bethesda, MD 20817
800-843-7323
http://www.woodbinehouse.com/Tourette-
Syndrome.21.0.0.2.htm
Disability Served: Tourette Syndrome
This informative handbook for parents of children
and teenagers with Tourette Syndrome provides
information on this often misunderstood
neurological disorder.

Children with Traumatic Brain Injury
Woodbine House
6510 Bells Mill Road

Bethesda, MD 20817

800-843-7323

http://www.woodbinehouse.com/Traumatic-Brain-
    Injury.22.0.0.2.htm

Disability Served: traumatic brain injury

This book provides parents with the support and
    information they need to help their child recover
    from a closed-head injury and prevent further
    incidents.

Children with Visual Impairments

Woodbine House

6510 Bells Mill Road

Bethesda, MD 20817

800-843-7323

http://www.woodbinehouse.com/Visual-
    Impairments.23.0.0.2.htm

Disability Served: vision

This book serves as a primer for parents, offering
    information and support on diagnosis and treatment,
    family adjustment, orientation and mobility, literacy,
    legal issues, and more.

Children with Visual Impairments: A Parent's Guide

National Association for Parents of Children with Visual
    Impairments Inc.

PO Box 317

Watertown, MA 02471

admin@spedex.com

http://www.spedex.com/napvi/order.html

Disability Served: vision

This book covers diagnosis and treatment; family life and
    adjustment; child development; early intervention
    and special education; literacy; orientation and
    mobility; multiple and visual disabilities; legal issues;
    and the years ahead.

Choices in Deafness

Woodbine House

6510 Bells Mill Road

Bethesda, MD 20817

800-843-7323

http://www.woodbinehouse.com/
    Communication.45.0.0.2.htm

Disability Served: hearing

This useful aid in choosing communication options
    for a child with deafness or a hearing loss presents
    information from experts using the following
    approaches: auditory-verbal, bilingual-bicultural,
    cued speech, oral, and total communication.

Choices in Deafness: A Parent's Guide to Communication Options

Alexander Graham Bell Association of the Deaf

3417 Volta Place, NW

Washington, DC 20007

866-337-5220, 202-337-5221 (TTY)

publications@agbell.org

http://www.agbell.org

Disability Served: hearing

This offers advice on communication options for parents
    of deaf children.

Choosing a Cleft Palate or Craniofacial Team

Cleft Palate Foundation

1504 East Franklin Street, Suite 102

Chapel Hill, NC 27514-2820

919-933-9044, 800-24CLEFT

info@cleftline.org

http://www.cleftline.org/publications

Disability Served: physically disabled

This free booklet provides an overview of the health care
    professionals who treat children with cleft lip and
    palate as well as other craniofacial anomalies.

Classroom Acoustics

Alexander Graham Bell Association of the Deaf

3417 Volta Place, NW

Washington, DC 20007

202-337-5220

publications@agbell.org

http://www.agbell.org

Disability Served: hearing

This book discusses the problems of acoustics in schools
    and classrooms and how they affect students with
    hearing impairments.

Classroom Listening and Speaking: Early Childhood

Pro-Ed Inc.

8700 Shoal Creek Boulevard

Austin, TX 78757-6897

800-897-3202

http://www.proedinc.com

Disability Served: learning disabled

This book helps teachers target reinforced learning for
    students in early childhood via the following eight
    units: kitchen, colors, farm animals, vegetables,
    shapes, water, numbers, and bedtime.

Cleft Lip and Palate: The Adult Patient

Cleft Palate Foundation

1504 East Franklin Street, Suite 102

Chapel Hill, NC 27514-2820
919-933-9044, 800-24CLEFT
info@cleftline.org
http://www.cleftline.org/publications
Disability Served: physically disabled
This free booklet is designed to empower adults to make informed decisions about what additional treatment, if any, they want to seek out in relation to their clefts.

Cleft Lip and Palate: The First Four Years
Cleft Palate Foundation
1504 East Franklin Street, Suite 102
Chapel Hill, NC 27514-2820
919-933-9044, 800-24CLEFT
info@cleftline.org
http://www.cleftline.org/publications
Disability Served: physically disabled
This free booklet provides a basic explanation of cleft lip and palate and an overview of the care that a baby born with a cleft requires.

Cleft Lip and Palate: The School Aged Child
Cleft Palate Foundation
1504 East Franklin Street, Suite 102
Chapel Hill, NC 27514-2820
919-933-9044, 800-24CLEFT
info@cleftline.org
http://www.cleftline.org/publications
Disability Served: physically disabled
This free booklet addresses both the medical concerns of school-aged child born with a cleft and the school experience for these children.

Closing the Gap
526 Main Street, PO Box 68
Henderson, MN 56044
507-248-3294
http://www.closingthegap.com
Disability Served: various
This bimonthly newsletter focuses on assistive technology and its relevance in the lives of persons with disabilities.

Cochlear Implants
Alexander Graham Bell Association of the Deaf
3417 Volta Place, NW
Washington, DC 20007
866-337-5220, 202-337-5221 (TTY)
publications@agbell.org
http://www.agbell.org

Disability Served: hearing
This is a reference guide that covers every aspect of cochlear implantation.

Cochlear Implants: A Handbook
Alexander Graham Bell Association of the Deaf
3417 Volta Place, NW
Washington, DC 20007
866-337-5220, 202-337-5221 (TTY)
publications@agbell.org
http://www.agbell.org
Disability Served: hearing
This provides a comprehensive overview, history, and evolution of cochlear implants.

Cochlear Implants In Children: Ethics and Choices
Alexander Graham Bell Association of the Deaf
3417 Volta Place, NW
Washington, DC 20007
866-337-5220, 202-337-5221 (TTY)
publications@agbell.org
http://www.agbell.org
Disability Served: hearing
This addresses the controversy of early cochlear implants via survey responses gathered from 439 parents of children with cochlear implants.

Collaborative Teams for Students with Severe Disabilities: Integrating Therapy and Educational Services
Paul H. Brookes Publishing Company
PO Box 10624
Baltimore, MD 21285-0624
410-337-9580, 800-638-3775
custserv@brookespublishing.com
http://www.pbrookes.com
Disability Served: various
This book provides guidance on teaching, curriculum development, and assessment of students with severe disabilities.

College Bound: A Guide for Students with Visual Impairments
American Foundation for the Blind
11 Penn Plaza, Suite 300
New York, NY 10001
212-502-7600, 800-232-5463
afbinfo@afb.net
http://www.afb.org
Disability Served: vision

This guidebook gives students the tools they need to select and apply to college and move forward with skill and confidence. It includes everything a student needs to know from developing organizational, note taking, test taking, and study skills to managing living space, student-teacher relationships, social and academic life, and extracurricular and leisure time activities.

College Freshmen with Disabilities

HEATH Resource Center
George Washington University
2121 K Street, NW, Suite 220
Washington, DC 20037
202-973-0904 (Voice/TTY), 800-544-3284
askheath@gwu.edu
http://www.heath.gwu.edu/PDFs/collegefreshmen.pdf
Disability Served: various
This is a biennial statistical profile of college freshmen who have disabilities.

College Funding Strategies for Students with Disabilities

DO-IT (Disabilities, Opportunities, Internetworking and Technology)
PO Box 355670
Seattle, WA 98195-5670
206-685-3648, 800-972-3648
doit@u.washington.edu
http://www.washington.edu/doit/Brochures/Academics
Disability Served: various
This free, downloadable brochure provides information on funding sources for students with disabilities.

Colleges for Students with Learning Disabilities or Attention Deficit Disorders

Peterson's Guides
2000 Lenox Drive, PO Box 67005
Lawrenceville, NJ 08648
800-338-3282, ext. 5660
custsvc@petersons.com
http://www.petersons.com
Disability Served: attention deficit disorder, learning disabled
This guide is geared toward high school students with learning disabilities/attention deficit disorder and helps prepare them for the transition to college.

College Students Who Are Deaf or Hard of Hearing

Association on Higher Education and Disability
PO Box 540666
Waltham, MA 02454
781-788-0004
ahead@ahead.org
http://www.ahead.org/publications/index.htm
Disability Served: hearing
This brochure—which addresses types of hearing loss, cultural and communication specifics, hearing loss in the academic environment, reasonable accommodation strategies, and universal design and hearing loss—is useful to have on hand to give to students, teachers, administrators, parents, peers.

College Students Who Have ADHD

Association on Higher Education and Disability
PO Box 540666
Waltham, MA 02454
781-788-0004
ahead@ahead.org
http://www.ahead.org/publications/index.htm
Disability Served: attention deficit disorder
This brochure defines attention deficit/hyperactivity disorder and discusses when it is considered a disability condition, reasonable accommodations, and important points to remember. It also provides a resource list for further information.

College Students Who Have Chronic Diseases or Medical Conditions

Association on Higher Education and Disability
PO Box 540666
Waltham, MA 02454
781-788-0004
ahead@ahead.org
http://www.ahead.org/publications/index.htm
Disability Served: various
This brochure defines what a disability is and addresses medical and chronic disabilities in the academic environment, reasonable accommodations, and universal design concepts.

College Students with Learning Disabilities

Association on Higher Education and Disability
PO Box 540666
Waltham, MA 02454
781-788-0004
ahead@ahead.org
http://www.ahead.org/publications/index.htm
Disability Served: learning disabled
This brochure offers a wealth of information on issues related to learning disabilities in higher education.

It addresses several crucial topics including definitions of what a learning disability is (and is not) and characteristics of college students with learning disabilities, as well as provides suggestions for faculty and students.

College Students with Learning Disabilities: A Handbook
Learning Disabilities Association of America
4156 Library Road
Pittsburgh, PA 15234-1349
412-341-1515
http://www.ldanatl.org/aboutld/resources/index.asp
Disability Served: learning disabled
This handbook provides a wealth of information for college students with learning disabilities.

College Survival Skills
DO-IT (Disabilities, Opportunities, Internetworking and Technology)
PO Box 355670
Seattle, WA 98195-5670
206-685-3648, 800-972-3648
doit@u.washington.edu
http://www.washington.edu/doit/Brochures/Academics
Disability Served: various
This free, downloadable brochure offers tips for students with disabilities to increase their success in college.

College: You Can DO IT!
DO-IT (Disabilities, Opportunities, Internetworking and Technology)
PO Box 355670
Seattle, WA 98195-5670
206-685-3648, 800-972-3648
doit@u.washington.edu
http://www.washington.edu/doit/Brochures/Academics
Disability Served: various
This free, downloadable publication addresses issues surrounding the transition from high school to college and beyond for people with disabilities.

Coming to Terms with Cancer
American Cancer Society
1599 Clifton Road, PO Box 49528
Atlanta, GA 30359-0528
800-ACS-2346
http://www.cancer.org/docroot/PUB/PUB_1.asp?sitearea=PUB
Disability Served: cancer patients and survivors
This reference book provides the most concise and accurate definitions for more than 1,000 cancer-related medical terms, including drug names, used throughout the course of the disease from diagnosis to recovery.

Commitment
Cystic Fibrosis Foundation
6931 Arlington Road
Bethesda, MD 20814
301-951-4422, 800-344-4823
commitment@cff.org
http://www.cff.org/publications/commitment
Disability Served: cystic fibrosis
This free, downloadable newsletter is the official news publication of the Cystic Fibrosis Foundation.

The Communicator
Amputee Coalition of America
900 East Hill Avenue, Suite 285
Knoxville, TN 37915-2568
888-267-5669, 865-525-4512 (TTY)
http://www.amputee-coalition.org
Disability Served: amputees
This is a bimonthly newsletter for amputee support group leaders.

Communiqué
National Association of School Psychologists
4340 East West Highway, Suite 402
Bethesda, MD 20814
301-657-0270
publications@naspweb.org
http://www.nasponline.org/publications/index.html
Disability Served: mental health
This official newspaper of the association is published eight times a year. It covers the latest news, events, innovative practice, legislative developments, parent/teacher handouts, book and test reviews, employment notices, and more.

Community Colleges and Students with Disabilities
HEATH Resource Center
George Washington University
2121 K Street, NW, Suite 220
Washington, DC 20037
202-973-0904 (Voice/TTY), 800-544-3284
askheath@gwu.edu
http://www.heath.gwu.edu/FactSheets.htm
Disability Served: various

This is a short primer for disabled students on the pros of attending a community college. Available for free online.

Complementary and Alternative Medicine for People with Multiple Sclerosis

Multiple Sclerosis Foundation Inc.
6350 North Andrews Avenue
Fort Lauderdale, FL 33309-2130
954-776-6805, 888-MSFOCUS
support@msfocus.org
http://www.msfacts.org/publications/pub_booklets.html
Disability Served: multiple sclerosis
This free booklet explores the many diverse and unique therapies that fall outside the scope of conventional medical treatment.

The Complete Directory for Pediatric Disorders

Grey House Publishing
185 Millerton Road, PO Box 860
Millerton, NY 12546
518-789-8700, 800-562-2139
http://www.greyhouse.com/peddisorders.htm
Disability Served: various
This comprehensive online database, available by subscription, provides information for more than 200 pediatric conditions, disorders, diseases, and disabilities.

The Complete Directory for People with Chronic Illness

Grey House Publishing
185 Millerton Road, PO Box 860
Millerton, NY 12546
518-789-8700, 800-562-2139
http://www.greyhouse.com/illness.htm
Disability Served: various
This online database, available by subscription, provides access to a comprehensive overview of the support services and information resources available for people diagnosed with a chronic illness. It covers more than 80 different chronic illnesses—everything from asthma to cancer to Wilson's Disease.

The Complete Directory for People with Disabilities

Grey House Publishing
185 Millerton Road, PO Box 860
Millerton, NY 12546
518-789-8700, 800-562-2139
http://www.greyhouse.com/disabilities.htm

Disability Served: various
This online database, available by subscription, offers a wealth of information on physical disabilities. Its listings include independent living centers, rehabilitation facilities, state and federal agencies, associations, support groups, and much more.

The Complete Directory for People with Rare Disorders

Grey House Publishing
185 Millerton Road, PO Box 860
Millerton, NY 12546
518-789-8700, 800-562-2139
http://www.greyhouse.com/raredisorders.htm
Disability Served: various
This publication provides comprehensive information on more than 1,100 rare disorders.

The Complete Learning Disabilities Directory

Grey House Publishing
Pocket Knife Square
Lakeville, CT 06039
860-435-0868, 800-562-2139
http://www.greyhouse.com/learningdisabilities.htm
Disability Served: learning disabled
This directory is published annually and lists associations, organizations, schools, camps, books, and government agencies that offer resources for the learning disabled.

The Complete Mental Health Directory

Grey House Publishing
185 Millerton Road, PO Box 860
Millerton, NY 12546
518-789-8700, 800-562-2139
http://www.greyhouse.com/health.htm
Disability Served: mental health
This online database, available by subscription, provides information about the field of behavioral health. It offers more than 5,000 information resources for both the layman and the mental health professional.

Comprehensive Receptive and Expressive Vocabulary Test

Pro-Ed Inc.
8700 Shoal Creek Boulevard
Austin, TX 78757-6897
800-897-3202
http://www.proedinc.com
Disability Served: learning disabled

This test for students with learning disabilities is designed to assess receptive and expressive vocabulary skills.

Computer Resources for People with Disabilities

Hunter House Publishers
PO Box 2914
Alameda, CA 94501-0914
510-865-5282
sales@hunterhouse.com
http://www.hunterhouse.com
Disability Served: physically disabled
This book helps people with disabilities choose, buy, adapt, and use the most appropriate technologies available to them. It includes worksheets and tools for planning and decision-making, 150 pages of easy-to-use charts that describe all current products, and a new keyword index organized by disability.

Connections, Advocacy, Resources, and Empowerment Newsletter

National Stuttering Association
119 West 40th Street, 14th Floor
New York, NY 10018
800-937-8888
info@westutter.org
http://www.nsastutter.org/material/index.
php?matid=112
Disability Served: communication
This quarterly newsletter is designed to address questions, concerns, and experiences of parents and family members of children who stutter. Each issue contains articles written by experts in the area of stuttering and fluency disorders.

Consumer Choice News

National Council on the Aging
300 D Street, SW, Suite 801
Washington, DC 20024
202-479-1200
info@ncoa.org
http://www.ncoa.org/content.cfm?sectionID=30
Disability Served: elderly
This free quarterly newsletter gives the latest news and trends in consumer choice.

A Consumer Handbook—Hearing Loss and Hearing Aids: A Bridge to Healing

American Tinnitus Association
PO Box 5
Portland, OR 97207-0005

503-248-9985, 800-634-8978
dan@ata.org
http://www.ata.org/resources/order.html
Disability Served: hearing
This book examines the stress experienced by tinnitus patients who also do not hear well and the realistic effects that improved hearing through hearing aid use has had on their lives.

Consumer's Guide to Hearing Aids

Self Help for Hard of Hearing People Inc.
7910 Woodmont Avenue, Suite 1200
Bethesda, MD 20814
301-657-2248, 301-657-2249 (TTY)
bookstore@hearingloss.org
http://hearingloss.sidestreetshop.com/default.cfm
Disability Served: hearing
This guide illustrates the different styles of hearing aids and compares different models and features. The technology pyramid and hearing aid pricing are also included.

A Consumer's Guide to Home Adaptation

Adaptive Environments
374 Congress Street, Suite 301
Boston, MA 02210
617-695-1225
http://www.adaptenv.org
Disability Served: physically disabled
This publication helps those who wish to modify their homes to make them accessible. It discusses how to lower countertops, widen doorways, install switches, and more.

A Consumer's Guide to TS Medications

Tourette Syndrome Association
42-40 Bell Boulevard
Bayside, NY 11361
718-224-2999
http://tsa-usa.org/Merchant2/merchant.
mvc?Screen=CTGY&Store_Code=TOS&Category_
Code=E
Disability Served: Tourette Syndrome
This brochure details the most commonly prescribed medications for tic control, obsessive traits, and attention difficulties. Tables provide dosages and side effects for all medications discussed.

Consumer Times: Living Better with Vision Loss

Lighthouse International
111 East 59th Street

New York, NY 10002-1202
212-821-9200, 800-829-0500
http://www.lighthouse.org/scripts/newsletter
Disability Served: vision
This free, downloadable newsletter provides timely
articles and links to useful resources for anyone who
receives services from New York Lighthouse Vision
Rehabilitation Services.

Contemporary Rehab
National Rehabilitation Association
633 South Washington Street
Alexandria, VA 22314
703-836-0850
info@nationalrehab.org
http://www.nationalrehab.org/website/pubs/index.html
Disability Served: various
This newsletter for members of the National
Rehabilitation Association is filled with the latest
rehabilitation and membership news.

Controlling Your Risk Factors: Our Guide to Reducing Your Risk of Heart Attack and Stroke
American Heart Association
7272 Greenville Avenue
Dallas, TX 75231
800-242-8721
http://www.americanheart.org/presenter.
jhtml?identifier=3001740
Disability Served: physically disabled, stroke
This free brochure defines each of the risk factors
(cholesterol, smoking, hypertension, physical
inactivity, obesity, diabetes, family history, sex, age,
and race) for heart attack and stroke and explains
the American Heart Association's recommendations.
It also discusses the effects of stress and excessive
alcohol intake.

Cook Well, Stay Well with Parkinson's Disease
National Parkinson Foundation
1501 Northwest Ninth Avenue/Bob Hope Road
Miami, FL 33136-1454
305-243-6666, 800-327-4545
contact@parkinson.org
http://www.parkinson.org/site/pp.asp?c=9dJFJLPwB&b
=116364
Disability Served: Parkinson's Disease
This book specializes in the dietary needs unique to
Parkinson's, featuring delicious recipes that are rich in
the nutrients most needed by those with Parkinson's
Disease.

Coping with Mood Changes Later in Life
Depressive and Bipolar Support Alliance
730 North Franklin Street, Suite 501
Chicago, IL 60610-7224
800-826-3632
bookstore@dbsalliance.org
http://www.dbsalliance.org/store
Disability Served: mental health
This free brochure discusses symptoms, causes,
and treatment options for depression.

Council for Exceptional Children Catalog
Council for Exceptional Children
1110 North Glebe Road, Suite 300
Arlington, VA 22201-5704
888-CEC-SPED, 866-915-5000 (TTY)
service@cec.sped.org
http://www.cec.sped.org
Disability Served: various
This semiannual catalog lists products such as books,
teaching materials, guides, and more.

Countdown for Kids
Juvenile Diabetes Foundation
120 Wall Street
New York, NY 10005-4001
800-533-2873
info@jdrf.org
http://www.jdf.org/index.cfm?page_id=100688
Disability Served: diabetes
This quarterly magazine for members of the
Juvenile Diabetes Research Foundation provides
information, fun, role models, and pen pals for kids
with diabetes.

Countdown Magazine
Juvenile Diabetes Foundation
120 Wall Street
New York, NY 10005-4001
800-533-2873
info@jdrf.org
http://www.jdf.org/index.cfm?page_id=100688
Disability Served: diabetes
This magazine, published quarterly and offered free
with a donation to the Juvenile Diabetes Research
Foundation, offers in-depth analysis of cutting-edge
research and new treatments, and also features
poignant stories from people who have juvenile
diabetes and their families.

Count Us In: A Demographic Overview of Childhood and Disability in Canada
L'Institut Roeher Institute
York University
4700 Keele Street
Toronto, ON M3J 1P3
Canada
416-661-9611, 800-856-2207
info@roeher.ca
http://www.roeher.ca
Disability Served: various
This provides statistical information about children with disabilities in Canada.

Creating Options: Financial Aid for Students with Disabilities 2005
HEATH Resource Center
George Washington University
2121 K Street, NW, Suite 220
Washington, DC 20037
202-973-0904 (Voice/TTY), 800-544-3284
askheath@gwu.edu
http://www.heath.gwu.edu/PDFs/FinancialAid05.pdf
Disability Served: various
This free, online publication offers an overview of financial aid for students with disabilities.

Creativity and Collaborative Learning: A Practical Guide to Empowering Students, Teachers, and Families
Paul H. Brookes Publishing Company
PO Box 10624
Baltimore, MD 21285-0624
410-337-9580, 800-638-3775
custserv@brookespublishing.com
http://www.pbrookes.com
Disability Served: various
This book provides teaching strategies, lesson plans, case studies, and materials to help instructors facilitate learning.

Creutzfeldt-Jakob Disease Fact Sheet
National Institute of Neurological Disorders and Stroke
PO Box 5801
Bethesda, MD 20824
301-496-5751, 800-352-9424
http://www.ninds.nih.gov/disorders/alzheimersdisease/alzheimersdisease.htm#Publications
Disability Served: physically disabled
This free fact sheet provides information about the symptoms and diagnosis of Creutzfeldt-Jakob Disease.

Current Perspectives on the Culture of Schools
Brookline Books
34 University Road
Brookline, MA 02445
617-734-6772
http://www.brooklinebooks.com
Disability Served: various
This book provides information on restructuring schools.

Cystic Fibrosis Fact Sheet
American Lung Association
61 Broadway
New York, NY 10006
212-315-8700, 800-LUNG
http://www.lungusa.org/site/apps/s/content.asp?c=dvLUK9O0E&b=34706&ct=910859
Disability Served: cystic fibrosis
This free Web resource provides facts and statistics on cystic fibrosis.

Deaf and Hearing Impaired Pupils in Mainstream Schools
Taylor & Francis Group
270 Madison Avenue
New York, NY 10016
212-216-7800
http://www.taylorandfrancisgroup.com
Disability Served: hearing
This offers information and advice on how to mainstream deaf and hard-of-hearing students.

Deaf-Blind American Magazine
American Association of the Deaf-Blind
8630 Fenton Street, Suite 121
Silver Spring, MD 20910-4500
301-495-4403, 301-495-4402 (TTY)
info@aadb.org
http://www.aadb.org
Disability Served: hearing, vision
This publication, distributed to members of the American Association of the Deaf-Blind, contains articles of interest to deaf-blind individuals, their families, and service providers who work with deaf-blind people.

Deafness/Hearing Loss
National Dissemination Center for Children with Disabilities
PO Box 1492
Washington, DC 20013
800-695-0285

nichcy@aed.org
http://nichcy.org/publist.asp
Disability Served: hearing
This free fact sheet defines the condition and provides information on incidence, characteristics, educational implications, additional resources, and associated organizations.

Dealing with Your Insurance Company/HMO
Cleft Palate Foundation
1504 East Franklin Street, Suite 102
Chapel Hill, NC 27514-2820
919-933-9044, 800-24CLEFT
info@cleftline.org
http://www.cleftline.org/publications
Disability Served: physically disabled
This free fact sheet offers advice on patients' rights and what to do if an insurance company denies coverage for cleft lip and palate related surgeries.

Deciphering the System: A Guide for Families of Young Disabled Children
Brookline Books
34 University Road
Brookline, MA 02445
617-734-6772
http://www.brooklinebooks.com
Disability Served: various
This guide is designed for parents of young disabled children and discusses their rights and provides strategies for accessing suitable educational programs.

Dementia
National Mental Health Association
2001 North Beauregard Street, 12th Floor
Alexandria, VA 22311
703-684-7722, 800-969-6642
http://www.nmha.org/infoctr/factsheets
Disability Served: dementia, elderly
This free fact sheet offers information under the following subject areas on dementia: causes, who is affected, symptoms, diagnosis, treatment, and additional resources.

The Dementias: Hope through Research
National Institute of Neurological Disorders and Stroke
PO Box 5801
Bethesda, MD 20824
301-496-5751, 800-352-9424
http://www.ninds.nih.gov/disorders/alzheimersdisease/alzheimersdisease.htm#Publications

Disability Served: dementia
This information booklet about Alzheimer's disease, vascular dementia, and other types of dementia provides data on diagnosis, treatment, and prevention.

Depression
Federal Citizen Information Center
1800 F Street, NW
Washington, DC 20405
888-878-3256
firstgov1@mail.fedinfo.gov
http://www.pueblo.gsa.gov/results.tpl?id1=16&startat=1&--woSECTIONSdatarq=16&--SECTIONSword=ww
Disability Served: mental health
This free brochure outlines the three main types of depression along with their causes and symptoms, and provides additional resources.

Depression and Anxiety in Youth Scale
Pro-Ed Inc.
8700 Shoal Creek Boulevard
Austin, TX 78757-6897
800-897-3202
http://www.proedinc.com
Disability Served: mental health
These tests help identify depressive disorders in children and adolescents.

Depression Is the Pits, but I'm Getting Better: A Guide for Adolescents
Magination Press
750 First Street, NE
Washington, DC 20002-4242
800-374-2721
magination@apa.org
http://www.maginationpress.com
Disability Served: mental health
This guide helps teens understand depression and the best treatments for it.

Design for Hospitality
6 Grant Avenue
Takoma Park, MD 20912
301-270-2470
UDandC@UniversalDesign.com
http://www.universaldesign.com/store.php
Disability Served: various
This book provides design suggestions to the hospitality industry for creating accessible lodgings for people with disabilities.

Developing Cross-Cultural Competence: A Guide for Working with Children and Their Families
Paul H. Brookes Publishing Company
PO Box 10624
Baltimore, MD 21285-0624
410-337-9580, 800-638-3775
custserv@brookespublishing.com
http://www.pbrookes.com
Disability Served: various
This book is designed for therapists and others who work with disabled children and discusses cultural, ethnic, and language diversity.

Developmental Observation Checklist System
Pro-Ed Inc.
8700 Shoal Creek Boulevard
Austin, TX 78757-6897
800-897-3202
http://www.proedinc.com
Disability Served: various
This kit is designed to assess the general development of very young children.

Developmental Problems in Children
American Occupational Therapy Association Inc.
4720 Montgomery Lane, PO Box 31220
Bethesda, MD 20824-1220
301-652-2682, 800-377-8555
http://www.aota.org/featured/area6/links/link02.asp
Disability Served: developmentally disabled
This free tip sheet offers information for parents of children with developmental disabilities and provides an overview of how occupational therapists can provide assistance.

Diabetes
American Occupational Therapy Association Inc.
4720 Montgomery Lane, PO Box 31220
Bethesda, MD 20824-1220
301-652-2682, 800-377-8555
http://www.aota.org/featured/area6/links/link02.asp
Disability Served: diabetes
This free tip sheet offers information to help diabetics cope with their illness and provides an overview of how occupational therapists can provide assistance.

Diabetes
Federal Citizen Information Center
1800 F Street, NW
Washington, DC 20405

888-878-3256
firstgov1@mail.fedinfo.gov
http://www.pueblo.gsa.gov/results.tpl?id1=16&startat=1&--woSECTIONSdatarq=16&--SECTIONSword=ww
Disability Served: diabetes
This free booklet outlines the risk factors, warning signs, and treatments for diabetes.

Diabetes: A Practical Guide to Managing Your Health
American Diabetes Association
1701 North Beauregard Street
Alexandria, VA 22311
800-342-2383
AskADA@diabetes.org
http://www.diabetes.org
Disability Served: diabetes
This comprehensive guide provides everything you need to know about living with diabetes, whatever type of diabetes you have and whatever your age.

Diabetes A to Z
American Diabetes Association
1701 North Beauregard Street
Alexandria, VA 22311
800-342-2383
AskADA@diabetes.org
http://www.diabetes.org
Disability Served: diabetes
This book covers everything from alcohol to vitamins to weight loss and includes the most up-to-date information on diabetes-related topics such as insurance, medications, and controlling blood pressure.

Diabetes Care for Babies, Toddlers, and Preschoolers
Juvenile Diabetes Foundation
120 Wall Street
New York, NY 10005-4001
800-533-2873
info@jdrf.org
http://www.jdrf.org/index.cfm?page_id=100250
Disability Served: diabetes
This guidebook for parents explains how diabetes impacts a child's growth and development, and provides plenty of ideas for dealing with routine diabetes care.

Diabetes Dateline
National Diabetes Information Clearinghouse
5 Information Way

Bethesda, MD 20892-3568
800-860-8747
catalog@niddk.nih.gov
http://catalog.niddk.nih.gov/AlphaList.cfm?CH=NDIC
Disability Served: diabetes
This biannual publication features news about current issues in diabetes research and control, special events, patient and professional meetings, and new publications available from the NDIC and other organizations. Single copies are free.

Diabetes Dictionary
National Diabetes Information Clearinghouse
5 Information Way
Bethesda, MD 20892-3568
800-860-8747
catalog@niddk.nih.gov
http://catalog.niddk.nih.gov/AlphaList.cfm?CH=NDIC
Disability Served: diabetes
This brochure defines more than 300 diabetes-related terms. Single copies are free.

Diabetes Overview
National Diabetes Information Clearinghouse
5 Information Way
Bethesda, MD 20892-3568
800-860-8747
catalog@niddk.nih.gov
http://catalog.niddk.nih.gov/AlphaList.cfm?CH=NDIC
Disability Served: diabetes
This brochure defines the various types of diabetes and various treatments, and provides information on the impact and cost of the disease, its increasing prevalence, and research being conducted by the government and private organizations. Single copies are free.

Diabetes Self-Management
R.A. Rapaport Publishing Inc.
PO Box 52890
Boulder, CO 80322
800-234-0923
http://www.diabetesselfmanagement.com
Disability Served: diabetes
This bimonthly report provides news stories and feature articles of interest to persons living with diabetes.

The Diabetes Self-Management Answer Book
R.A. Rapaport Publishing Inc.
PO Box 11066

Des Moines, IA 50336-1066
800-664-9269
https://www.diabetesselfmanagement.com/eds/books.cfm
Disability Served: diabetes
This book groups the most frequently asked questions about diabetes into broad subject areas. Physicians, educators, dieticians, exercise specialists, researchers, and medical writers offer practical, easy-to-apply advice to help people with diabetes live happier and healthier lives.

The Diabetic Athlete
Juvenile Diabetes Foundation
120 Wall Street
New York, NY 10005-4001
800-533-2873
info@jdrf.org
http://www.jdrf.org/index.cfm?page_id=100250
Disability Served: diabetes
This book, written by a diabetic athlete with a Ph.D. in exercise physiology, draws on the experiences of hundreds of diabetic athletes to provide great advice for people with Type 1 and Type 2 diabetes.

The Diabetic Gourmet
R.A. Rapaport Publishing Inc.
PO Box 11066
Des Moines, IA 50336-1066
800-664-9269
https://www.diabetesselfmanagement.com/eds/books.cfm
Disability Served: diabetes
This book, with 203 quick and easy recipes, provides healthy meal ideas that are low in fat, so users can easily add gourmet variety to their meal planning.

Diagnosis and Treatment of Hearing Impairment in Children
Alexander Graham Bell Association of the Deaf
3417 Volta Place, NW
Washington, DC 20007
866-337-5220, 202-337-5221 (TTY)
publications@agbell.org
http://www.agbell.org
Disability Served: hearing
This covers a variety of issues pertaining to hearing loss in children.

A Dictionary of Catholic Religious Words for Deaf People
National Catholic Office for the Deaf
7202 Buchanan Street
Landover Hills, MD 20784-2236
301-577-1684, 301-577-4184 (TTY)
ncod@erols.com
http://www.ncod.org
Disability Served: hearing
This dictionary contains 170 words with pictures.

Dictionary of Special Education and Rehabilitation
Love Publishing Company
9101 East Kenyon Avenue, Suite 2200
Denver, CO 80237
303-221-7333
lpc@lovepublishing.com
http://www.lovepublishing.com
Disability Served: various
This comprehensive guide provides definitions of more than 2,000 terms unique to special education and rehabilitation.

Did You Know . . .
Stuttering Foundation of America
3100 Walnut Grove Road, Suite 603, PO Box 11749
Memphis, TN 38111-0749
901-452-7342, 800-992-9392
info@stutteringhelp.org
http://www.stutteringhelp.org/Default.aspx?tabid=131
Disability Served: communication
This free fact sheet provides statistics on stuttering.

Digestive Diseases Dictionary
National Digestive Diseases Information Clearinghouse
2 Information Way
Bethesda, MD 20892-3570
800-891-5389
nddic@info.niddk.nih.gov
http://catalog.niddk.nih.gov/PubType.cfm?Type=174
    &CH=NDDIC
Disability Served: various
This free, online dictionary, designed for people who have digestive diseases and their families and friends, defines words that are often used when talking or writing about digestive diseases.

Digestive Diseases Patient Education Fact Sheets
National Digestive Diseases Information Clearinghouse
2 Information Way

Bethesda, MD 20892-3570
800-891-5389
nddic@info.niddk.nih.gov
http://catalog.niddk.nih.gov/PubType.
    cfm?Type=175&CH=NDDIC
Disability Served: various
These free fact sheets provide facts and fallacies about various digestive diseases.

Directions: Technology in Special Education
DREAMMS for Kids Inc.
273 Ringwood Road
Freeville, NY 13068-5606
607-539-3027
http://dreamms.org
Disability Served: various
This quarterly journal discusses technology as it relates to education, including the use of software and hardware, videotapes, and online services.

Directory for Exceptional Children
Porter Sargent Publishers Inc.
11 Beacon Street
Boston, MA 02108
617-523-1679
orders@portersargent.com
http://www.portersargent.com
Disability Served: various
This directory provides a listing of schools, organizations, and facilities that serve youth with disabilities.

Directory of Accessible Building Projects
National Association of Home Builders Research Center
400 Prince George's Boulevard
Upper Marlboro, MD 20774
301-249-4000, 800-638-8556
http://www.nahbrc.org/bookstore2.asp?TrackID=&Cate
    goryID=1652
Disability Served: various
This manual provides descriptions of more than 200 commercially available products designed for use by people with disabilities.

The Directory of Drug and Alcohol Residential Rehabilitation Facilities
Grey House Publishing
185 Millerton Road, PO Box 860
Millerton, NY 12546
518-789-8700, 800-562-2139
http://www.greyhouse.com/rehab.htm

Disability Served: chemical dependency,

This directory contains listings for more than 6,000 facilities, with detailed contact information for each one, including their mission statements, types of treatment programs, cost, average length of stay, numbers of residents and counselors, accreditation, insurance plans accepted, type of environment, religious affiliation, and education components.

The Directory of Independent Ambulatory Care Centers

Grey House Publishing
185 Millerton Road, PO Box 860
Millerton, NY 12546
518-789-8700, 800-562-2139
http://www.greyhouse.com/ambulatory.htm
Disability Served: various

This online database, available by subscription, provides a comprehensive database of 8,000 ambulatory centers, surgery centers, diagnostic imaging centers, and urgent care centers. It includes a listing of key personnel, purchasing agents, contact information, specialties, services, and more.

Directory of Summer Camps

National Dissemination Center for Children with Disabilities
PO Box 1492
Washington, DC 20013
800-695-0285
nichcy@aed.org
http://nichcy.org/publist.asp
Disability Served: various

This free directory provides a listing of summer camps for children with disabilities.

Disability and Social Performance: Using Drama to Achieve Successful Acts of Being

Brookline Books
34 University Road
Brookline, MA 02445
617-734-6772
http://www.brooklinebooks.com
Disability Served: various

This book discusses how theatrical performance can enhance the creativity and lives of people with disabilities.

Disability Compliance Bulletin

LRP Publications
747 Dresher Road, Suite 500, PO Box 980

Horsham, PA 19044
800-341-7874, 215-658-0938 (TTY)
http://www.shoplrp.com/disability/cat-Newsletters.html
Disability Served: various

This biweekly publication provides the latest information on Americans With Disabilities Act compliance and legislation.

Disability Employment 101

Office of Special Education and Rehabilitative Services
400 Maryland Avenue, SW
Washington, DC 20202-7100
202-245-7468
http://www.ed.gov/about/offices/list/osers/reports.html
Disability Served: various

This free, downloadable guide for business leaders includes information about how to find qualified workers with disabilities, how to put disability and employment research into practice, and how to model what other businesses have done to successfully integrate individuals with disabilities into the workforce.

Disability Etiquette

United Spinal Association
75-20 Astoria Boulevard
Jackson Heights, NY 11370
718-803-3782, 800-444-0120
publications@unitedspinal.org
http://www.unitedspinal.org/pages.php?catid=7
Disability Served: various

This free booklet is for anyone who wants to interact more effectively with people with disabilities.

Disability Publishers

National Dissemination Center for Children with Disabilities
PO Box 1492
Washington, DC 20013
800-695-0285
nichcy@aed.org
http://nichcy.org/publist.asp
Disability Served: various

This free resource guide provides a list of commercial publishers who offer books, videos, and journals on specific disabilities, special education, parenting, and other disability and special needs topics.

Disability Resources Monthly

Disability Resources Inc.
Department IN, Four Glatter Lane

Centereach, NY 11720-1032
631-585-0290
pubs@disabilityresources.org
http://disabilityresources.org
Disability Served: various
This monthly publication is geared for educators, librarians, social workers, and other professionals and provides information on new disability-related publications, services, and resources.

Disability Studies Quarterly

Society for Disability Studies
University of Illinois at Chicago (MC 626)
Department of Disability and Human Development
1640 Roosevelt Road, #236
Chicago, IL 60608-6904
http://www.dsq-sds.org
Disability Served: various
This publication provides articles on disability issues as well as resources for disabled people.

Disabled American Veterans Magazine

Disabled American Veterans
3725 Alexandria Pike
Cold Spring, KY 41076
859-441-7300
http://www.dav.org/magazine
Disability Served: various
This magazine features news and events for members of Disabled American Veterans.

Disabled Dealer Magazine

426 Island Cay Way
Apollo Beach, FL 33572
888-521-8778
disdeal@aol.com
http://www.disableddealer.com
Disability Served: various
This is a print and online resource for buying and selling adapted equipment.

Disabled We Stand

Brookline Books
34 University Road
Brookline, MA 02445
617-734-6772
http://www.brooklinebooks.com
Disability Served: various
This book discusses the rights of persons with disabilities.

Discipline and the Child with TS: A Guide For Parents and Teachers

Tourette Syndrome Association
42-40 Bell Boulevard
Bayside, NY 11361
718-224-2999
http://tsa-usa.org/Merchant2/merchant.mvc?Screen=CTGY&Store_Code=TOS&Category_Code=E
Disability Served: Tourette Syndrome
This publication offers advice on how to help children redirect impulses and compulsions by teaching cause/effect relationships. Included are techniques for disciplining without aggression or intimidation.

Disclosure: The Basic Facts

National Multiple Sclerosis Society
733 Third Avenue
New York, NY 10017
800-344-4867
http://www.nationalmssociety.org/Newly%20Diagnosed.asp
Disability Served: multiple sclerosis
This free brochure discusses whom, when, and how to tell that you have multiple sclerosis in both personal and work situations.

The Do-Able Renewable Home

6 Grant Avenue
Takoma Park, MD 20912
301-270-2470
UDandC@UniversalDesign.com
http://www.universaldesign.com/store.php
Disability Served: elderly
This free, online booklet provides advice on remodeling residential spaces so that they are accessible for the elderly.

Do I Have Lupus?

Federal Citizen Information Center
1800 F Street, NW
Washington, DC 20405
888-878-3256
firstgov1@mail.fedinfo.gov
http://www.pueblo.gsa.gov/results.tpl?id1=16&startat=1&--woSECTIONS
datarq=16&--SECTIONSword=ww
Disability Served: immune deficiency disorders
This free booklet describes the three main types of lupus, their symptoms, who is affected, and how lupus is diagnosed and treated.

Don't Lose Sight of Glaucoma
Federal Citizen Information Center
1800 F Street, NW
Washington, DC 20405
888-878-3256
firstgov1@mail.fedinfo.gov
http://www.pueblo.gsa.gov/results.
    tpl?id1=16&startat=1&--woSECTIONSdatarq
    =16&--SECTIONSword=ww
Disability Served: vision
This brochure offers some facts on who is at risk, what
    the symptoms are, how it is detected, and what
    treatments are available.

Don't Lose Your Balance
Multiple Sclerosis Society of Canada
175 Bloor Street East, Suite 700, North Tower
Toronto, ON M4W 3R8
Canada
416-922-6065, 800-268-7582
info@mssociety.ca
http://www.mssociety.ca/en/information/references.htm
Disability Served: multiple sclerosis
This illustrated booklet is a collection of stories from
    adolescents who have a parent with multiple
    sclerosis. It can act as a communication tool between
    parents and teens and also be useful in group
    workshops.

Down's Syndrome and Stuttering
Stuttering Foundation of America
3100 Walnut Grove Road, Suite 603, PO Box 11749
Memphis, TN 38111-0749
901-452-7343, 800-992-9392
info@stutteringhelp.org
http://www.stutteringhelp.org/Default.aspx?tabid=131
Disability Served: communication, Down Syndrome
This free, downloadable brochure discusses the effect of
    Down Syndrome on speech fluency and how to help
    people with Down Syndrome.

Down Syndrome
National Dissemination Center for Children with
    Disabilities
PO Box 1492
Washington, DC 20013
800-695-0285
nichcy@aed.org
http://nichcy.org/publist.asp
Disability Served: Down Syndrome

This free fact sheet defines the disease and provides
    information on incidence, characteristics, educational
    implications, additional resources, and associated
    organizations.

Down Syndrome: Birth To Adulthood
Love Publishing Company
9101 East Kenyon Avenue, Suite 2200
Denver, CO 80237
303-221-7333
lpc@lovepublishing.com
http://www.lovepublishing.com
Disability Served: Down Syndrome
This is a guide for families and professionals that traces
    Down Syndrome from birth to adulthood.

Down Syndrome News
National Down Syndrome Congress
1370 Center Drive, Suite 102
Atlanta, GA 30338
800-232-6372
http://www.ndsccenter.org
Disability Served: Down Syndrome
This newsletter is published approximately every
    two months and is available to members of the
    organization.

Drug Interactions: What You Should Know
Federal Citizen Information Center
1800 F Street, NW
Washington, DC 20405
888-878-3256
firstgov1@mail.fedinfo.gov
http://www.pueblo.gsa.gov/results.
    tpl?id1=16&startat=1&--woSECTIONSdatarq
    =16&--SECTIONSword=ww
Disability Served: various
This free brochure tells you how to protect yourself and
    your family from potentially dangerous interactions
    of prescription drugs, over-the-counter drugs, food,
    and medical conditions.

Dual Diagnosis and Recovery
Depressive and Bipolar Support Alliance
730 North Franklin Street, Suite 501
Chicago, IL 60610-7224
800-826-3632
bookstore@dbsalliance.org
http://www.dbsalliance.org/store
Disability Served: chemical dependency, mental health

This free brochure helps readers identify whether or not they may have a dependency problem, as well as offers information and suggestions for dealing with a dual diagnosis.

Dyscalculia
National Center for Learning Disabilities
381 Park Avenue South, Suite 1401
New York, NY 10016
212-545-7510
http://www.ld.org/LDInfoZone/InfoZone_
    FactSheetIndex.cfm
Disability Served: learning disabled
This free fact sheet provides an introduction to learning disabilities in math.

Dysgraphia
National Center for Learning Disabilities
381 Park Avenue South, Suite 1401
New York, NY 10016
212-545-7510
http://www.ld.org/LDInfoZone/InfoZone_
    FactSheetIndex.cfm
Disability Served: learning disabled
This free fact sheet provides an introduction to learning disabilities in writing.

Dyslexia
National Center for Learning Disabilities
381 Park Avenue South, Suite 1401
New York, NY 10016
212-545-7510
http://www.ld.org/LDInfoZone/InfoZone_
    FactSheetIndex.cfm
Disability Served: dyslexic
This free fact sheet offers an introduction to learning disabilities in reading.

Dyslexia and Related Disorders
International Dyslexia Association
8600 LaSalle Road, Chester Building, Suite 382
Baltimore, MD 21286-2044
410-296-0232
http://www.interdys.org
Disability Served: attention deficit disorder, dyslexic
This online brochure helps parents determine if their child has dyslexia or related disorders, such as dysgraphia, dyscalculia, and attention deficit/hyperactivity disorder.

Dyslexia Basics
International Dyslexia Association
Chester Building, 8600 LaSalle Road, Suite 382
Baltimore, MD 21286-2044
410-296-0232
http://www.interdys.org
Disability Served: dyslexic
This online brochure provides an overview of dyslexia. A Spanish-language version is also available.

Dyspraxia
National Center for Learning Disabilities
381 Park Avenue South, Suite 1401
New York, NY 10016
212-545-7510
http://www.ld.org/LDInfoZone/InfoZone_
    FactSheetIndex.cfm
Disability Served: learning disabled
This free fact sheet provides an introduction to learning disabilities in motor skills.

Ear Facts
Ear Foundation
PO Box 330867
Nashville, TN 37203
615-627-2724, 800-545-HEAR
info@earfoundation.org
http://www.earfoundation.org/articles.asp
Disability Served: hearing
This online article offers fact about the ear and hearing loss.

Early Childhood Deafness
Alexander Graham Bell Association of the Deaf
3417 Volta Place, NW
Washington, DC 20007
866-337-5220, 202-337-5221 (TTY)
publications@agbell.org
http://www.agbell.org
Disability Served: hearing
This covers the diagnostic process, hearing aid fitting strategies, and developments in the field.

Eating Well, Staying Well During and After Cancer
American Cancer Society
1599 Clifton Road, PO Box 49528
Atlanta, GA 30359-0528
800-ACS-2346
http://www.cancer.org/docroot/PUB/PUB_
    1.asp?sitearea=PUB

Disability Served: cancer patients and survivors
This publication details what you should eat and what you should avoid in order to stay strong and benefit from cancer treatment.

Educating Children with Multiple Disabilities: A Collaborative Approach
Paul H. Brookes Publishing Company
PO Box 10624
Baltimore, MD 21285-0624
410-337-9580, 800-638-3775
custserv@brookespublishing.com
http://www.pbrookes.com
Disability Served: various
This textbook provides strategies for teaching children with mental retardation and other impairments.

Educating Deaf Students: Global Perspectives
Gallaudet University Press
800 Florida Avenue, NE
Washington, DC 20002
202-651-5488 (Voice/TTY)
valencia.simmons@gallaudet.edu
http://gupress.gallaudet.edu
Disability Served: hearing
This covers a cross-section of issues discussed at The 19th International Congress on Education of the Deaf.

Educational Audiology for the Limited-Hearing Infant and Preschooler: An Auditory-Verbal Program
Charles C. Thomas, Publisher
2600 South First Street
Springfield, IL 62704
800-258-8980
books@ccthomas.com
http://www.ccthomas.com
Disability Served: hearing
This book is designed to assist preschool educators of deaf children.

Educational Audiology Handbook
Alexander Graham Bell Association of the Deaf
3417 Volta Place, NW
Washington, DC 20007
866-337-5220, 202-337-5221 (TTY)
publications@agbell.org
http://www.agbell.org
Disability Served: hearing
This is a training tool for audiology students who work in educational settings.

Educational Dimensions of Acquired Brain Injury
Pro-Ed Inc.
8700 Shoal Creek Boulevard
Austin, TX 78757-6897
800-897-3202
http://www.proedinc.com
Disability Served: traumatic brain injury
This collection of articles discusses issues regarding the education of those with acquired brain injuries.

Education and Training in Developmental Disabilities
Council for Exceptional Children
1110 North Glebe Road, Suite 300
Arlington, VA 22201-5704
888-CEC-SPED, 866-915-5000 (TTY)
service@cec.sped.org
http://www.cec.sped.org
Disability Served: developmentally disabled
This quarterly publication provides scholarly articles on the education of students with developmental disabilities.

An Educator's Guide to Tourette Syndrome
Tourette Syndrome Association
42-40 Bell Boulevard
Bayside, NY 11361
718-224-2999
http://tsa-usa.org/Merchant2/merchant.mvc?Screen=CTGY&Store_Code=TOS&Category_Code=E
Disability Served: Tourette Syndrome
This publication for educators discusses the symptoms of the disease, answers teachers' commonly asked questions, and offers suggestions for classroom management.

Effective Listening
The Speech Bin
1965 25th Avenue
Vero Beach, FL 32960
800-477-3324
info@speechbin.com
http://www.speechbin.com
Disability Served: communication
This text seeks to help people improve their auditory processing skills.

Elderly Health Services Letter
Health Resources Publishing
PO Box 456

Allenwood, NJ 08720
800-516-4343
info@healthresourcesonline.com
http://www.healthresourcesonline.com/
elderly_health/10nl.htm
Disability Served: elderly
This monthly publication focuses on health care
provisions for the elderly.

Emotional Disturbance
National Dissemination Center for Children with
Disabilities
PO Box 1492
Washington, DC 20013
800-695-0285
nichcy@aed.org
http://nichcy.org/publist.asp
Disability Served: emotionally disabled adolescents
This free fact sheet defines the condition and provides
information on incidence, characteristics, educational
implications, additional resources, and associated
organizations.

Encounters with Reality: 1001 Interpreter Scenarios
Registry of the Interpreters for the Deaf
333 Commerce Street
Alexandria, VA 22314
703-838-0030, 703-838-0459 (TTY)
info@rid.org
http://www.rid.org/pubs.html
Disability Served: hearing
The text discusses how interpreters must be mentally
prepared for the unexpected. It includes ethical,
cross-cultural, and communication challenging
scenarios with sample responses from both deaf
consumers and experienced interpreters.

E-Newsletters
National Organization on Disability
910 16th Street, NW, Suite 600
Washington, DC 20006
202-293-5960
http://www.nod.org
Disability Served: various
This organization offers several e-newsletters on
disability issues such as education, health care
access, and emergency preparedness.

EnVision
Lighthouse International
111 East 59th Street

New York, NY 10022-1202
212-821-9200, 800-829-0500
http://www.lighthouse.org/scripts/newsletter
Disability Served: vision
This free, online newsletter is targeted to parents
and educators of children with impaired vision.

Epilepsy
National Dissemination Center for Children
with Disabilities
PO Box 1492
Washington, DC 20013
800-695-0285
nichcy@aed.org
http://nichcy.org/publist.asp
Disability Served: epilepsy
This free fact sheet defines the condition and provides
information on incidence, characteristics, educational
implications, additional resources, and associated
organizations.

Epilepsy: Hope through Research
National Institute of Neurological Disorders and Stroke
PO Box 5801
Bethesda, MD 20824
301-496-5751, 800-352-9424
http://www.ninds.nih.gov/disorders/epilepsy/epilepsy.
htm#Publications
Disability Served: epilepsy
This free information booklet on seizures, seizure
disorders, and epilepsy explains diagnosis,
preventative measures, treatments, effects on
daily life, and current research findings.

**Equals in Partnership: Basic Rights for Families
of Children with Blindness or Visual Impairment**
National Association for Parents of Children
with Visual Impairments.
PO Box 317
Watertown, MA 02471
admin@spedex.com
http://www.spedex.com/napvi/order.html
Disability Served: vision
This comprehensive compilation of educational
advocacy materials helps parents better
understand the special needs of their children
who have visual impairments and assists them in
accessing appropriate services.

Even Little Kids Get Diabetes
Juvenile Diabetes Foundation
120 Wall Street

New York, NY 10005-4001
800-533-2873
info@jdrf.org
http://www.jdrf.org/index.cfm?page_id=100250
Disability Served: diabetes
This is a storybook parents can read to their child about a little girl with diabetes. It's an excellent resource for helping a child deal with the psychological effects of diabetes.

Everyone Likes to Eat: How Children Can Eat Most of the Foods They Enjoy and Still Take Care of Their Diabetes
Juvenile Diabetes Foundation
120 Wall Street
New York, NY 10005-4001
800-533-2873
info@jdrf.org
http://www.jdrf.org/index.cfm?page_id=100250
Disability Served: diabetes
This guidebook is filled with activities, puzzles, and problem-solving exercises that show kids how to control their diabetes, yet eat at school, parties, holiday time, and fast food restaurants.

Exceptional Children
Council for Exceptional Children
1110 North Glebe Road, Suite 300
Arlington, VA 22201-5704
888-CEC-SPED, 866-915-5000 (TTY)
service@cec.sped.org
http://www.cec.sped.org
Disability Served: various
This quarterly publication provides information regarding students with special needs and special education.

Exceptional Parent Magazine
EP Global Communications
65 East Route 4
River Edge, NJ 07661
877-372-7368
EPAR@kable.com
http://www.eparent.com
Disability Served: various
This magazine is designed for parents of children with disabilities.

Expectations: Parenting Children and Teens with Limb Differences
Amputee Coalition of America
900 East Hill Avenue, Suite 285

Knoxville, TN 37915-2568
888-267-5669, 865-525-4512 (TTY)
http://www.amputee-coalition.org
Disability Served: amputees
This free, online publication offers advice to parents of young amputees. Issues discussed include adjustment issues, prosthetics, funding, peer support, advocacy, insurance reimbursement, technology, and prevention of secondary conditions.

Facilitating Hearing and Listening in Young Children
Alexander Graham Bell Association of the Deaf
3417 Volta Place, NW
Washington, DC 20007
866-337-5220, 202-337-5221 (TTY)
publications@agbell.org
http://www.agbell.org
Disability Served: hearing
This popular guide that offers advice to parents of children with hearing difficulties, covers recent developments in amplification technology, cochlear implants, federal legislation, and listening strategies.

Facing AD/HD A Survival Guide for Parents of Children with Attention Deficit Hyperactivity Disorder
Research Press
Department 25W, PO Box 9177
Champaign, IL 61826
217-352-3273, 800-519-2707
rp@researchpress.com
http://www.researchpress.com
Disability Served: attention deficit disorder
This text for parents addresses structure, routines, setting goals, using charts, persistency with consistency, teamwork, treatment options, medication, and more.

Facts about ALS
Muscular Dystrophy Association
3300 East Sunrise Drive
Tucson, AZ 85718
800-572-1717
publications@mdausa.org
http://www.mdausa.org/publications
Disability Served: physically disabled
This free booklet discusses the history, description, and causes of Amytrophic Lateral Sclerosis. It also covers the search for treatments and cures.

Facts about Disease Booklets
Muscular Dystrophy Association
3300 East Sunrise Drive

Tucson, AZ 85718
800-572-1717
publications@mdausa.org
http://www.mdausa.org/publications
Disability Served: various
These free brochures offer detailed introductory
explanations of the more than 40 neuromuscular
diseases in the association's program.

Facts about Down Syndrome

National Institute of Child Health and Human
Development
PO Box 2006
Rockville, MD 20847
800-370-2943
NICHDInformationResourceCenter@mail.nih.gov
http://www.nichd.nih.gov/publications/pubs.cfm
Disability Served: Down Syndrome
This free booklet for parents and families explains
Down Syndrome, its cause, its symptoms, diagnosis,
its associated disorders, and the treatments available
for those with the syndrome.

Facts about Lung Cancer

American Lung Association
61 Broadway
New York, NY 10006
212-315-8700
http://www.lungusa.org/site/apps/s/content.asp?
c=dvLUK9O0E&b=34706&ct=67325
Disability Served: cancer patients and survivors
This free Web resource offers answers to the following
questions: What is lung cancer?, What causes lung
cancer?, How is lung cancer detected?, How is lung
cancer treated?, and How can you prevent lung
cancer?

Fact Sheet on Depression and Anxiety in Individuals with Spina Bifida

Spina Bifida Association of America
4590 MacArthur Boulevard, NW, Suite 250
Washington, DC 20007-4226
202-944-3285, 800-621-3141
sbaa@sbaa.org
http://www.sbaa.org/site/PageServer?pagename=
asb_facts
Disability Served: mental health, spina bifida
This free fact sheet lists symptoms, causes, and
treatment for depression and how it relates
to persons with spina bifida.

Fact Sheet on Educational Issues Among Children with Spina Bifida

Spina Bifida Association of America
4590 MacArthur Boulevard, NW, Suite 250
Washington, DC 20007-4226
202-944-3285, 800-621-3141
sbaa@sbaa.org
http://www.sbaa.org/site/PageServer?pagename=
asb_facts
Disability Served: learning disabilities, spina bifida
This free fact sheet describes how the physical aspects
of spina bifida relate to a child's intelligence and
learning ability.

Fact Sheet on Genetics and Spina Bifida

Spina Bifida Association of America
4590 MacArthur Boulevard, NW, Suite 250
Washington, DC 20007-4226
202-944-3285, 800-621-3141
sbaa@sbaa.org
http://www.sbaa.org/site/PageServer?pagename=
asb_facts
Disability Served: spina bifida
This free fact sheet describes causes of this birth defect
as well as information on how to help prevent it.

Fact Sheet on Travel with a Disability: Easier than Ever

Spina Bifida Association of America
4590 MacArthur Boulevard, NW, Suite 250
Washington, DC 20007-4226
202-944-3285, 800-621-3141
sbaa@sbaa.org
http://www.sbaa.org/site/PageServer?pagename=
asb_facts
Disability Served: spina bifida
This free fact sheet offers useful tips for people with
spina bifida when traveling by air, land, or sea, and
staying in a hotel.

Fact Sheets

Amytrophic Lateral Sclerosis Association
27001 Agoura Road, Suite 150
Calabasas Hills, CA 91301-5104
818-880-9007
info@alsa-national.org
http://www.alsa.org/resources/fyi.cfm?CFID=1048742
&CFTOKEN=97497558
Disability Served: physically disabled
The Amytrophic Lateral Sclerosis Association offers fact
sheets, free of charge, on a variety of topics under the

following headings: caregivers, benefits, research/clinics, newly diagnosed patients, patients, and speech/swallowing.

Fact Sheets
Blind Babies Foundation
1814 Franklin Street, 11th Floor
Oakland, CA 94612
510-446-2229
bbfinfo@blindbabies.org
http://blindbabies.typepad.com/resources
Disability Served: vision
This collection of fact sheets contains information on six common visual diagnoses, as well as information on eye specialists and vision assessments. Content topics include "Visual and Behavioral Characteristics", "Myths", and "Teaching Strategies." Individual fact sheets are available free of charge, full packets for a minimal donation.

Fact Sheets
United States Department of Health and Human Services
200 Independence Avenue, SW
Washington, DC 20201
202-690-6343
http://www.hhs.gov/news/facts
Disability Served: various
This agency provides free, downloadable fact sheets on a variety of health and human services topics from aging to teen pregnancy to protecting the health of minority communities.

Fact Sheets for Spinocerebellar Ataxias
National Ataxia Foundation
2600 Fernbrook Lane, Suite 119
Minneapolis, MN 55447
naf@ataxia.org
http://www.ataxia.org
Disability Served: physically disabled
These free fact sheets explain each of the 10 types of spino-cerebellar ataxias.

Fair Housing: How to Make the Law Work for You
Paralyzed Veterans of America
801 Eighteenth Street, NW
Washington, DC 20006-3517
301-932-7834, 888-860-7244
info@pva.org
http://www.pva.org/cgi-bin/pvastore/products.cgi?id=2
Disability Served: various

This free publication explains the rights of all individuals with disabilities when they seek housing, and the remedies they can pursue if they encounter discrimination because of their disability.

Fall Prevention
American Occupational Therapy Association Inc.
4720 Montgomery Lane, PO Box 31220
Bethesda, MD 20824-1220
301-652-2682, 800-377-8555
http://www.aota.org/featured/area6/links/link02.asp
Disability Served: various
This free tip sheet offers information to people on how to prevent falls.

The Family Guide to Surviving Stroke and Communication Disorders
Pro-Ed Inc.
8700 Shoal Creek Boulevard
Austin, TX 78757-6897
800-897-3202
http://www.proedinc.com
Disability Served: communication, stroke
This offers advice for families dealing with victims of stroke and related illnesses that cause difficulty with communication. It features questions and answers, case studies, and examples for easy readability and comprehension.

Family Resource Guides
Association for Retarded Citizens of the United States
1010 Wayne Avenue, Suite 650
Silver Spring, MD 20910
301-565-3842
Info@thearc.org
http://www.thearc.org/info-mr.html
Disability Served: developmentally disabled, mental retardation
These resource guides (which vary by state according to state guidelines) provide an overview of benefits, supports, and services for families raising children with mental retardation and related developmental disabilities.

Fast Facts Series: What To Do When You Have Type 2 Diabetes
American Diabetes Association
1701 North Beauregard Street
Alexandria, VA 22311
800-342-2383

AskADA@diabetes.org
http://www.diabetes.org
Disability Served: diabetes
This booklet offers advice on nutrition, exercise, and medications, and fast facts on meal planning, carbohydrate counting, and psychological issues.

A Field Guide to Type 1 Diabetes
American Diabetes Association
1701 North Beauregard Street
Alexandria, VA 22311
800-342-2383
AskADA@diabetes.org
http://www.diabetes.org
Disability Served: diabetes
This book provides checklists of resources for people with Type 1 diabetes.

A Field Guide to Type 2 Diabetes
American Diabetes Association
1701 North Beauregard Street
Alexandria, VA 22311
800-342-2383
AskADA@diabetes.org
http://www.diabetes.org
Disability Served: diabetes
This book is a valuable resource to the diabetes educator who is trying to explain a complicated disease in simple terms.

Fighting Cancer
R.A. Bloch Cancer Foundation Inc.
4400 Main Street
Kansas City, MO 64111
816-932-8453, 800-433-0464
http://www.blochcancer.org
Disability Served: cancer patients and survivors
This is a free, online, step-by-step guide to help fight cancer.

Financial Aid for Individuals with Learning Disabilities
HEATH Resource Center
George Washington University
2121 K Street, NW, Suite 220
Washington, DC 20037
202-973-0904 (Voice/TTY), 800-544-3284
askheath@gwu.edu
http://www.heath.gwu.edu/factsheet.htm
Disability Served: learning disabled
This is a free, online resource that details financial aid options for students with learning disabilities.

Financial Aid for the Disabled and Their Families
Reference Service Press
5000 Windplay Drive, Suite 4
El Dorado Hills, CA 95762
916-939-9620
findaid@aol.com
http://www.rspfunding.com
Disability Served: various
This reference book for applicants at any level— from high school through postdoctorate and professional—lists nearly 1,200 available funding programs for the disabled and describes them in the following categories: program title, sponsoring organization address and telephone number (including toll-free and TDD), email and Web address, purpose, eligibility, financial data, duration, special features, limitations, number of awards, and deadline.

Financial Help for Diabetes Care
National Diabetes Information Clearinghouse
5 Information Way
Bethesda, MD 20892-3568
800-860-8747
catalog@niddk.nih.gov
http://catalog.niddk.nih.gov/AlphaList.cfm?CH=NDIC
Disability Served: diabetes
This brochure reviews the two government-funded health care assistance programs, Medicare and Medicaid, as well as other health care services available for people with diabetes. Single copies are free.

Finding a Mental Health Professional: A Personal Guide
Depressive and Bipolar Support Alliance
730 North Franklin Street, Suite 501
Chicago, IL 60610-7224
800-826-3632
bookstore@dbsalliance.org
http://www.dbsalliance.org/store
Disability Served: mental health
This free brochure provides answers to many of the questions people have regarding mental health including what kind of professional to choose, what to expect during a first appointment, and how to handle the financial side of treatment.

Finding Out about Epilepsy: A Guide to Treatment
Epilepsy Foundation
4351 Garden City Drive
Landover, MD 20785-7223
800-332-1000
http://www.epilepsyfoundation.org

Disability Served: epilepsy

This pamphlet describes different types of seizures and what one can do to control them.

Finding Peace of Mind: Treatment Strategies for Depression and Bipolar Disorder

Depressive and Bipolar Support Alliance

730 North Franklin Street, Suite 501

Chicago, IL 60610-7224

800-826-3632

bookstore@dbsalliance.org

http://www.dbsalliance.org/store

Disability Served: mental health

This free brochure can help people build a cooperative relationship with their doctors by explaining some of the treatments for mood disorders and how they work.

Fingerspelling in American Sign Language

Registry of the Interpreters for the Deaf

333 Commerce Street

Alexandria, VA 22314

703-838-0030, 703-838-0459 (TTY)

info@rid.org

http://www.rid.org/pubs.html

Disability Served: hearing

This text, for beginning to intermediate American Sign Language classes and study groups, offers an innovative approach to finger spelling practice by incorporating lessons on history, use, receptive and expressive pointers, lexicalized finger spelling, and more.

Fire Safety for Wheelchair Users at Work and at Home

United Spinal Association

75-20 Astoria Boulevard

Jackson Heights, NY 11370

718-803-3782, 800-444-0120

publications@unitedspinal.org

http://www.unitedspinal.org/pages.php?catid=7

Disability Served: physically disabled

Created in response to the events of September 11, 2011, this free brochure covers the special evacuation needs of wheelchair users during an emergency and outlines the efforts of the United Spinal Association to ensure up-to-date state and building codes to improve the safety of mobility-impaired persons.

First Aid Fast

American Red Cross

2025 E Street, NW

Washington, DC 20006

202-303-4498

http://www.redcross.org/pubs

Disability Served: physically disabled

This reference guide provides step-by-step guidance for the following emergencies: breathing emergencies, cardiac emergencies, injuries to muscles, bones, and joints; poisonings; and much more.

First Aid for Epilepsy Card

Epilepsy Foundation

4351 Garden City Drive

Landover, MD 20785-7223

800-332-1000

http://www.epilepsyfoundation.org

Disability Served: epilepsy

This wallet-size card contains first aid information for managing different seizure types.

First Step: A Guide for Adapting to Limb Loss

Amputee Coalition of America

900 East Hill Avenue, Suite 285

Knoxville, TN 37915-2568

888-267-5669, 865-525-4512 (TTY)

http://www.amputee-coalition.org

Disability Served: amputees

This guide provides support and advice to people who have recently lost a limb.

The Fitness Prescription

Multiple Sclerosis Foundation Inc.

6350 North Andrews Avenue

Fort Lauderdale, FL 33309-2130

954-776-6805, 888-MSFOCUS

support@msfocus.org

http://www.msfacts.org/publications/pub_booklets.html

Disability Served: multiple sclerosis

This free publication offers the most up-to-date research on exercise and multiple sclerosis.

Focus on Autism and Other Developmental Disabilities

Pro-Ed Inc.

8700 Shoal Creek Boulevard

Austin, TX 78757-6897

800-897-3202

http://www.proedinc.com

Disability Served: autism

This quarterly journal discusses the treatment and education of students with autism and other developmental disabilities.

Focus on Exceptional Children
9101 East Kenyon Avenue, Suite 2200
Denver, CO 80237
303-221-7333
lpc@lovepublishing.com
http://www.lovepublishing.com
Disability Served: *various*
This monthly newsletter is designed for special
education instructors, administrators, and
professionals and provides articles and news on
special education issues.

Food and Drug Administration Consumer
Federal Citizen Information Center
1800 F Street, NW
Washington, DC 20405
888-878-3256
firstgov1@mail.fedinfo.gov
http://www.pueblo.gsa.gov/results.
   tpl?id1=16&startat=1&--woSECTIONSdata
   rq=16&--SECTIONSword=ww
Disability Served: *various*
This bimonthly magazine, available by subscription,
offers the latest in medical news.

Foods and Moods
Depressive and Bipolar Support Alliance
730 North Franklin Street, Suite 501
Chicago, IL 60610-7224
800-826-3632
bookstore@dbsalliance.org
http://www.dbsalliance.org/store
Disability Served: *mental health*
This free brochure explains how foods impact mood.

For Parents of Newborn Babies with Cleft Lip/Palate
Cleft Palate Foundation
1504 East Franklin Street, Suite 102
Chapel Hill, NC 27514-2820
919-933-9044, 800-24CLEFT
info@cleftline.org
http://www.cleftline.org/publications
Disability Served: *physically disabled*
This free fact sheet provides basic information for
parents who have just had a baby with a cleft lip
and/or palate.

4 Steps to Control Your Diabetes for Life
National Diabetes Information Clearinghouse
5 Information Way

Bethesda, MD 20892-3568
800-860-8747
catalog@niddk.nih.gov
http://catalog.niddk.nih.gov/AlphaList.cfm?CH=NDIC
Disability Served: *diabetes*
This booklet helps health care providers educate patients
in vital self-care principles. The four steps help people
with diabetes understand, monitor, and take control
of their diabetes. The first 25 copies are free.

***Fragile Success: Ten Autistic Children, Childhood
   to Adulthood***
Paul H. Brookes Publishing Company Inc.
PO Box 10624
Baltimore, MD 21285-0624
800-638-3775
custserv@brookespublishing.com
http://www.pbrookes.com
Disability Served: *autism*
A former teacher follows the lives of her autistic students
over 30 years.

***Free Appropriate Public Education: The Law and
   Children with Disabilities***
Love Publishing Company
9101 East Kenyon Avenue, Suite 2200
Denver, CO 80237
303-221-7333
lpc@lovepublishing.com
http://www.lovepublishing.com
Disability Served: *various*
This text discusses legislative issues and regulations in
regard to the education of students who are disabled.

Frequently Asked Questions about Spina Bifida
Spina Bifida Association of America
4590 MacArthur Boulevard, NW, Suite 250
Washington, DC 20007-4226
202-944-3285, 800-621-3141
sbaa@sbaa.org
http://www.sbaa.org/site/PageServer?pagename=
   asb_facts
Disability Served: *spina bifida*
This free fact sheet offers a general overview of spina
bifida including the different types of spina bifida,
treatments, prevention, and related conditions.

Future Reflections
National Federation of the Blind
1800 Johnson Street

Baltimore, MD 21230
410-659-9314
nfbstore@nfb.org
http://www.nfb.org/publications.html
Disability Served: vision
This quarterly magazine for parents and teachers of blind children covers the issues surrounding blind children as they grow from birth through college.

Generations
National Ataxia Foundation
2600 Fernbrook Lane, Suite 119
Minneapolis, MN 55447
naf@ataxia.org
http://www.ataxia.org
Disability Served: physically disabled
This quarterly news publication offers up-to-date information and articles on ataxia.

Generic Drugs
Federal Citizen Information Center
1800 F Street, NW
Washington, DC 20405
888-878-3256
firstgov1@mail.fedinfo.gov
http://www.pueblo.gsa.gov/results.
   tpl?id1=16&startat=1&--woSECTIONS
   datarq=16&--SECTIONSword=ww
Disability Served: various
This free brochure covers the effectiveness, appearance, and safety of generic drugs.

Geriatrics
Advanstar Communications
131 West First Street
Duluth, MN 55802-2065
888-527-7008
fullfill@superfill.com
http://www.geri.com/geriatrics
Disability Served: elderly
This monthly publication discusses medical care of the aged.

Get Connected! Linking Older Adults With Medication, Alcohol, and Mental Health Resources: A Toolkit
National Council on the Aging
300 D Street, SW, Suite 801
Washington, DC 20024
202-479-1200
info@ncoa.org
http://www.ncoa.org/content.cfm?sectionID=30
Disability Served: chemical dependency, elderly, mental health
This free downloadable publication is designed to help older adults gain access to needed substance abuse and mental health services by promoting new linkages between well-known, trusted providers of aging, substance abuse, and mental health services.

Get Real! You Don't Have to Knock Yourself Out to Prevent Diabetes
National Diabetes Information Clearinghouse
5 Information Way
Bethesda, MD 20892-3568
800-860-8747
catalog@niddk.nih.gov
http://catalog.niddk.nih.gov/AlphaList.cfm?CH=NDIC
Disability Served: diabetes
This fact sheet encourages people at risk for type 2 diabetes to take small steps to prevent the disease. The first 25 copies are free.

Getting Into College: Strategies for the Student with TS
Tourette Syndrome Association
42-40 Bell Boulevard
Bayside, NY 11361
718-224-2999
http://tsa-usa.org/Merchant2/merchant.
   mvc?Screen=CTGY&Store_Code=TOS
   &Category_Code=E
Disability Served: Tourette Syndrome
This publication focuses on matching the school to the student, SATs, accommodations, and the challenges faced when transitioning from high school to college.

Getting the Best IEP for Your Child
International Dyslexia Association
Chester Building, 8600 LaSalle Road, Suite 382
Baltimore, MD 21286-2044
410-296-0232
http://www.interdys.org
Disability Served: dyslexic
This is an online brochure that features advice for parents on setting up an Individualized Education Plan.

The Girls' Guide to AD/HD
Woodbine House
6510 Bells Mill Road
Bethesda, MD 20817

800-843-7323
http://www.woodbinehouse.com/ADD-&-
ADHD.9.0.0.2.htm
Disability Served: attention deficit disorder
This book offers candid and funny facts, advice, and
encouragement for teen girls with attention deficit/
hyperactivity disorder.

Going to College: Expanding Opportunities for People with Disabilities
Paul H. Brookes Publishing Company Inc.
PO Box 10624
Baltimore, MD 21285-0624
800-638-3775
custserv@brookespublishing.com
http://www.pbrookes.com
Disability Served: various
Useful advice and information for the disabled who plan
to go to college.

Grief Digest
Centering Corporation
7230 Maple Street
Omaha, NE 68134
402-533-1200
https://www.centeringcorp.com
Disability Served: various
This magazine includes articles on coping and dealing
with grief.

Guide for Cancer Supporters
R.A. Bloch Cancer Foundation Inc.
4400 Main Street
Kansas City, MO 64111
816-932-8453, 800-433-0464
http://www.blochcancer.org
Disability Served: cancer patients and survivors
This free, step-by-step book offers ways to help a relative
or friend fight cancer.

A Guide for Women and Girls with Bleeding Disorders
National Hemophilia Foundation
116 West 32nd Street, 11th Floor
New York, NY 10001
212-328-3700, 800-42-HANDI
handi@hemophilia.org
http://www.hemophilia.org/resources/handi_pubs.htm
Disability Served: inherited bleeding disorders
This booklet for women and girls with bleeding disorders

discusses the safety of blood products as well as
obstetric and gynecologic concerns. Single copies
are free to members.

Guide to Children's Literature and Disability
National Dissemination Center for Children
with Disabilities
PO Box 1492
Washington, DC 20013
800-695-0285
nichcy@aed.org
http://nichcy.org/publist.asp
Disability Served: various
This free guide includes a long list of mysteries,
adventure stories, dramas, and real life stories for
children and youth written by or featuring individuals
with disabilities.

Guide to Choosing a Nursing Home
Centers for Medicare and Medicaid Services
7500 Security Boulevard
Baltimore, MD 21244-1850
800-633-4227
http://www.medicare.gov
Disability Served: various
This publication provides information and tips
for selecting a nursing home.

A Guide to High School Success for Students with Disabilities
Greenwood Publishing Group Inc.
88 Post Road West
Westport, CT 06881
203-226-3571
http://www.greenwood.com
Disability Served: various
This book, written largely by students with disabilities,
provides unique insights into how to navigate
adolescence if one happens to have special needs.
It covers issues such as handling difficult teachers,
advocating for yourself, extracurricular activities,
dating and sexuality, and life after high school.

Guide to Selecting and Monitoring Brain Injury Rehabilitation Services
Brain Injury Association of America
8201 Greensboro Drive, Suite 611
McLean, VA 22102
703-761-0750, 800-444-6443

familyhelpline@biausa.org
http://www.biausa.org/Pages/guide_to_selecting.html
Disability Served: traumatic brain injury
This free, downloadable brochure provides information regarding brain injury rehabilitation programs and services.

Guide to the Diagnosis and Treatment of Tourette Syndrome

Tourette Syndrome Association
42-40 Bell Boulevard
Bayside, NY 11361
718-224-2999
http://tsa-usa.org/Merchant2/merchant.
mvc?Screen=CTGY&Store_Code=TOS&
Category_Code=E
Disability Served: Tourette Syndrome
This medical overview for professionals and families offers in-depth coverage of Tourette Syndrome and other tic disorders. Treatment, monitoring, education, academic and occupational interventions, and family dynamics are featured.

A Guide to Toys for Children with Special Needs

American Foundation for the Blind
11 Penn Plaza, Suite 300
New York, NY 10001
212-502-7600, 800-232-5463
afbinfo@afb.net
http://www.afb.org
Disability Served: various
This free guidebook is a one-of-a-kind resource for parents, grandparents, and teachers that contains information about commercially available toys and games that are fun, safe, and appropriate for children of all ages with special needs—including those who are blind or visually impaired

Guide to Your Child's Allergies and Asthma

American Academy of Pediatrics
141 Northwest Point Boulevard
Elk Grove Village, IL 60007-3808
847-949-6064, 888-290-0878
info@arttherapy.org
http://www.aap.org/bookstorepubs.html
Disability Served: asthma
This guide includes real-life questions and answers, highlighted tips, and tables to help parents raise healthy, active children.

Handbook of Career Planning for Students with Special Needs

Pro-Ed Inc.
8700 Shoal Creek Boulevard
Austin, TX 78757-6897
800-897-3202
http://www.proedinc.com
Disability Served: various
This handbook provides strategies for teaching vocational skills to students with special needs.

Handbook of Services for the Deaf and the Hard-of-Hearing: A Bridge to Accessibility

Elsevier Inc.
30 Corporate Drive, Suite 400
Burlington, MA 01803
http://www.apnet.com
Disability Served: hearing
This is a comprehensive overview of issues affecting the lives of deaf and hard of hearing people.

Handbook on Disability Discrimination Law

American Bar Association Commission on Mental and Physical Disability Law
740 15th Street, NW
Washington, DC 20005-1019
202-662-1000
orders@abanet.org
http://www.abanet.org/disability/pubs1.html
Disability Served: various
This handbook for lawyers, judges, disability professionals, advocates, and law students provides a concise, but comprehensive, summary and analysis of the federal and state statutes and case law that govern disability discrimination.

Handbook on Mental Disability Law

American Bar Association Commission on Mental and Physical Disability Law
740 15th Street, NW
Washington, DC 20005-1019
202-662-1000
orders@abanet.org
http://www.abanet.org/disability/pubs1.html
Disability Served: mentally disabled
This handbook for lawyers, judges, disability professionals, advocates, and law students is a primer on mental disability law from both clinical and legal perspectives.

Hands-on Reading
Ablenet
2808 Fairview Avenue
Roseville, MN 55113-1308
800-322-0956
customerservice@ablenetinc.com
http://www.ablenetinc.com
Disability Served: learning disabled
This interactive, whole language approach to reading
and learning is based on favorite children's stories,
including *Put Me in the Zoo, The Runaway Bunny,
Caps for Sale*, and 11 more titles.

Health Technology Trends
ECRI
5200 Butler Pike
Plymouth Meeting, PA 19462-1298
610-825-6000, ext. 5891
communications@ecri.org
http://www.ecri.org/Products_and_Services/Products/
Health_Technology_Trends/Default.aspx
Disability Served: various
This monthly journal reports on health technology
trends and is geared toward health care professionals.

Healthy and Hearty Diabetic Cooking
R.A. Rapaport Publishing Inc.
PO Box 11066
Des Moines, IA 50336-1066
800-664-9269
https://www.diabetesselfmanagement.com/eds/
books.cfm
Disability Served: diabetes
This book contains more than 300 healthy recipes that
are quick and easy to make.

Healthy Eating
Multiple Sclerosis Society of Canada
175 Bloor Street East, Suite 700, North Tower
Toronto, ON M4W 3R8
Canada
416-922-6065, 800-268-7582
info@mssociety.ca
http://www.mssociety.ca/en/information/references.htm
Disability Served: multiple sclerosis
This booklet, free in downloadable form, describes some
of the special diets claimed, though never proven, to
be beneficial for multiple sclerosis. It also presents a
clear guide to what makes up a healthy diet based on
Canada's food guide.

**Hearing Impaired Infants: Support In The First Eighteen
Months**
Alexander Graham Bell Association of the Deaf
3417 Volta Place, NW
Washington, DC 20007
866-337-5220, 202-337-5221 (TTY)
publications@agbell.org
http://www.agbell.org
Disability Served: hearing
This offers a roadmap of how parents and hearing
professionals can work together to provide the best
support for hearing-impaired children up to 18
months of age.

Hearing Loss and Hearing Aids: A Bridge to Healing
Self Help for Hard of Hearing People Inc.
7910 Woodmont Avenue, Suite 1200
Bethesda, MD 20814
301-657-2248, 301-657-2249 (TTY)
bookstore@hearingloss.org
http://hearingloss.sidestreetshop.com/default.cfm
Disability Served: hearing
This handbook for consumers explores the emotions
and issues surrounding hearing loss and offers ideas
on how to improve quality of life. It also includes
questions and answers posed by experts, as well as
information on a variety of other issues related to
hearing loss.

**Hearing Loss: The Journal of Self Help for Hard
of Hearing People**
Self Help for Hard of Hearing People Inc.
7910 Woodmont Avenue, Suite 1200
Bethesda, MD 20814
301-657-2248
http://www.hearingloss.org
Disability Served: hearing
This journal is designed for persons with hearing
impairments and provides information, emotional
support, reviews on assistive technology, and more.

Heart Disease
Federal Citizen Information Center
1800 F Street, NW
Washington, DC 20405
888-878-3256
firstgov1@mail.fedinfo.gov
http://www.pueblo.gsa.gov/results.tpl?id1=16&startat=1
&--woSECTIONSdatarq=16&--SECTIONSword=ww
Disability Served: physically disabled

This free booklet outlines the signs of heart disease, including the silent symptoms, and offers tips on how to lower your risk.

HEATH National Resource Directory on Postsecondary Education and Disability
HEATH Resource Center
George Washington University
2121 K Street, NW, Suite 220
Washington, DC 20037
202-973-0904 (Voice/TTY), 800-544-3284
askheath@gwu.edu
http://www.heath.gwu.edu/bookstore/pdf/heath_resource_directory.pdf
Disability Served: various
This features more than 180 organizations that assist disabled students pursue higher education. It is available as a free, online resource.

Helping Children at Home and School II: Handouts for Families and Educators
National Association of School Psychologists
4340 East West Highway, Suite 402
Bethesda, MD 20814
301-657-0270
publications@naspweb.org
http://www.nasponline.org/publications/index.html
Disability Served: behavioral disorders, learning disabled
This resource includes more than 250 new or completely revised reproducible handouts for parents, educators, child advocates, and teens on a wide range of issues affecting learning and behavior.

Helping Teens Cope with Death
Centering Corporation
7230 Maple Street
Omaha, NE 68134
402-533-1200
https://www.centeringcorp.com
Disability Served: various
This book discusses how the death of a loved one can impact a teen. It covers the common grief reactions of teenagers, specific challenges grieving teenagers face, when to seek professional help, and advice from other parents.

Helping the Student with Diabetes Succeed
National Diabetes Information Clearinghouse
5 Information Way
Bethesda, MD 20892-3568

800-860-8747
catalog@niddk.nih.gov
http://catalog.niddk.nih.gov/AlphaList.cfm?CH=NDIC
Disability Served: diabetes
This comprehensive resource guide helps school personnel ensure a safe learning environment and equal access to educational opportunities for students with diabetes. Single copies are free.

Help with Hearing Aids: A Three-Part Series
Self Help for Hard of Hearing People Inc.
7910 Woodmont Avenue, Suite 1200
Bethesda, MD 20814
301-657-2248, 301-657-2249 (TTY)
bookstore@hearingloss.org
http://hearingloss.sidestreetshop.com/default.cfm
Disability Served: hearing
This three-part series includes *Preparing for and Getting the Most Out of a Visit to a Hearing Aid Dispenser, Selecting and Purchasing a Hearing Aid,* and *Troubleshooting Your Hearing Aid.*

HemAware
National Hemophilia Foundation
116 West 32nd Street, 11th Floor
New York, NY 10001
212-328-3700, 800-42-HANDI
handi@hemophilia.org
http://www.hemophilia.org/resources/handi_pubs.htm
Disability Served: inherited bleeding disorders
This magazine is published six times a year and offers updates on the advances in treatments, information on the foundation, and human-interest stories.

Hemophilia, Sports, and Exercise
National Hemophilia Foundation
116 West 32nd Street, 11th Floor
New York, NY 10001
212-328-3700, 800-42-HANDI
handi@hemophilia.org
http://www.hemophilia.org/resources/handi_pubs.htm
Disability Served: inherited bleeding disorders
This guidebook presents valuable information for the person with a bleeding disorder who is considering participation in sports activities. Single copies are free to members.

High Blood Pressure: Treat It for Life
Federal Citizen Information Center
1800 F Street, NW

Washington, DC 20405
888-878-3256
firstgov1@mail.fedinfo.gov
http://www.pueblo.gsa.gov/results.
    tpl?id1=16&startat=1&--woSECTIONS
    datarq=16&--SECTIONSword=ww
Disability Served: physically disabled
This book describes how high blood pressure can lead
    to heart failure, kidney failure, or stroke and teaches
    how it can be controlled through diet, exercise, and
    medication.

Hip Replacement
American Occupational Therapy Association Inc.
4720 Montgomery Lane, PO Box 31220
Bethesda, MD 20824-1220
301-652-2682, 800-377-8555
http://www.aota.org/featured/area6/links/link02.asp
Disability Served: physically disabled
This free tip sheet offers information for patients
    undergoing hip replacement surgery, and details
    how occupational therapists can assist these patients.

HIV/AIDS Fact Book
American Red Cross
2025 East Street, NW
Washington, DC 20006
202-303-4498
http://www.redcross.org/pubs
Disability Served: AIDS
This book provides basic information about HIV and
    AIDS in a question-and-answer format suitable for
    laypersons and health professionals.

HomeCare
Primedia Business Magazines and Media
PO Box 2100
Skokie, IL 60076-7800
866-505-7173
hzcs@pbsub.com
http://homecaremag.com/index.html
Disability Served: various
This monthly magazine focuses on the home health care
    industry.

Home Health Care Services Quarterly
The Haworth Press
10 Alice Street
Binghamton, NY 13904
607-722-5857, 800-342-9678

http://www.haworthpressinc.com/journals/default.asp
Disability Served: various
This quarterly journal provides articles and news to the
    home health care professional.

How Children Learn Language
Alexander Graham Bell Association of the Deaf
3417 Volta Place, NW
Washington, DC 20007
866-337-5220, 202-337-5221 (TTY)
publications@agbell.org
http://www.agbell.org
Disability Served: hearing, learning disabled
This is an introductory text for professionals in non-
    language fields and students in education/special
    education courses.

How Do I Teach This Kid?
Future Horizons
721 West Abram Street
Arlington, TX 76013
800-489-0727
info@futurehorizons-autism.com
http://www.futurehorizons-autism.com
Disability Served: autism
This is the first in a series of books with ideas for
    using visual strategies to teach children with
    autism. This resource provides special education
    teachers, therapists, and parents with practical,
    easy-to-implement ideas to teach students to work
    independently.

How's Your Hearing? A Self-Quiz
Ear Foundation
PO Box 330867
Nashville, TN 37203
615-627-2724, 800-545-HEAR
info@earfoundation.org
http://www.earfoundation.org/articles.asp
Disability Served: hearing
This online quiz will help you discover whether or not
    your hearing is fine or if you should see a doctor or
    specialist.

How to Find Medical Information
Federal Citizen Information Center
1800 F Street, NW
Washington, DC 20405
888-878-3256
firstgov1@mail.fedinfo.gov

http://www.pueblo.gsa.gov/results.tpl?id1=16&startat=1
&--woSECTIONSdatarq=16&--SECTIONSword=ww

Disability Served: various

This free booklet offers advice on how to use your local library, the federal government, and the Internet to get information on an illness or disorder.

How to Keep Your Heart Healthy

Federal Citizen Information Center
1800 F Street, NW
Washington, DC 20405
888-878-3256
firstgov1@mail.fedinfo.gov
http://www.pueblo.gsa.gov/results.tpl?id1=16&startat=1
&--woSECTIONSdatarq=16&--SECTIONSword=ww

Disability Served: physically disabled

This free brochure helps people learn to recognize heart attack symptoms and make lifestyle changes to reduce the risk of heart attack.

How to Pick the Right Alternative Keyboard

LRP Publications
747 Dresher Road, Suite 500, PO Box 980
Horsham, PA 19044-0980
215-784-0860, 800-341-7874
http://www.shoplrp.com/disability/cat-
Ergonomics Workplace_Safety.html

Disability Served: physically disabled

This tip sheet explains the difference between fixed-split keyboards and adjustable-split keyboards and includes key points to consider before purchasing a keyboard.

The HUB

SPOKES Unlimited
415 Main Street
Klamath Falls, OR 97601
541-883-7547 (Voice/TTY)
infonojunkmail@spokesunlimited.org
http://www.spokesunlimited.org/hub.html

Disability Served: various

This publication provides information on various disabilities, rehabilitation, peer counseling, and more.

I Can Sign My ABC's

Gallaudet University Press
800 Florida Avenue, NE
Washington, DC 20002
202-651-5488 (Voice/TTY)
valencia.simmons@gallaudet.edu

http://gupress.gallaudet.edu

Disability Served: hearing

This picture book is designed to teach the letters of the alphabet in American Sign Language.

If You Think Your Child Is Stuttering

Stuttering Foundation of America
3100 Walnut Grove Road, Suite 603, PO Box 11749
Memphis, TN 38111-0749
901-452-7342, 800-992-9392
info@stutteringhelp.org
http://www.stutteringhelp.org/Default.aspx?tabid=131

Disability Served: communication

This free, downloadable brochure explains the difference between normal speech development and stuttering in the young child and gives nine tips on how to help the child with stuttering problems.

I'm an Adult with Spina Bifida. What's Out There to Help Me?

Spina Bifida Association of America
4590 MacArthur Boulevard, NW, Suite 250
Washington, DC 20007-4226
202-944-3285, 800-621-3141
sbaa@sbaa.org
http://www.sbaa.org/site/PageServer?pagename=
asb_facts

Disability Served: spina bifida

This resource illustrates the challenges that are unique to adults with spina bifida. Subject areas include employment, government assistance, clinics that treat adults, support groups, accessible housing, and sexuality.

Immune Deficiency Foundation Advocate

Immune Deficiency Foundation
40 West Chesapeake Avenue, Suite 308
Towson, MD 21204
800-296-4433
idf@primaryimmune.org
http://www.primaryimmune.org/pubs/newsletter/
newsletter.htm

Disability Served: immune deficiency disorders

This quarterly newsletter provides news and information on immune deficiencies.

Immune Deficiency Foundation Patient and Family Handbook For The Primary Immune Deficiency Diseases

Immune Deficiency Foundation
40 West Chesapeake Avenue, Suite 308

Towson, MD 21204
800-296-4433
idf@primaryimmune.org
http://www.primaryimmune.org/pubs/pubs.htm
Disability Served: immune deficiency disorders
This handbook provides up-to-date information on
10 specific primary immune deficiency diseases,
inheritance, general care, specific medical therapy,
health insurance, and lifestyle issues affecting
children, teens, and adults.

In Control: A Guide for Teens with Diabetes
Juvenile Diabetes Foundation
120 Wall Street
New York, NY 10005-4001
800-533-2873
info@jdrf.org
http://www.jdrf.org/index.cfm?page_id=100250
Disability Served: diabetes
This guide helps teenagers learn to take care of their
diabetes without letting it get in the way of their
lives, by dispelling myths and tackling the issues
teens with diabetes face.

Infinite Difference: An Interactive Online Literary Journal
VSA arts
818 Connecticut Avenue, NW, Suite 600
Washington, DC 20006
800-933-8721, 202-737-0645 (TDD)
info@vsarts.org
http://www.vsarts.org/x621.xml
Disability Served: various
This online literary journal showcases creative writing by
students ages 11-18, with a connection to disability.
It also offers educators an interactive tool to tackle
national writing standards and promote literacy in
the classroom.

Information, Tips, and Strategies for Individuals Interested in Pursuing a College Education
Institute on Disability
University of New Hampshire
10 Ferry Street, Unit 14
Concord, NH 03301
http://iod.unh.edu/publications/pdf/tips-
PostSecondaryEd.pdf
Disability Served: various
This free, downloadable resource provides information
for individuals with disabilities who are interested in
pursing a college education.

Information Processing Disorders
National Center for Learning Disabilities
381 Park Avenue South, Suite 1401
New York, NY 10016
212-545-7510
http://www.ld.org/LDInfoZone/InfoZone_
FactSheetIndex.cfm
Disability Served: learning disabled
This free fact sheet offers a basic introduction to the
general category of information processing disorders,
including the different types of auditory and visual
processing disorders.

Information Services for People with Developmental Disabilities
Greenwood Publishing Group Inc.
88 Post Road West
Westport, CT 06881
203-226-3571
http://www.greenwood.com
Disability Served: developmentally disabled
This book provides information for librarians so they can
better serve clients with developmental disabilities.

Information Technology and Disabilities
Equal Access to Software and Information
PO Box 818
Lake Forest, CA 92609
949-916-2837
http://www.rit.edu/%7Eeasi/itd.htm
Disability Served: various
This e-zine provides information on information
technology as it relates to people with disabilities.

Informed Decisions
American Cancer Society
1599 Clifton Road, PO Box 49528
Atlanta, GA 30359-0528
800-ACS-2346
http://www.cancer.org/docroot/PUB/PUB_
1.asp?sitearea=PUB
Disability Served: cancer patients and survivors
This book offers the latest information on every aspect
of cancer, from detection to recovery.

Inheritance of Hemophilia
National Hemophilia Foundation
116 West 32nd Street, 11th Floor
New York, NY 10001
212-328-3700, 800-42-HANDI
handi@hemophilia.org

http://www.hemophilia.org/resources/handi_pubs.htm

Disability Served: *inherited bleeding disorders*

This free booklet provides an explanation of the genetic transmission of hemophilia. It also describes tests used to find out if the hemophilia gene is present, particularly in women who may carry the gene but who show no signs of excessive bleeding.

Injured Mind, Shattered Dreams: Brian's Survival from a Severe Head Injury to a New Dream

Brookline Books
34 University Road
Brookline, MA 02445
617-734-6772
http://www.brooklinebooks.com

Disability Served: *traumatic brain injury*

This book tells the story of a young man who suffers a severe head injury and how he and his family dealt with the injury and his recovery.

In Motion

Amputee Coalition of America
900 East Hill Avenue, Suite 285
Knoxville, TN 37915-2568
888-267-5669, 865-525-4512 (TTY)
http://www.amputee-coalition.org

Disability Served: *amputees*

This is a bimonthly magazine for amputees, caregivers, and healthcare professionals.

Inside MS

National Multiple Sclerosis Society
733 Third Avenue
New York, NY 10017
800-344-4867
http://www.nationalmssociety.org/Newly%20
   Diagnosed.asp

Disability Served: *multiple sclerosis*

This lifestyle magazine for people with multiple sclerosis, their families, and healthcare professionals is packed with news and features on symptom management, daily living, research, financial and employment issues, travel, achievements, and book and video reviews.

inSight

Association for Retarded Citizens of the United States
1010 Wayne Avenue, Suite 650
Silver Spring, MD 20910
301-565-3842
Info@thearc.org
http://www.thearc.org/info-mr.html

Disability Served: *developmentally disabled, mental retardation*

This newspaper for people with cognitive, intellectual, and development disabilities and their families is available as a free download from the organization's Web site.

Instructional Methods for Secondary Students with Learning and Behavior Problems

Allyn & Bacon
75 Arlington Street, Suite 300
Boston, MA 02116
800-852-8024
http://www.ablongman.com

Disability Served: *learning disabled*

This guide provides teaching methods for use with learning disabled students.

Integrating Transition Planning Into the IEP Process

Council for Exceptional Children
1110 North Glebe Road, Suite 300
Arlington, VA 22201-5704
888-CEC-SPED, 866-915-5000 (TTY)
service@cec.sped.org
http://www.cec.sped.org

Disability Served: *various*

This book is designed to help students with disabilities make a successful transition from student life to adulthood.

International Association of Laryngectomees News

International Association of Laryngectomees
Box 691060
Stockton, CA 95269-1060
866-425-3678
ialhq@larynxlink.com
http://www.larynxlink.com/Main/ial.htm

Disability Served: *communication*

This publication provides information for people who have had laryngectomies.

International Rehabilitation Review

Rehabilitation International
25 East 21st Street
New York, NY 10010
RI@riglobal.org
http://www.rehab-international.org/publications/
   index.html

Disability Served: *various*

This publication provides news and information on vocational and medical rehabilitation.

Intervention in School and Clinic
Pro-Ed Inc.
8700 Shoal Creek Boulevard
Austin, TX 78757-6897
800-897-3202
http://www.proedinc.com
Disability Served: various
This journal is published five times a year and discusses topics related to special education.

Intimacy and Sexuality with Multiple Sclerosis
Multiple Sclerosis Foundation Inc.
6350 North Andrews Avenue
Fort Lauderdale, FL 33309-2130
954-776-6805, 888-MSFOCUS
support@msfocus.org
http://www.msfacts.org/publications/pub_booklets.html
Disability Served: multiple sclerosis
This free booklet offers a thorough and candid approach to the sexual concerns of individuals with multiple sclerosis.

Introduction to Communicative Disorders
Pro-Ed Inc.
8700 Shoal Creek Boulevard
Austin, TX 78757-6897
800-897-3202
http://www.proedinc.com
Disability Served: communication
This is an introductory text for undergraduate students who are contemplating careers in communication disorders.

Introduction to Depression and Bipolar Disorder
Depressive and Bipolar Support Alliance
730 North Franklin Street, Suite 501
Chicago, IL 60610-7224
800-826-3632
bookstore@dbsalliance.org
http://www.dbsalliance.org/store
Disability Served: mental health
This free brochure is a quick and easy-to-read brochure describing symptoms and treatments for mood disorders.

An Introduction to Spinal Cord Injury
Paralyzed Veterans of America
801 Eighteenth Street, NW
Washington, DC 20006-3517
301-932-7834, 888-860-7244

info@pva.org
http://www.pva.org/cgi-bin/pvastore/products.cgi?id=2
Disability Served: spinal-cord injury
This pamphlet provides some basic information about spinal cord injury and some of the resources available to help you plan your recovery.

It's Time to Learn about Diabetes
Juvenile Diabetes Foundation
120 Wall Street
New York, NY 10005-4001
800-533-2873
info@jdrf.org
http://www.jdrf.org/index.cfm?page_id=100250
Disability Served: diabetes
This workbook helps school age kids learn everything they need to know about diabetes, and dispels much of the fear associated with insulin shots and blood tests.

JADARA: The Journal for Professionals Networking for Excellence in Service Delivery with Individuals who are Deaf and Hard of Hearing
American Deafness and Rehabilitation Association
PO Box 480
Myersville, MD 21773
http://www.adara.org/pages/publications.shtml
Disability Served: hearing
This quarterly journal focuses on research studies and news articles regarding deafness and rehabilitation.

JAMA: The Journal of the American Medical Association
American Medical Association
PO Box 10946
Chicago, IL 60610-0946
312-670-7827, 800-262-2350
ama-subs@ama-assn.org
http://pubs.ama-assn.org
Disability Served: various
This professional journal reports on medical research and clinical medicine.

Joslin's Diabetes Deskbook: A Guide for Healthcare Providers
Joslin Diabetes Center
One Joslin Place
Boston, MA 02215
617-732-2400
https://store.joslin.org
Disability Served: diabetes

This guide provides a comprehensive overview of diabetes.

Journal for Vocational Special Needs Education

National Association of Vocational Education Special Needs Personnel
5405 Boucher Drive
Orient, OH 43146
http://www.specialpopulations.org/journ.htm
Disability Served: various
This journal reports on vocational education for persons with disabilities.

Journal of Addictions and Offender Counseling

American Counseling Association
5999 Stevenson Avenue
Alexandria, VA 22304
800-347-6647, 703-823-6862 (TDD)
http://www.counseling.org/Content/NavigationMenu/
PUBLICATIONS/JOURNALS/JOURNALS.htm
Disability Served: chemical dependency,
This publication is geared toward substance abuse counselors.

Journal of Adolescent Health Care

Society for Adolescent Medicine
1916 Copper Oaks Circle
Blue Springs, MO 64015
816-224-8010
sam@adolescenthealth.org
http://www.adolescenthealth.org
Disability Served: various
This journal provides articles on adolescent medicine.

Journal of Autism and Developmental Disabilities

Springer
233 Spring Street
New York, NY 10013
800-SPRINGER
service-ny@springer-sbm.com
http://www.springerlink.com
Disability Served: autism, developmentally disabled
This bimonthly journal focuses on childhood psychopathologies.

Journal of Chronic Fatigue Syndrome

The Haworth Press
10 Alice Street
Binghamton, NY 13904
607-722-5857, 800-342-9678
http://www.haworthpressinc.com/journals/default.asp
Disability Served: physically disabled
This quarterly journal provides medical articles regarding chronic fatigue syndrome.

Journal of Clinical Psychology

Wiley Periodicals Inc.
111 River Street
Hoboken, NJ 07030
800-825-7550
http://www3.interscience.wiley.com/cgi-bin/
jhome/31171
Disability Served: mental health
This professional journal provides articles on clinical psychology.

Journal of Cognitive Rehabilitation

NeuroScience Publishers
6555 Carrollton Avenue
Indianapolis, IN 46220
317-257-9672
info@JofCR.net
http://www.jofcr.com/enter.php
Disability Served: traumatic brain injury
This publication for therapists, families, and patients is designed to provide information relevant to the diagnosis and rehabilitation of cognitive impairment due to neurological causes.

Journal of Communication Disorders

Elsevier Inc.
655 Avenue of the Americas
New York, NY 10010
212-989-5800
http://www.sciencedirect.com/science/
journal/00219924
Disability Served: communication
This journal provides articles on topics related to communication disorders.

Journal of Community Psychology

Wiley Periodicals Inc.
111 River Street
Hoboken, NJ 07030
800-825-7550
http://www3.interscience.wiley.com/cgi-bin/
jhome/32213
Disability Served: mental health
This publication provides scholarly articles on the study of human behavior in community settings.

Journal of Developmental and Physical Disabilities
Springer
233 Spring Street
New York, NY 10013
800-SPRINGER
service-ny@springer-sbm.com
http://www.springerlink.com
Disability Served: various
This quarterly journal reports case studies and research findings on all disabilities.

Journal of Disability Policy Studies
Pro-Ed
8700 Shoal Creek Boulevard
Austin, TX 78757-6897
800-897-3202
http://www.proedinc.com/jdps.html
Disability Served: various
This journal focuses on disability policy issues.

Journal of Emotional and Behavioral Disorders
Pro-Ed Inc.
8700 Shoal Creek Boulevard
Austin, TX 78757-6897
800-897-3202
http://www.proedinc.com
Disability Served: behavioral disorders, mental health
This quarterly journal focuses on behavioral disorders and provides updates on the latest in research, practice, and theory.

Journal of Interpretation
Registry of the Interpreters for the Deaf
333 Commerce Street
Alexandria, VA 22314
703-838-0030, 703-838-0459 (TTY)
info@rid.org
http://www.rid.org/pubs.html
Disability Served: hearing
This professional journal contains up-to-date articles and research in the field of interpreting.

Journal of Learning Disabilities
Pro-Ed Inc.
8700 Shoal Creek Boulevard
Austin, TX 78757-6897
800-897-3202
http://www.proedinc.com
Disability Served: learning disabled

This bimonthly journal provides articles on the research, practice, and theory of learning disabilities.

Journal of Mental Health Counseling
American Mental Health Counselors Association
801 North Fairfax Street, Suite 3
Alexandria, VA 22314
703-548-6002
http://www.amhca.org/journal
Disability Served: mental health
This quarterly journal provides articles on mental health issues in counseling.

Journal of Musculoskeletal Pain
The Haworth Press
10 Alice Street
Binghamton, NY 13904
607-722-5857, 800-342-9678
http://www.haworthpressinc.com/journals/default.asp
Disability Served: chronic pain
This quarterly journal provides information for the medical professional on musculoskeletal pain.

Journal of Postsecondary Education and Disability
Association on Higher Education and Disability
PO Box 540666
Waltham, MA 02454
781-788-0003
ahead@ahead.org
http://www.ahead.org/publications/index.htm
Disability Served: various
This journal explores educational policies, programs, and issues regarding the postsecondary education of students with disabilities.

Journal of Prosthetics and Orthotics
American Academy of Orthotics and Prosthetics
526 King Street, Suite 201
Alexandria, VA 22314
703-836-0788
academy@oandp.org
http://www.oandp.org/jpo
Disability Served: physically disabled
This quarterly journal provides research articles and news on orthotics and prosthetics.

Journal of Rehabilitation
National Rehabilitation Association
633 South Washington Street

Alexandria, VA 22314
703-836-0850
info@nationalrehab.org
http://www.nationalrehab.org/website/pubs/index.html
Disability Served: various
This quarterly journal is an internationally acclaimed scholarly journal on the cutting-edge of rehabilitation research.

Journal of Religion, Disability, and Health

The Haworth Press
10 Alice Street
Binghamton, NY 13904
607-722-5857, 800-342-9678
http://www.haworthpressinc.com/journals/default.asp
Disability Served: various
This quarterly journal is geared toward religious professionals serving persons with disabilities and provides information about rehabilitation techniques and trends.

Journal of Special Education

Pro-Ed Inc.
8700 Shoal Creek Boulevard
Austin, TX 78757-6897
800-897-3202
http://www.proedinc.com
Disability Served: various
This quarterly publication contains research articles on special education.

Journal of the Academy of Rehabilitation Audiology

Academy of Rehabilitative Audiology
PO Box 26532
Minneapolis, MN 55426
952-920-0484
ara@incnet.com
http://www.audrehab.org
Disability Served: hearing
This professional journal offers articles and news on the field of audiology.

Journal of Visual Impairment and Blindness

American Foundation for the Blind
11 Penn Plaza, Suite 300
New York, NY 10001
212-502-7600, 800-232-5463
afbinfo@afb.net
http://www.afb.org

Disability Served: vision
This annual journal provides articles on various subjects related to blindness, including rehabilitation, education, employment, health issues, and more.

Journal of Vocational Behavior

Elsevier Inc.
655 Avenue of the Americas
New York, NY 10010
212-989-5800
http://www.sciencedirect.com/science/journal/00018791
Disability Served: various
This professional journal provides articles on research findings, theories, and more regarding vocational behavior.

Just Diagnosed

Arthritis Foundation
PO Box 7669
Atlanta, GA 30357
800-568-4045
http://www.arthritis.org/afstore/storehome.asp
Disability Served: physically disabled
This free magazine offers information tailored to the newly diagnosed person with arthritis.

KALEIDOSCOPE Magazine

United Disability Services
701 South Main Street
Akron, OH 44311-1019
330-762-9755
http://www.udsakron.org/kaleidoscope.htm
Disability Served: various
This magazine provides feature articles, art, poetry, and fiction regarding disability.

K & W Guide to Colleges for Students with Learning Disabilities or Attention Deficit Disorder

Princeton Review
2315 Broadway
New York, NY 10024
http://www.princetonreview.com
Disability Served: attention deficit disorder, learning disabled
This book provides an overview of top colleges for students with learning disabilities or attention deficit disorder.

Kernel Books
National Federation of the Blind
1800 Johnson Street
Baltimore, MD 21230
410-659-9314
nfbstore@nfb.org
http://www.nfb.org/publications.html
Disability Served: vision
This is a series of large print, Braille, and tape booklets that include inspirational stories written by blind people about themselves.

Kid-Friendly Parenting with Deaf and Hard of Hearing Children: A Treasury of Fun Activities Toward Better Behavior
Gallaudet University Press
800 Florida Avenue, NE
Washington, DC 20002
202-651-5488 (Voice/TTY)
valencia.simmons@gallaudet.edu
http://gupress.gallaudet.edu
Disability Served: hearing
This book provides hundreds of ideas and methods for parents with deaf or hard-of-hearing children, ages three to 12.

Kindergarten Language Screening Test
Pro-Ed Inc.
8700 Shoal Creek Boulevard
Austin, TX 78757-6897
800-897-3202
http://www.proedinc.com
Disability Served: communication
This test is designed to identify students with potential language disabilities and target them for additional tests.

Kitchen Design for the Wheelchair User
Paralyzed Veterans of America
801 Eighteenth Street, NW
Washington, DC 20006-3517
301-932-7834, 888-860-7244
info@pva.org
http://www.pva.org/cgi-bin/pvastore/products.cgi?id=2
Disability Served: physically disabled
This free, downloadable brochure tells how the kitchen can be tailored to meet the needs and challenges of its users.

Know Stroke. Know the Signs. Act in Time.
National Institute of Neurological Disorders and Stroke
PO Box 5801
Bethesda, MD 20824
301-496-5751, 800-352-9424
http://www.ninds.nih.gov/disorders/stroke/stroke.htm#Publications
Disability Served: stroke
This free educational booklet defines stroke and explains the causes, signs, and symptoms. It also offers advice regarding what to do when someone is having a stroke and how to prevent stroke.

Know the Facts, Get the Stats
American Heart Association
7272 Greenville Avenue
Dallas, TX 75231
800-242-8721
http://www.americanheart.org/presenter.jhtml?identifier=3001740
Disability Served: physically disabled, stroke
This downloadable brochure provides basic information about heart attack and stroke, including risk factors and warning signs.

Large-Print Loan Library
National Association for the Visually Handicapped
22 West 21st Street, 6th Floor
New York, NY 10010
212-889-3141
navh@navh.org
http://www.navh.org/faq.html#large
Disability Served: vision
This free-by-mail library offers more than 7,000 titles in large print and is accessible to anyone in the United States.

Learning Disabilities
National Dissemination Center for Children with Disabilities
PO Box 1492
Washington, DC 20013
800-695-0285
nichcy@aed.org
http://nichcy.org/publist.asp
Disability Served: learning disabled
This free fact sheet defines the condition and provides information on its signs, symptoms, and characteristics. It also provides tips for parents, teachers, and schools; additional resources; and associated organizations.

Learning Disabilities
National Mental Health Association
2001 North Beauregard Street, 12th Floor

Alexandria, VA 22311
703-684-7722, 800-969-6642
http://www.nmha.org/infoctr/factsheets
Disability Served: learning disabled
This free fact sheet offers information regarding learning
disabilities with the following subcategories: causes,
early detection and treatment, warning signs,
prevalence, and additional resources for parents.

Learning Disabilities: A Multidisciplinary Journal
Learning Disabilities Association of America
4156 Library Road
Pittsburgh, PA15234-1349
412-341-1515
http://www.ldanatl.org/aboutld/resources/guide.asp
Disability Served: learning disabled
This comprehensive resource provides information on
a full range of learning disorders.

Learning Disabilities and the Arts
National Center for Learning Disabilities
381 Park Avenue South, Suite 1401
New York, NY 10016
212-545-7510
http://www.ld.org/LDInfoZone/InfoZone_
FactSheetIndex.cfm
Disability Served: learning disabled
This free fact sheet provides an introduction to how
the arts can be used to help children with learning
disabilities.

Learning Disabilities at a Glance
National Center for Learning Disabilities
381 Park Avenue South, Suite 1401
New York, NY 10016
212-545-7510
http://www.ld.org/LDInfoZone/InfoZone_
FactSheetIndex.cfm
Disability Served: learning disabled
This free fact sheet offers an introduction to learning
disabilities and how they affect people at different
ages.

Learning Disabilities Fast Facts
National Center for Learning Disabilities
381 Park Avenue South, Suite 1401
New York, NY 10016
212-545-7510
http://www.ld.org/LDInfoZone/InfoZone_
FactSheetIndex.cfm
Disability Served: learning disabled

This free fact sheet provides facts and statistics on
learning disabilities and the educational system.

Learning Problems and the Student with Tourette Syndrome
Tourette Syndrome Association
42-40 Bell Boulevard
Bayside, NY 11361
718-224-2999
http://tsa-usa.org/Merchant2/merchant.
mvc?Screen=CTGY&Store_Code=TOS&
Category_Code=E
Disability Served: learning disabled, Tourette Syndrome
This brochure explores the symptoms and conditions
associated with Tourette Syndrome that affect
learning. Topics covered include difficulties in
acquiring the basic skills of reading, writing, spelling,
and math, and classroom modifications pertaining
to auditory processing, fine motor, visual-motor, and
executive function deficits.

Learning Strategies for Students with Learning Disabilities
National Dissemination Center for Children with
Disabilities
PO Box 1492
Washington, DC 20013
800-695-0285
nichcy@aed.org
http://nichcy.org/publist.asp
Disability Served: learning disabled
This free resource provides educators with teaching
resources for students with learning disabilities.

Learning to Slow Down and Pay Attention: A Book for Kids about ADD
Magination Press
750 First Street, NE
Washington, DC 20002-4242
800-374-2721
magination@apa.org
http://www.maginationpress.com
Disability Served: attention deficit disorder
This book is geared toward children who have attention
deficit disorder.

Learn: Playful Techniques to Accelerate Learning
Zephyr Press
814 North Franklin
Chicago, IL 60610
800-232-2187

zephyrpress@zephyrpress.com
http://www.zephyrpress.com/index.cfm
Disability Served: learning disabled
This book contains learning strategies for students who learn differently.

Legacy of the Blue Heron: Living with Learning Disabilities

Learning Disabilities Association of America
4156 Library Road
Pittsburgh, PA15234-1349
412-341-1515
http://www.ldanatl.org/aboutld/resources/index.asp
Disability Served: learning disabled
This book chronicles Harry Sylvester's inspirational story beginning with his devastating educational experiences, his diagnosis of a learning disability, and the incredible work he has done from that pivotal moment.

Legal Rights for the Deaf and Hard of Hearing

Self Help for Hard of Hearing People Inc.
7910 Woodmont Avenue, Suite 1200
Bethesda, MD 20814
301-657-2248, 301-657-2249 (TTY)
bookstore@hearingloss.org
http://hearingloss.sidestreetshop.com/default.cfm
Disability Served: hearing
This book is a comprehensive analysis of recent laws passed to protect the rights of and guarantee equal access for people with hearing loss. The book explains in layman's terminology how legislation affects individuals with disabilities in everyday life.

Legal Rights of Persons with Disabilities: An Analysis of Federal Law

LRP Publications
747 Dresher Road, Suite 500, PO Box 980
Horsham, PA 19044
800-341-7874, 215-658-0938 (TTY)
http://www.shoplrp.com/disability/cat-Books_Pamphlets.html
Disability Served: various
This text provides background information regarding the legal rights of persons with disabilities and is appropriate for those with disabilities and professionals working with them.

Legislative Network for Nurses

Business Publishers Inc.
8737 Colesville Road, 10th Floor

Silver Spring, MD 20910-3928
301-589-5103, 800-274-6737
custserv@bpinews.com
http://www.bpinews.com
Disability Served: various
This biweekly publication provides news pertinent to nurses.

Lesson Plans for Deaf Children

National Catholic Office for the Deaf
7202 Buchanan Street
Landover Hills, MD 20784-2236
301-577-1684, 301-577-4184 (TTY)
ncod@erols.com
http://www.ncod.org/pages/book1.html
Disability Served: hearing
These Christian-based lesson plans for deaf children include titles such as "All About Me, My Family and Jesus," "Preparation for Holy Communion," "Preparation for the Sacrament of Reconciliation," and "In the Beginning-Activity Book."

Let's Talk about Depression

Federal Citizen Information Center
1800 F Street, NW
Washington, DC 20405
888-878-3256
firstgov1@mail.fedinfo.gov
http://www.pueblo.gsa.gov/results.tpl?id1=16&startat=1&--woSECTIONS
datarq=16&--SECTIONSword=ww
Disability Served: mental health
This free brochure helps teenagers learn the symptoms of depression and where to get help.

Let's Talk Facts about Anxiety Disorders

American Psychiatric Association
1000 Wilson Boulevard, Suite 1825
Arlington, VA 22209
703-907-7300, 888-35-PSYCH
apa@psych.org
http://www.healthyminds.org/letstalkfacts.cfm
Disability Served: mental health
This free, downloadable brochure explains that anxiety disorders are the most common of emotional disorders and affect more than 25 million Americans. It provides information on two popular types of treatment: psychotherapy and medication.

Let's Talk Facts about Bipolar Disorder (Manic Depression)
American Psychiatric Association
1000 Wilson Boulevard, Suite 1825
Arlington, VA 22209
703-907-7300, 888-35-PSYCH
apa@psych.org
http://www.healthyminds.org/letstalkfacts.cfm
Disability Served: mental health
This free, downloadable brochure defines bipolar disorder and details treatment options.

Let's Talk Facts about Choosing a Psychiatrist
American Psychiatric Association
1000 Wilson Boulevard, Suite 1825
Arlington, VA 22209
703-907-7300, 888-35-PSYCH
apa@psych.org
http://www.healthyminds.org/letstalkfacts.cfm
Disability Served: mental health
This free, downloadable brochure discusses the profession of psychiatry and offers advice on how to choose a psychiatrist.

Let's Talk Facts about Depression
American Psychiatric Association
1000 Wilson Boulevard, Suite 1825
Arlington, VA 22209
703-907-7300, 888-35-PSYCH
apa@psych.org
http://www.healthyminds.org/letstalkfacts.cfm
Disability Served: mental health
This free, downloadable brochure defines depression and discusses its causes, symptoms, and treatments.

Let's Talk Facts about What Is Mental Illness?
American Psychiatric Association
1000 Wilson Boulevard, Suite 1825
Arlington, VA 22209
703-907-7300, 888-35-PSYCH
apa@psych.org
http://www.healthyminds.org/letstalkfacts.cfm
Disability Served: mental health
This free, downloadable brochure promotes factual discussion on mental illness and its treatments. It provides answers to commonly asked questions on mental health issues and disorders.

Letter to Medical Professional
Charcot-Marie-Tooth Association
2700 Chestnut Street

Chester, PA 19013-4867
800-606-2682
info@charcot-marie-tooth.org
https://secure.charcot-marie-tooth.org/publications.php
Disability Served: Charcot-Marie-Tooth Disease
This free form letter informs doctors and other medical professionals that a person has been diagnosed with Charcot-Marie-Tooth Disease and that certain drugs may worsen his or her symptoms.

Life Beyond the Classroom: Transition Strategies for Young People With Disabilities
Paul H. Brookes Publishing Company
PO Box 10624
Baltimore, MD 21285-0624
410-337-9580, 800-638-3775
custserv@brookespublishing.com
http://www.pbrookes.com
Disability Served: various
This textbook discusses how to plan, design, and implement transition programs for students with disabilities.

Lifelines
Disabled and Alone
61 Broadway, Suite 510
New York, NY 10006
212-532-6740, 800-995-0066
info@disabledandalone.org
http://www.disabledandalone.org/lifelines.html
Disability Served: various
This is a publication of Disabled and Alone/Life Services for the Handicapped Inc., a national not-for-profit organization whose purpose is to assure the well being of disabled individuals, particularly those whose families wish to plan for the time when they will no longer be able to provide care.

Life Without Limits
United Cerebral Palsy
1660 L Street, NW, Suite 700
Washington, DC 20036
202-776-0406, 800-872-5827
http://www.ucp.org/ucp_general.cfm/1/12591
Disability Served: cerebral palsy
This is the monthly newsletter of United Cerebral Palsy.

Listen Learn and Talk-Cochlear Limited
Alexander Graham Bell Association of the Deaf
3417 Volta Place, NW
Washington, DC 20007

866-337-5220, 202-337-5221 (TTY)
publications@agbell.org
http://www.agbell.org
Disability Served: communication, hearing
This three-volume videotape and guidebook set
provides guiding theory, support materials, and
age-appropriate strategies.

Literacy Resource Guide for Families and Educators
Federation for Children with Special Needs
1135 Tremont Street, Suite 420
Boston, MA 02120
617-236-7210, 800-331-0688
fcsninfo@fcsn.org
http://www.fcsn.org/publications_resources/
publications.html
Disability Served: various
This book for parents, educators, and caregivers
highlights current research-based literacy resources
available through the U.S. Department of Education
and its funded projects.

Living an Idea: Empowerment and the Evolution of an Alternative School
Brookline Books
34 University Road
Brookline, MA 02445
617-734-6772
http://www.brooklinebooks.com
Disability Served: various
This book details the history and creation of an
alternative, inner-city high school and the reasons
behind its success.

Living in the State of Stuck
Brookline Books
34 University Road
Brookline, MA 02445
617-734-6772
http://www.brooklinebooks.com
Disability Served: physically disabled
This book takes a look at adaptive technologies and
how they can affect the lives of the disabled.

Living with Alzheimer's Disease
American Occupational Therapy Association Inc.
4720 Montgomery Lane, PO Box 31220
Bethesda, MD 20824-1220
301-652-2682, 800-377-8555
http://www.aota.org/featured/area6/links/link02.asp

Disability Served: dementia
This free tip sheet offers information on Alzheimer's
Disease and provides an overview of how
occupational therapists can help patients and
their families cope with the illness.

Living with Ataxia
National Ataxia Foundation
2600 Fernbrook Lane, Suite 119
Minneapolis, MN 55447
naf@ataxia.org
http://www.ataxia.org
Disability Served: physically disabled
This book offers a compassionate, easy to understand
explanation of ataxia and ideas on how to live with
the disease.

Living with Congestive Heart Failure
American Heart Association
7272 Greenville Avenue
Dallas, TX 75231
800-242-8721
http://www.americanheart.org/presenter.
jhtml?identifier=3001740
Disability Served: physically disabled
This free brochure describes the causes, signs, and
treatments of congestive heart failure and offers
recommendations for exercise and healthy eating
for those who have been diagnosed.

Living with Heart Problems
American Occupational Therapy Association Inc.
4720 Montgomery Lane, PO Box 31220
Bethesda, MD 20824-1220
301-652-2682, 800-377-8555
http://www.aota.org/featured/area6/links/link02.asp
Disability Served: physically disabled
This free tip sheet offers information for patients
with heart problems and details the services of
occupational therapists as they relate to the illness.

Living with Juvenile Diabetes: A Practical Guide for Parents and Caregivers
Juvenile Diabetes Foundation
120 Wall Street
New York, NY 10005-4001
800-533-2873
info@jdrf.org
http://www.jdrf.org/index.cfm?page_id=100250
Disability Served: diabetes

This book for parents and caregivers presents the latest scientific information and provides answers and coping strategies for families who are struggling with Type 1 juvenile diabetes.

Living with Lowe Syndrome: A Guide for Families, Friends, and Professionals

Lowe Syndrome Association
18919 Voss Road
Dallas, TX 75287
612-869-5693
info@lowesyndrome.org
http://www.lowesyndrome.org/Lowe%20Syndrome/Publications/index.html
Disability Served: Lowe Syndrome
This booklet provides medical and developmental information about Lowe Syndrome, including genetics, research, and effect on the family. The first copy is offered free of charge.

Living with Low Vision: A Resource Guide for People with Sight Loss

Resources for Rehabilitation
22 Bonad Road
Winchester, MA 01890
781-368-9094
info@rfr.org
http://www.rfr.org
Disability Served: vision
This valuable self-help guide provides people with sight loss due to macular degeneration, glaucoma, diabetic retinopathy, retinitis pigmentosa, and other conditions with the information they need to keep reading, working, and enjoying life.

Living with Parkinson's Disease

American Occupational Therapy Association Inc.
4720 Montgomery Lane, PO Box 31220
Bethesda, MD 20824-1220
301-652-2682, 800-377-8555
http://www.aota.org/featured/area6/links/link02.asp
Disability Served: Parkinson's Disease
This free tip sheet offers information to help people with Parkinson's Disease cope, as well as an overview of how occupational therapists can help treat patients with this illness.

Living with Rheumatoid Arthritis

Arthritis Foundation
PO Box 7669

Atlanta, GA 30357
800-568-4045
http://www.arthritis.org/AFstore/SubCatHome.asp?idCat=8&idSubCat=150
Disability Served: physically disabled
This free brochure provides an overview of rheumatoid arthritis and tips for living with the disease.

Living with Spinal Cord Injury

American Occupational Therapy Association Inc.
4720 Montgomery Lane, PO Box 31220
Bethesda, MD 20824-1220
301-652-2682, 800-377-8555
http://www.aota.org/featured/area6/links/link02.asp
Disability Served: spinal-cord injury
This free tip sheet offers information to help people with spinal cord injuries cope, as well as an overview of how occupational therapists can help treat patients with this illness.

Long-Term Disability Income Insurance

Federal Citizen Information Center
1800 F Street, NW
Washington, DC 20405
888-878-3256
firstgov1@mail.fedinfo.gov
http://www.pueblo.gsa.gov/results.tpl?id1=13&startat=1&--woSECTIONS datarq=13&--SECTIONSword=ww
Disability Served: various
This free guide outlines the features and costs of individual disability income insurance and offers tips and a checklist on purchasing the right policy.

Low Back Pain Fact Sheet

National Institute of Neurological Disorders and Stroke
PO Box 5801
Bethesda, MD 20824
301-496-5751, 800-352-9424
http://www.ninds.nih.gov/disorders/chronic_pain/chronic_pain.htm#Publications
Disability Served: back pain, chronic pain
This free fact sheet provides information on the diagnosis, treatment, and prevention of back pain.

Lung Cancer

Federal Citizen Information Center
1800 F Street, NW
Washington, DC 20405
888-878-3256

firstgov1@mail.fedinfo.gov
http://www.pueblo.gsa.gov/results.tpl?id1=16&startat=1
&--woSECTIONSdatarq=16&--SECTIONSword=ww
Disability Served: cancer patients and survivors
This free brochure describes how lung cancer is
diagnosed, the types and stages of lung cancer,
warning signs, and more.

Lung Cancer Fact Sheet
American Lung Association
61 Broadway
New York, NY 10006
212-315-8700, 800-LUNG
http://www.lungusa.org/site/apps/s/content.asp?c=dvL
UK9O0E&b=34706&ct=910873
Disability Served: cancer patients and survivors
This free Web resource provides facts and statistics
on lung cancer.

Lupus
Federal Citizen Information Center
1800 F Street, NW
Washington, DC 20405
888-878-3256
firstgov1@mail.fedinfo.gov
http://www.pueblo.gsa.gov/results.
tpl?id1=16&startat=1&--woSECTIONSdatarq=16&--
SECTIONSword=ww
Disability Served: immune deficiency disorders
This free brochure describes the disease of lupus,
including warning signs and available treatments.

Maintaining Good Nutrition with ALS
Amytrophic Lateral Sclerosis Association
27001 Agoura Road, Suite 150
Calabasas Hills, CA 91301-5104
818-880-9007
info@alsa-national.org
http://www.alsa.org/resources/brochures.cfm?CFID=
1048742&CFTOKEN=97497558
Disability Served: physically disabled
This free, downloadable brochure helps people with
Amyotrophic Lateral Sclerosis overcome the obstacles
to eating well. It discusses the importance of nutrition
and offers suggestions for dealing with various eating
problems.

Maintaining Quality of Life with Low Vision
American Occupational Therapy Association Inc.
4720 Montgomery Lane, PO Box 31220

Bethesda, MD 20824-1220
301-652-2682, 800-377-8555
http://www.aota.org/featured/area6/links/link02.asp
Disability Served: vision
This free tip sheet offers information for patients on
maintaining their quality of life with low vision, as
well as an overview of how occupational therapists
can help treat patients with this condition.

Making a Place for Kids with Disabilities
Greenwood Publishing Group Inc.
88 Post Road West
Westport, CT 06881
203-226-3571
http://www.greenwood.com
Disability Served: various
This book describes the author's quest to learn as much
as possible about one community's experience with
the inclusion of children with special needs in youth
programs such as Girl Scouts, Boy Scouts, and park
and recreation programs.

Making Connections
Ablenet
2808 Fairview Avenue
Roseville, MN 55113-1308
800-322-0956
customerservice@ablenetinc.com
http://www.ablenetinc.com
Disability Served: communication
This is an idea book for assistive technology trainers,
speech language pathologists, and educators.
Topics include strategies for introducing voice
output communication to students of all abilities,
ideas for effective messages, and more.

Making Plans: A Financial Guide for People with Down Syndrome and Their Families
National Down Syndrome Society
666 Broadway
New York, NY 10012
800-221-4602
info@ndss.org
http://www.ndss.org/content.cfm?fuseaction=InfoRes.
SrchResMat
Disability Served: Down Syndrome
This free booklet helps families move toward
independence by making plans for the future,
managing money so that plans can become a
reality, and learning how to use the resources and

laws that enable people with disabilities to lead fulfilling lives.

Making Self-Employment Work for People with Disabilities
Paul H. Brookes Publishing Company Inc.
PO Box 10624
Baltimore, MD 21285-0624
800-638-3775
custserv@brookespublishing.com
http://www.pbrookes.com
Disability Served: various
Provides a comprehensive overview of self-employment options for people with disabilities. Includes a discussion of business plans, marketing tactics, financing, and other topics.

Making the 'No Child Left Behind Act' Work for Children Who Struggle to Learn: A Parent's Guide
National Center for Learning Disabilities
381 Park Avenue South, Suite 1401
New York, NY 10016
212-545-7510
http://www.ld.org/LDInfoZone/InfoZone_
    FactSheetIndex.cfm
Disability Served: learning disabled
This free fact sheet is provided by the National Center for Learning Disabilities and Schwab Learning.

Making Wise Medical Decisions: How to Get the Information You Need
Resources for Rehabilitation
22 Bonad Road
Winchester, MA 01890
781-368-9094
info@rfr.org
http://www.rfr.org
Disability Served: various
This book includes a wealth of information about where to go and what to read in order to make informed, rational, medical decisions. The book describes a plan for obtaining relevant health information and evaluating medical tests and procedures, health care providers, and health facilities.

Mammography Today
Federal Citizen Information Center
1800 F Street, NW
Washington, DC 20405
888-878-3256
firstgov1@mail.fedinfo.gov
http://www.pueblo.gsa.gov/results.
    tpl?id1=16&startat=1&--woSECTIONS
    datarq=16&--SECTIONSword=ww
Disability Served: cancer patients and survivors
This free brochure describes how to tell if you are getting a high-quality mammogram, what to do if you need to change mammogram facilities, and more.

Managing Chronic Pain
American Occupational Therapy Association Inc.
4720 Montgomery Lane, PO Box 31220
Bethesda, MD 20824-1220
301-652-2682, 800-377-8555
http://www.aota.org/featured/area6/links/link02.asp
Disability Served: chronic pain
This free tip sheet offers information to how to help people manage their chronic pain and cope with specific situations. It also provides an overview of how occupational therapists can help.

Managing Chronic Pain
Federal Citizen Information Center
1800 F Street, NW
Washington, DC 20405
888-878-3256
firstgov1@mail.fedinfo.gov
http://www.pueblo.gsa.gov/results.
    tpl?id1=16&startat=1&--woSECTIONS
    datarq=16&--SECTIONSword=ww
Disability Served: various
This free brochure describes how to cope with chronic pain, including back pain, headaches, arthritis, cancer pain, and neuropathic pain.

Managing Gestational Diabetes: A Patient's Guide to a Healthy Pregnancy
National Institute of Child Health and Human Development
PO Box 2006
Rockville, MD 20847
800-370-2943
NICHDInformationResourceCenter@mail.nih.gov
http://www.nichd.nih.gov/publications/pubs.cfm
Disability Served: diabetes
This free booklet for pregnant women who have been diagnosed with gestational diabetes explains the symptoms, outcomes, and treatments of the condition.

Managing Incontinence: A Guide to Living with Loss of Bladder Control
Simon Foundation for Continence
PO Box 815
Wilmette, IL 60091
800-237-4666
cbgartley@simonfoundation.org
http://www.simonfoundation.org/AboutIncontinence/
educational_materials.htm
Disability Served: physically disabled
This is a book of hope and counsel for those who suffer
urinary incontinence.

Managing Your Pain
Arthritis Foundation
PO Box 7669
Atlanta, GA 30357
800-568-4045
http://www.arthritis.org/AFstore/SubCatHome.
asp?idCat=8&idSubCat=130
Disability Served: chronic pain
This free brochure tells patients how to manage pain
with medication, exercise, relaxation and other
treatments.

Managing Your Stress
Arthritis Foundation
PO Box 7669
Atlanta, GA 30357
800-568-4045
http://www.arthritis.org/AFstore/SubCatHome.
asp?idCat=8&idSubCat=11
Disability Served: physically disabled
This free brochure defines stress, including how the body
reacts to physical and emotional changes. It offers
skills to reduce the effects on the body and tips for
managing stress.

A Man's Guide to Coping with Disability
Resources for Rehabilitation
22 Bonad Road
Winchester, MA 01890
781-368-9094
info@rfr.org
http://www.rfr.org
Disability Served: various
This book includes information about men's responses to
disability, with a special emphasis on the values men
place on independence, occupational achievement,
and physical activity. Information on finding local

services, self-help groups, laws that affect men with
disabilities, sports and recreation, and employment is
also included.

Many Ways to Learn: Young People's Guide to Learning Disabilities
Magination Press
750 First Street, NE
Washington, DC 20002-4242
800-374-2721
magination@apa.org
http://www.maginationpress.com
Disability Served: learning disabled
This book educates children about learning disabilities
and provides encouragement to help them overcome
challenges associated with these disabilities.

Matilda Ziegler Magazine for the Blind
80 Eighth Avenue, Room 1304
New York, NY 10011
212-242-0263
http://www.zieglermag.org
Disability Served: vision
This monthly magazine reprints articles from
newspapers and periodicals on a variety of topics,
including travel, nature, history, music, health, and
science. The magazine is available in Grade 2 Braille
and on cassette tape.

Mayo Clinic on Managing Incontinence
Simon Foundation for Continence
PO Box 815
Wilmette, IL 60091
800-237-4666
cbgartley@simonfoundation.org
http://www.simonfoundation.org/AboutIncontinence/
educational_materials.htm
Disability Served: physically disabled
This book explains the causes of incontinence and
provides information on medications and devices,
behavior, and surgery for the treatment of both
urinary and fecal incontinence.

Me and My World Storybook
Epilepsy Foundation
4351 Garden City Drive
Landover, MD 20785-7223
800-332-1000
http://www.epilepsyfoundation.org
Disability Served: epilepsy

This storybook helps parents discuss epilepsy with their children, ages four to eight, and their friends. Other children's reactions to seizures are explored together with effects on family members.

Medicare Health Plan Choices: Consumer Update
National Council on the Aging
300 D Street, SW, Suite 801
Washington, DC 20024
202-479-1200
info@ncoa.org
http://www.ncoa.org/content.cfm?sectionID=30
Disability Served: various
This pamphlet, updated annually, contains important information about options that are available to Medicare beneficiaries.

Medicines for Epilepsy
Epilepsy Foundation
4351 Garden City Drive
Landover, MD 20785-7223
800-332-1000
http://www.epilepsyfoundation.org
Disability Served: epilepsy
This pamphlet describes medication types, why people react differently to medication, and how the patient can help the physician find the right medicine.

Meeting the Needs of Employees with Disabilities
Resources for Rehabilitation
22 Bonad Road
Winchester, MA 01890
781-368-9094
info@rfr.org
http://www.rfr.org
Disability Served: various
This book provides background information for persons with disabilities in the workplace, including federal regulations, training programs, accessible work areas, and more.

Mental and Physical Disability Law Reporter
American Bar Association Commission on Mental and Physical Disability Law
740 15th Street, NW
Washington, DC 20005-1019
202-662-1000
cmpdl@abanet.org
http://www.abanet.org/disability/pubs1.html
Disability Served: various

This bimonthly newsletter provides information on legal issues and court cases regarding persons with mental or physical disabilities.

Mental Health Law Reporter
Business Publishers Inc.
8737 Colesville Road, 10th Floor
Silver Spring, MD 20910-3928
301-589-5103, 800-274-6737
custserv@bpinews.com
http://www.bpinews.com
Disability Served: mental health
This monthly publication discusses the latest legal issues regarding mental health.

The Mental Health Resource Guide
Resources for Rehabilitation
22 Bonad Road
Winchester, MA 01890
781-368-9094
info@rfr.org
http://www.rfr.org
Disability Served: mental health
This guidebook is designed to help individuals who are mentally ill, their families, and health professionals understand the issues surrounding mental illness, and find services and advocates that can help.

Mental Retardation
Allyn & Bacon
75 Arlington Street, Suite 300
Boston, MA 02116
800-852-8024
http://www.ablongman.com
Disability Served: mental retardation
This book provides an overview of mental retardation, including legal aspects and social issues.

Mental Retardation
National Dissemination Center for Children with Disabilities
PO Box 1492
Washington, DC 20013
800-695-0285
nichcy@aed.org
http://nichcy.org/publist.asp
Disability Served: mental retardation
This free fact sheet defines the condition and provides information on its signs, symptoms, and characteristics. It also provides tips for parents,

teachers, and schools, additional resources, and associated organizations.

Mental Retardation
Prentice Hall/Pearson Education
One Lake Street
Upper Saddle River, NJ 07458
http://www.pearsoned.com
Disability Served: mental retardation
This text provides information on mental retardation, including research findings and information for educators.

Mental Retardation: A Life-Cycle Approach
Prentice Hall/Pearson Education
One Lake Street
Upper Saddle River, NJ 07458
http://www.pearsoned.com
Disability Served: mental retardation
This text provides information on the life cycle of the mentally retarded individual and his or her needs at each stage.

Miracles
March of Dimes
1275 Mamaroneck Avenue
White Plains, NY 10605
http://www.msfacts.org/publications/pub_booklets.html
Disability Served: physically disabled
This free monthly email newsletter offers a personal spotlight story along with information related to the mission of the March of Dimes, to improve the health of babies by preventing birth defects and infant mortality.

The Misunderstood Child: Understanding and Coping with Your Child's Learning Disabilities
Learning Disabilities Association of America
4156 Library Road
Pittsburgh, PA 15234-1349
412-341-1515
http://www.ldanatl.org/aboutld/resources/index.asp
Disability Served: learning disabled
This book for parents on understanding and coping with a child's learning disabilities provides a thorough overview of how these conditions are evaluated and treated.

Modern Healthcare
Crain Communications
360 North Michigan Avenue, 5th Floor
Chicago, IL 60601-3806
888-446-1422
subs@crain.com
http://modernhealthcare.com
Disability Served: various
This weekly publication is designed for health care professionals interested in the business of medicine.

Modifying Your Home for Independence
American Occupational Therapy Association Inc.
4720 Montgomery Lane, PO Box 31220
Bethesda, MD 20824-1220
301-652-2682, 800-377-8555
http://www.aota.org/featured/area6/links/link02.asp
Disability Served: physically disabled
This free tip sheet offers information for patients and families who are modifying their homes to create the highest level of independence. It also provides an overview of what types of recommendations occupational therapists might give to improve access.

The Moisture Seekers
Sjogren's Syndrome Foundation Inc.
8120 Woodmont Avenue, Suite 530
Bethesda, MD 20814
301-718-0300
http://www.sjogrens.org/servlet/Cart.catalog?categoryId=40
Disability Served: immune deficiency disorders
This monthly newsletter reports on Sjogren's Syndrome.

MOOSE: A Very Special Person
Brookline Books
34 University Road
Brookline, MA 02445
617-734-6772
http://www.brooklinebooks.com
Disability Served: Down Syndrome
This book is a story of a boy born with Down Syndrome whose parents decide to ignore medical advice and raise him at home.

More Than 50 Ways to Prevent Diabetes
National Diabetes Information Clearinghouse
5 Information Way
Bethesda, MD 20892-3568
800-860-8747
catalog@niddk.nih.gov
http://catalog.niddk.nih.gov/AlphaList.cfm?CH=NDIC
Disability Served: diabetes
This fact sheet encourages people at risk for type 2

diabetes to take small steps to prevent the disease. Up to 25 copies free.

MSFocus
Multiple Sclerosis Foundation Inc.
6305 North Andrews Avenue
Fort Lauderdale, FL 33309-2130
954-776-6805, 888-MSFOCUS
support@msfocus.org
http://www.msfacts.org/publications/pub_subscriptions.html
Disability Served: multiple sclerosis
This free quarterly magazine is available to multiple sclerosis patients, relatives, caregivers, and healthcare professionals. It provides practical information on research, alternative healthcare, coping techniques, and quality of life issues.

MSFYi
Multiple Sclerosis Foundation Inc.
6350 North Andrews Avenue
Fort Lauderdale, FL 33309-2130
954-776-6805, 888-MSFOCUS
support@msfocus.org
http://www.msfacts.org/publications/pub_subscriptions.html
Disability Served: multiple sclerosis
This online newsletter presents the latest developments in multiple sclerosis research, alternative approaches to traditional treatment, prescription drug treatment, and tips for dealing with the daily challenges of this chronic illness.

Multidisciplinary Second Opinion Centers
R.A. Bloch Cancer Foundation Inc.
4400 Main Street
Kansas City, MO 64111
816-932-8453, 800-433-0464
http://www.blochcancer.org
Disability Served: cancer patients and survivors
This free, online publication provides a comprehensive listing and background information on institutions offering second opinions for people who have been diagnosed with cancer.

Multiple Sclerosis: A Guide for Families
Multiple Sclerosis Foundation Inc.
6350 North Andrews Avenue
Fort Lauderdale, FL 33309-2130
954-776-6805, 888-MSFOCUS
support@msfocus.org

http://www.msfacts.org/publications/pub_booklets.html
Disability Served: multiple sclerosis
This free publication addresses the feelings and emotions that accompany the diagnosis and adjustment period. It included information on talking to children, frequently asked questions, and recommended reading.

Multiple Sclerosis and Employment
National Multiple Sclerosis Society
733 Third Avenue
New York, NY 10017
800-344-4867
http://www.nationalmssociety.org/Newly%20Diagnosed.asp
Disability Served: multiple sclerosis
This resource list of programs and materials will help those with multiple sclerosis make informed career decisions. Included is information on disclosure, making employment decisions, changing careers, and knowing one's rights.

Multiple Sclerosis: Facts for Persons Recently Diagnosed
Multiple Sclerosis Society of Canada
175 Bloor Street East, Suite 700, North Tower
Toronto, ON M4W 3R8
Canada
416-922-6065, 800-268-7582
info@mssociety.ca
http://www.mssociety.ca/en/information/references.htm
Disability Served: multiple sclerosis
This brochure, free in downloadable format, is aimed at newly diagnosed persons. It provides information on multiple sclerosis including the following: definition, causes, symptoms, types, expectations, treatment, research, and services provided by the society.

Multiple Sclerosis: Helpful Information for Patients and Families
Multiple Sclerosis Foundation Inc.
6305 North Andrews Avenue
Fort Lauderdale, FL 33309-2130
954-776-6805, 888-MSFOCUS
support@msfocus.org
http://www.msfacts.org/publications/pub_booklets.html
Disability Served: multiple sclerosis
This free publication provides helpful information on multiple sclerosis, including an overview of treatment and symptom management.

Multiple Sclerosis: Hope through Research
National Institute of Neurological Disorders and Stroke
PO Box 5801
Bethesda, MD 20824
301-496-5751, 800-352-9424
http://www.ninds.nih.gov/disorders/multiple_sclerosis/
multiple_sclerosis.htm#Publications
Disability Served: multiple sclerosis
This free information sheet provides information about
the diagnosis and treatment of multiple sclerosis
(MS). It also discusses recent research findings and
the outlook for people with MS.

**Multiple Sclerosis: Its Effects on You and Those
You Love**
Multiple Sclerosis Society of Canada
175 Bloor Street East, Suite 700, North Tower
Toronto, ON M4W 3R8
Canada
416-922-6065, 800-268-7582
info@mssociety.ca
http://www.mssociety.ca/en/information/references.htm
Disability Served: multiple sclerosis
This handbook for those newly diagnosed with multiple
sclerosis answers some of the most frequently asked
questions about the disease and describes effective
coping mechanisms.

Multiple Sclerosis Quarterly Report
Consortium of MS Centers
718 Teaneck Road
Teaneck, NJ 07666
201-837-0727
info@mscare.org
http://www.mscare.org/professional.cfm?doc_id=155
Disability Served: multiple sclerosis
This quarterly report features news articles on multiple
sclerosis.

**Muscular Dystrophy Association/Amyotrophic Lateral
Sclerosis Newsmagazine**
Muscular Dystrophy Association
3300 East Sunrise Drive
Tucson, AZ 85718
800-572-1717
publications@mdausa.org
http://www.mdausa.org/publications
Disability Served: physically disabled
This magazine offers the latest information on
Amyotrophic Lateral Sclerosis.

My Mommy Has Multiple Sclerosis
Multiple Sclerosis Society of Canada
175 Bloor Street East, Suite 700, North Tower
Toronto, ON M4W 3R8
Canada
416-922-6065, 800-268-7582
info@mssociety.ca
http://www.mssociety.ca/en/information/references.htm
Disability Served: multiple sclerosis
This free booklet for preschool children describes
multiple sclerosis and its effects in an easy to
understand manner.

Myths and Facts about Depression and Bipolar Disorder
Depressive and Bipolar Support Alliance
730 North Franklin Street, Suite 501
Chicago, IL 60610-7224
800-826-3632
bookstore@dbsalliance.org
http://www.dbsalliance.org/store
Disability Served: mental health
This free brochure outlines some common myths about
depression and bipolar disorder and the truths that
combat them.

**National Association for Down Syndrome:
Down Syndrome Facts**
National Association for Down Syndrome
PO Box 206
Wilmette, IL 60091
630-325-9112
http://www.nads.org/pages/facts.htm
Disability Served: Down Syndrome
This free, downloadable brochure for new parents,
students, or family members offers the basic facts
about Down Syndrome, its origins, and its affects on
those who have it.

National Cancer Institute Cancer Facts
Cancer Information Service
PO Box 24128
Baltimore, MD 21227
800-422-6237
http://cis.nci.nih.gov/fact/index.htm
Disability Served: cancer patients and survivors
These free fact sheets offer statistics and information on
specific forms of cancer.

National Captioning Institute Newsletter
National Captioning Institute
1900 Gallows Road, Suite 3000

Vienna, VA 22182
703-917-7600 (Voice/TTY)
http://www.ncicap.org/newsletter.asp
Disability Served: hearing
This publication provides news and information on closed captioning and the activities of the institute.

National Council on Disability Bulletin

National Council on Disability
1331 F Street, NW, Suite 850
Washington, DC 20004
202-272-2004, 202-272-2074 (TTY)
info@ncd.gov
http://www.ncd.gov
Disability Served: various
This monthly bulletin provides information and news for people with disabilities.

National Directory of Brain Injury Rehabilitation Services

Brain Injury Association of America
8201 Greensboro Drive, Suite 611
McLean, VA 22102
703-761-0750, 800-444-6443
familyhelpline@biausa.org
http://www.biausa.org/Pages/national_directory.html
Disability Served: traumatic brain injury
This comprehensive resource contains listings of more than 600 brain-injury-related providers in the United States and Canada, including rehabilitation centers, brain injury units, attorneys, and neuropsychologists.

National Organization for Rare Disorders Resource Guide

National Organization for Rare Disorders
55 Kenosia Avenue, PO Box 1968
Danbury, CT 06813-1968
203-744-0100, 203-797-9590 (TDD)
http://www.rarediseases.org
Disability Served: various
This publication provides information on 1,348 patient organizations, foundations, and registries that help individuals and families affected by rare diseases.

New Mobility

No Limits Communications Inc.
PO Box 220
Horsham, PA19044
215-675-9133
http://www.newmobility.com

Disability Served: various
This lifestyle magazine provides news articles, photographs, and more for persons with disabilities.

Newsletter

World Association of Persons with Disabilities
5016 Alan Lane
Oklahoma City, OK 73135
405-672-4440
info@wapd.org
http://www.wapd.org/news
Disability Served: various
This free, online weekly newsletter includes letters to the editor, articles, and information for people with disabilities.

New Technologies in the Treatment of Mood Disorders

Depressive and Bipolar Support Alliance
730 North Franklin Street, Suite 501
Chicago, IL 60610-7224
800-826-3632
bookstore@dbsalliance.org
http://www.dbsalliance.org/store
Disability Served: mental health
This free brochure describes technological advancements in the treatment of mood disorders.

New Ways of Looking at Learning Disabilities

Love Publishing Company
9101 East Kenyon Avenue, Suite 2200
Denver, CO 80237
303-221-7333
lpc@lovepublishing.com
http://www.lovepublishing.com
Disability Served: learning disabled
This text uses case studies and discussions to examine new educational approaches to students with learning disabilities.

No More Victims: Families' and Friends' Manual

L'institut Roeher Institute
4700 Keele Street
North York, ON M3J 1P3
Canada
416-661-9611
http://www.roeher.ca/english/about/about.htm
Disability Served: mentally disabled
This guide discusses the sexual abuse of persons with mental handicaps and what families and friends can do about it.

Non-Degree Postsecondary Options for Individuals with Disabilities
HEATH Resource Center
George Washington University
2121 K Street, NW, Suite 220
Washington, DC 20037
202-973-0904 (Voice/TTY), 800-544-3284
askheath@gwu.edu
http://www.heath.gwu.edu/FactSheets.htm
Disability Served: various
A free, online resource that covers non-degree postsecondary options for high school graduates who have disabilities.

Not Deaf Enough: Raising a Child Who Is Hard of Hearing With Hugs Humor and Imagination
Alexander Graham Bell Association of the Deaf
3417 Volta Place, NW
Washington, DC 20007
866-337-5220, 202-337-5221 (TTY)
publications@agbell.org
http://www.agbell.org
Disability Served: hearing
This profiles a family as they raise a child who has a mild-to-moderate hearing loss.

Numbering in American Sign Language
Registry of the Interpreters for the Deaf
333 Commerce Street
Alexandria, VA 22314
703-838-0030, 703-838-0459 (TTY)
info@rid.org
http://www.rid.org/pubs.html
Disability Served: hearing
This book, for beginning to intermediate American Sign Language students, incorporates lessons on a wide range of numbering topics, including both citation forms and common variations. Each topic is accompanied by a diverse assortment of practical and creative exercises, drills, and activities.

Occupational Therapy in Mental Health
The Haworth Press
10 Alice Street
Binghamton, NY 13904
607-722-5857, 800-342-9678
http://www.haworthpressinc.com/journals/default.asp
Disability Served: mental health
This quarterly journal is designed for occupational therapists working in the mental health field.

Occupational Therapy Practice
American Occupational Therapy Association Inc.
4720 Montgomery Lane, PO Box 31220
Bethesda, MD 20824-1220
301-652-2682, ext. 2866
otpractice@aota.org
http://www.aota.org
Disability Served: various
This publication provides information on occupational therapy services and more for people with disabilities.

101 Hints to "Help with Ease" for Patients with Neuromuscular Disease
Muscular Dystrophy Association
3300 East Sunrise Drive
Tucson, AZ 85718
800-572-1717
publications@mdausa.org
http://www.mdausa.org/publications
Disability Served: physically disabled
This free booklet was written to assist patients with neuromuscular disease in handling the tasks of daily living.

101 Weight Loss Tips for Preventing and Controlling Diabetes
American Diabetes Association
1701 North Beauregard Street
Alexandria, VA 22311
800-342-2383
AskADA@diabetes.org
http://www.diabetes.org
Disability Served: diabetes
This book provides tips on losing weight for people with diabetes.

100 Questions and Answers about Parkinson Disease
National Parkinson Foundation
1501 Northwest Ninth Avenue/Bob Hope Road
Miami, FL 33136-1454
305-243-6666, 800-327-4545
contact@parkinson.org
http://www.parkinson.org/site/pp.asp?c=9dJFJLPwB&b=116364
Disability Served: Parkinson's Disease
This book of questions and answers about Parkinson disease is available with a donation to the National Parkinson Foundation.

On The Beam
Lowe Syndrome Association
18919 Voss Road
Dallas, TX 75287
612-869-5693
info@lowesyndrome.org
http://www.lowesyndrome.org/Lowe%20Syndrome/
    Publications/index.html
Disability Served: Lowe Syndrome
This newsletter for parents, families, and friends features
    letters from parents, organizational news, research
    news, recommended resources, and other helpful
    information.

**1,000 Signs of Life: Basic ASL for Everyday
    Conversation**
Gallaudet University Press
800 Florida Avenue, NE
Washington, DC 20002
202-651-5488 (Voice/TTY)
valencia.simmons@gallaudet.edu
http://gupress.gallaudet.edu
Disability Served: hearing
Provides common signs for animals, food, clothes,
    people, health and body, the time, days of the week,
    seasons, colors, quantities, transportation and travel,
    and other topics.

**1001 Great Ideas for Teaching and Raising Children
    with Autism Spectrum**
Future Horizons
721 West Abram Street
Arlington, TX 76013
800-489-0727
info@futurehorizons-autism.com
http://www.futurehorizons-autism.com/search_result.
    asp
Disability Served: autism
This book offers solutions that have worked for
    thousands of children grappling with sensory,
    communication, social, behavior, and self-care issues,
    and more.

**Opening Doors: Technology and Communication
    Options for Children with Hearing Loss**
Office of Special Education and Rehabilitative Services
400 Maryland Avenue, SW
Washington, DC 20202-7100
202-245-7468
http://www.ed.gov/about/offices/list/osers/reports.html

Disability Served: hearing
This free, downloadable publication provides
    background on early intervention, the use of
    technology, and other support available to children
    with hearing difficulties, and their families.

Our Immune System
Immune Deficiency Foundation
40 West Chesapeake Avenue, Suite 308
Towson, MD 21204
800-296-4433
idf@primaryimmune.org
http://www.primaryimmune.org/pubs/pubs.htm
Disability Served: immune deficiency disorders
This booklet educates children on the immune system,
    including T cells, B cells, and phagocytes, through a
    series of illustrations and animated characters.

**Our Voices: Inspirational Insights from Young People
    who Stutter**
National Stuttering Association
119 West 40th Street, 14th Floor
New York, NY 10018
800-937-8888
info@westutter.org
http://www.nsastutter.org/material/index.
    php?matid=117
Disability Served: communication
This newsletter is a special insert for teens who stutter
    that comes with the association's monthly newsletter,
    Letting Go. Articles in *Our Voices* are contributed by
    kids who stutter from all over the country.

**Out of Harm's Way: A Safety Kit for People with
    Disabilities Who Feel Unsafe and Want to Do
    Something About It**
L'Institut Roeher Institute
York University, 4700 Keele Street
Toronto, ON M3J 1P3
Canada
416-661-9611, 800-856-2207
info@roeher.ca
http://www.roeher.ca
Disability Served: various
This text is geared to help the disabled assess safety
    issues at home, work, study, and play.

Overcoming Drug and Alcohol Abuse
American Occupational Therapy Association Inc.
4720 Montgomery Lane, PO Box 31220

Bethesda, MD 20824-1220
301-652-2682, 800-377-8555
http://www.aota.org/featured/area6/links/link02.asp
Disability Served: chemical dependency
This free tip sheet offers information to help people
overcoming drug and alcohol abuse cope with
specific situations. It also provides an overview of
how occupational therapists can assist people with
substance abuse problems.

Overcoming Dyslexia in Children, Adolescents, and Adults

Pro-Ed Inc.
8700 Shoal Creek Boulevard
Austin, TX 78757-6897
800-897-3202
http://www.proedinc.com
Disability Served: dyslexic
This book defines various forms of dyslexia and discusses
the impact of dyslexia on the emotional, social, and
personal development of individuals.

Pain: Hope through Research

National Institute of Neurological Disorders and Stroke
PO Box 5801
Bethesda, MD 20824
301-496-5751, 800-352-9424
http://www.ninds.nih.gov/disorders/chronic_pain/
chronic_pain.htm#Publications
Disability Served: chronic pain
This free brochure offers up-to-date research on acute
and chronic pain, including diagnosis and treatments.

The Palette

VSA arts
818 Connecticut Avenue, NW, Suite 600
Washington, DC 20006
800-933-8721, 202-737-0645 (TDD)
info@vsarts.org
http://www.vsarts.org/x621.xml
Disability Served: various
This free newsletter for disabled visual artists features
informative articles, technical assistance, and news,
as well as interviews and profiles.

Paralyzed Veterans of America Guide to Federal Health Programs

Paralyzed Veterans of America
801 Eighteenth Street, NW
Washington, DC 20006-3517

301-932-7834, 888-860-7244
info@pva.org
http://www.pva.org/cgi-bin/pvastore/products.cgi?id=2
Disability Served: various
This free guide provides a glossary of terms and a short
description of each federal program, eligibility
requirements, coverage and benefits provided, and
sources for more information.

Paraplegia News

Paralyzed Veterans of America
801 Eighteenth Street, NW
Washington, DC 20006-3517
602-246-9426
info@pva.org
http://www.pvamagazines.com/pnnews
Disability Served: spinal-cord injury
This publication provides news and information for
paraplegics.

The Paraprofessional's Guide to the Inclusive Classroom: Working as a Team

Paul H. Brookes Publishing Company
PO Box 10624
Baltimore, MD 21285-0624
410-337-9580, 800-638-3775
custserv@brookespublishing.com
http://www.pbrookes.com
Disability Served: various
This handbook for the paraprofessional working in
inclusive classrooms offers guidance and strategies
for assisting students.

Parenting a Child with Diabetes

Juvenile Diabetes Foundation
120 Wall Street
New York, NY 10005-4001
800-533-2873
info@jdrf.org
http://www.jdrf.org/index.cfm?page_id=100250
Disability Served: diabetes
This book teaches parents about caring for their diabetic
child in simple, but accurate, language.

Parenting a Child with Special Needs

National Dissemination Center for Children
with Disabilities
PO Box 1492
Washington, DC 20013
800-695-0285

nichcy@aed.org
http://nichcy.org/publist.asp
Disability Served: various
This free publication offers tips to parents of children
with special needs.

Parenting Children with Learning Disabilities
Greenwood Publishing Group Inc.
88 Post Road West
Westport, CT 06881
203-226-3571
http://www.greenwood.com
Disability Served: learning disabled
This book offers support to parents of children with
learning disabilities. It will provide parents with the
ability to provide the academic and personal support
their children need to thrive.

The Parents' Guide to Cochlear Implants
Alexander Graham Bell Association of the Deaf
3417 Volta Place, NW
Washington, DC 20007
866-337-5220, 202-337-5221 (TTY)
publications@agbell.org
http://www.agbell.org
Disability Served: hearing
This publication details each stage of the cochlear
implantation process.

A Parent's Guide to Down Syndrome: Toward a Brighter Future
Paul H. Brookes Publishing Company Inc.
PO Box 10624
Baltimore, MD 21285-0624
800-638-3775
custserv@brookespublishing.com
http://www.pbrookes.com
Disability Served: Down Syndrome
This is a useful guide for parents who have children
with Down Syndrome. It is also available in Spanish.

A Parent's Guide to Special Education
Federation for Children with Special Needs
1135 Tremont Street, Suite 420
Boston, MA 02120
617-236-7210, 800-331-0688
fcsninfo@fcsn.org
http://www.fcsn.org/publications_resources/
publications.html
Disability Served: various

This free, downloadable guide assists families in obtaining
the support and services that their children with
disabilities need to succeed in school.

Parkinson Disease: Caring and Coping
National Parkinson Foundation
1501 Northwest Ninth Avenue/Bob Hope Road
Miami, FL 33136-1454
305-243-6666, 800-327-4545
contact@parkinson.org
http://www.parkinson.org/site/pp.asp?c=9dJFJLPwB&b
=71407
Disability Served: Parkinson's Disease
This free booklet includes chapters on Parkinson's
partners, the extended family, activities of daily
living, taking care of business, and building a support
network.

Parkinson Disease: Fitness Counts
National Parkinson Foundation
1501 Northwest Ninth Avenue/Bob Hope Road
Miami, FL 33136-1454
305-243-6666, 800-327-4545
contact@parkinson.org
http://www.parkinson.org/site/pp.asp?c=9dJFJLPwB&b
=71407
Disability Served: Parkinson's Disease
This free booklet includes chapters on fitness, balance,
avoiding falls, posture, helpful therapies, and care
partner-assisted exercise.

Parkinson Disease: Medications
National Parkinson Foundation
1501 Northwest Ninth Avenue/Bob Hope Road
Miami, FL 33136-1454
305-243-6666, 800-327-4545
contact@parkinson.org
http://www.parkinson.org/site/pp.asp?c=9dJFJLPwB&b
=71407
Disability Served: Parkinson's Disease
This free booklet lists and describes all of the drugs
on the market today used for the treatment
of Parkinson's Disease. Included are dietary
considerations, special instructions, and side effects.

Parkinson Disease: Nutrition Matters
National Parkinson Foundation
1501 Northwest Ninth Avenue/Bob Hope Road
Miami, FL 33136-1454
305-243-6666, 800-327-4545

contact@parkinson.org

http://www.parkinson.org/site/pp.asp?c=9dJFJLPwB&b
=71407

Disability Served: Parkinson's Disease

This free booklet discusses issues regarding weight
maintenance, protein absorption in the patient who
takes levodopa, and other components of healthful
living.

Parkinson Disease: Speech and Swallowing

National Parkinson Foundation

1501 Northwest Ninth Avenue/Bob Hope Road

Miami, FL 33136-1454

305-243-6666, 800-327-4545

contact@parkinson.org

http://www.parkinson.org/site/pp.asp?c=9dJFJLPwB&b
=71407

Disability Served: Parkinson's Disease

This free booklet covers communication issues in
Parkinson's Disease, personal assessment tools,
memory and concentration, improving swallowing
function and communication practice sets.

The Parkinson Report

National Parkinson Foundation

1501 Northwest Ninth Avenue/Bop Hope Road

Miami, FL 33136-1454

305-243-6666, 800-327-4545

contact@parkinson.org

http://www.parkinson.org/site/pp.asp?c=9dJFJLPwB&b
=71407

Disability Served: Parkinson's Disease

This quarterly report provides the latest news on
Parkinson's Disease.

Parkinson's Disease: Challenges, Progress, and Promise

National Institute of Neurological Disorders and Stroke

PO Box 5801

Bethesda, MD 20824

301-496-5751, 800-352-9424

http://www.ninds.nih.gov/disorders/parkinsons_
disease/parkinsons_disease.htm#Publications

Disability Served: Parkinson's Disease

This free brochure offers the latest Parkinson's Disease
(PD) research update, providing information on current treatments, research findings, and new directions.

Parkinson's Disease: Hope through Research

National Institute of Neurological Disorders and Stroke

PO Box 5801

Bethesda, MD 20824

301-496-5751, 800-352-9424

http://www.ninds.nih.gov/disorders/parkinsons_
disease/parkinsons_disease.htm#Publications

Disability Served: Parkinson's Disease

This free fact sheet offers up-to-date information
on Parkinson's Disease-its signs and symptoms,
medications used to manage disease symptoms,
and current research findings.

Pathways to Competence: Encouraging Healthy Social and Emotional Development in Young Children

Paul H. Brookes Publishing Company

PO Box 10624

Baltimore, MD 21285-0624

410-337-9580, 800-638-3775

custserv@brookespublishing.com

http://www.pbrookes.com

Disability Served: various

This textbook provides information and proposes
intervention methods to enhance social competence
and skills in children with disabilities.

Patient's Check List

R.A. Bloch Cancer Foundation Inc.

4400 Main Street

Kansas City, MO 64111

816-932-8453, 800-433-0464

http://www.blochcancer.org

Disability Served: cancer patients and survivors

This free, online listing of factors that assist in fighting
cancer helps patients maintain a positive attitude
while in treatment.

Person to Person: A Guide for Professionals Working with People with Disabilities

Paul H. Brookes Publishing Company

PO Box 10624

Baltimore, MD 21285-0624

410-337-9580, 800-638-3775

custserv@brookespublishing.com

http://www.pbrookes.com

Disability Served: various

This book is designed to increase awareness of those
working with people who have disabilities.

Photo Articulation Test

Pro-Ed Inc.

8700 Shoal Creek Boulevard

Austin, TX 78757-6897

800-897-3202
http://www.proedinc.com
Disability Served: communication
This test is designed to assess speech skills through a series of 72 photographs.

Physical Activities Workbook
American Association of Retired Persons
601 East Street, NW
Washington, DC 20049
888-687-2277
http://www.aarp.org/health/fitness/get_motivated/
a2004-06-28-workbook-users.html
Disability Served: elderly
This free handbook shows how seniors can add physical activity into their daily routines based on their unique needs and lifestyle. It also teaches how to start safely, set goals, develop a support network, find motivation, and overcome barriers.

Physical Therapy
American Physical Therapy Association
1111 North Fairfax Street
Alexandria, VA 22314-1488
703-684-2782, 800-999-2782, 703-683-6748 (TDD)
http://www.apta.org
Disability Served: various
This publication provides scholarly articles on physical therapy topics.

Physical Therapy in Bleeding Disorders
National Hemophilia Foundation
116 West 32nd Street, 11th Floor
New York, NY 10001
212-328-3700, 800-42-HANDI
handi@hemophilia.org
http://www.hemophilia.org/resources/handi_pubs.htm
Disability Served: inherited bleeding disorders
This booklet provides up-to-date information regarding physical therapy evaluation, modalities, types of splints, forms of exercise, and developmental issues. Single copies are free to members.

Planning for Long-Term Care
National Council on the Aging
300 D Street, SW, Suite 801
Washington, DC 20024
202-479-1200
info@ncoa.org
http://www.ncoa.org/content.cfm?sectionID=30

Disability Served: various
This publication provides information on long-term care resources.

Post-Polio Health
Post-Polio Health International
4207 Lindell Boulevard, #110
St Louis, MO 63108-2915
314-534-0475
info@post-polio.org
http://www.post-polio.org
Disability Served: physically disabled
This newsletter focuses on issues affecting polio survivors.

Postsecondary Education and Transition for Students with Learning Disabilities
Pro-Ed Inc.
8700 Shoal Creek Boulevard
Austin, TX 78757-6897
800-897-3202
http://www.proedinc.com
Disability Served: learning disabled
This guide is designed to assist persons who work with college students with learning disabilities.

Post-Stroke Rehabilitation Fact Sheet
National Institute of Neurological Disorders and Stroke
PO Box 5801
Bethesda, MD 20824
301-496-5751, 800-352-9424
http://www.ninds.nih.gov/disorders/stroke/stroke.
htm#Publications
Disability Served: stroke
This free fact sheet defines post-stroke rehabilitation and describes the disabilities that can result from stroke. It also gives advice on where to go for rehabilitation treatment.

Practical Guidelines for Care of Individuals with Down's Syndrome and Dementia
A.J. Pappanikou Center for Developmental Disabilities
University of Connecticut
263 Farmington Avenue, MC 6222
Farmington, CT 06030
860-679-1500, 860-679-1502 (TTY)
http://www.uconnucedd.org
Disability Served: dementia, developmentally disabled, Down Syndrome
This online publication provides care guidelines for individuals with Down Syndrome and dementia.

Pregnancy for Women with MS
Multiple Sclerosis Foundation Inc.
6350 North Andrews Avenue
Fort Lauderdale, FL 33309-2130
954-776-6805, 888-MSFOCUS
support@msfocus.org
http://www.msfacts.org/publications/pub_booklets.html
Disability Served: multiple sclerosis
This free booklet helps separate fact from fiction and
provides the information you need to know about
pregnancy and multiple sclerosis.

**Preparing for an International Career: Pathways
for People with Disabilities**
Mobility International USA
PO Box 10767
Eugene, OR 97440
541-343-1284 (Voice/TTY)
http://www.miusa.org/publications
Disability Served: various
This free, online publication covers career opportunities
in international affairs, exchange, and development
for the disabled.

Preparing for College: An Online Tutorial
DO-IT (Disabilities, Opportunities, Internetworking
and Technology)
PO Box 355670
Seattle, WA 98195-5670
206-685-3648, 800-972-3648
doit@u.washington.edu
http://www.washington.edu/doit/Brochures/
Academics
Disability Served: various
This free publication lists Internet resources for college-
bound teens with disabilities.

**Preparing for College: Options for Students with
Learning Disabilities**
Association on Higher Education and Disability
PO Box 540666
Waltham, MA 02454
781-788-0004
ahead@ahead.org
http://www.ahead.org/publications/index.htm
Disability Served: learning disabled
This booklet is full of useful, practical information for
students, families, and others who have an interest
in facilitating successful secondary to postsecondary
transition for students with learning disabilities.

Preparing Your Child for Social Situations
Cleft Palate Foundation
1504 East Franklin Street, Suite 102
Chapel Hill, NC 27514-2820
919-933-9044, 800-24CLEFT
info@cleftline.org
http://www.cleftline.org/publications
Disability Served: physically disabled
This free fact sheet offers advice to parents about
nurturing their children so that they have a positive
sense of self and are prepared to handle negative
social interactions.

**Preschool Children Who Stutter: Information
and Support for Parents**
National Stuttering Association
119 West 40th Street, 14th Floor
New York, NY 10018
800-937-8888
info@westutter.org
http://www.nsastutter.org/material/index.php?matid=115
Disability Served: communication
This booklet provides helpful advice for parents who
are concerned about their preschool child's speech.

Preventing Discrimination in the Workplace
Paralyzed Veterans of America
801 Eighteenth Street, NW
Washington, DC 20006-3517
301-932-7834, 888-860-7244
info@pva.org
http://www.pva.org/cgi-bin/pvastore/products.cgi?id=2
Disability Served: various
This free brochure provides information useful for both
employers and employees concerning measures to
ensure accessible, discrimination-free workplaces.

Prevention in Community Mental Health
Brookline Books
34 University Road
Brookline, MA 02445
617-734-6772
http://www.brooklinebooks.com
Disability Served: mental health
This book explores prevention programs in community
mental health and how they work.

**Primary Immune Deficiency Diseases in America:
The First National Survey of Patients and Specialists**
Immune Deficiency Foundation
40 West Chesapeake Avenue, Suite 308

Towson, MD 21204
800-296-4433
idf@primaryimmune.org
http://www.primaryimmune.org/pubs/pubs.htm
Disability Served: immune deficiency disorders
This free, downloadable report outlines the first national survey of patients with and specialists in primary immune deficiency diseases in the United States.

A Promising Future Together: A Guide for New Parents of Children with Down Syndrome
National Down Syndrome Society
666 Broadway
New York, NY 10012
800-221-4602
info@ndss.org
http://www.ndss.org/content.cfm?fuseaction=InfoRes.SrchResMat
Disability Served: Down Syndrome
This free guide educates parents about their new or expected baby with Down Syndrome using the experiences of parents at different stages in their children's lives, developmental pediatricians, and other professionals.

Provider Magazine
American Health Care Association
1201 L Street, NW
Washington, DC 20005
202-842-4444
http://www.providermagazine.com
Disability Served: various
This monthly magazine is designed for the long-term health care professional.

Psychiatric Hospitalization: A Guide for Families
Depressive and Bipolar Support Alliance
730 North Franklin Street, Suite 501
Chicago, IL 60610-7224
800-826-3632
bookstore@dbsalliance.org
http://www.dbsalliance.org/store
Disability Served: mental health
This free brochure explains how to cope with someone in crisis, how to help your loved one prepare for hospitalization, how to get information about treatment, and how to support loved ones when they come home.

Psychiatric Rehabilitation Journal
Boston University
Center for Psychiatric Rehabilitation

940 Commonwealth Avenue
Boston, MA 02215
617/353-3549, 617-353-7701 (TTY)
http://www.bu.edu/prj
Disability Served: mental health
This quarterly journal offers articles on psychiatric rehabilitation, including research findings, programs, and current issues.

Psychology of Disability
Springer Publishing Company
11 West 42nd Street
New York, NY 10036
877-687-7476
http://www.springerpub.com
Disability Served: various
This book discusses the societal challenges encountered by persons with disabilities.

Psychotherapy: How it Works and How it Helps
Depressive and Bipolar Support Alliance
730 North Franklin Street, Suite 501
Chicago, IL 60610-7224
800-826-3632
bookstore@dbsalliance.org
http://www.dbsalliance.org/store
Disability Served: mental health
This free brochure explains the process and benefits of psychotherapy.

Public Health Reports
Association of Schools of Public Health
1101 15th Street, NW, Suite 910
Washington, DC 20005
202-296-1099
info@asph.org
http://www.publichealthreports.org
Disability Served: various
This bimonthly publication provides articles on public health issues.

Putting Creativity to Work: Careers in the Arts for People with Disabilities
VSA arts
818 Connecticut Avenue, NW, Suite 600
Washington, DC 20006
800-933-8721, 202-737-0645 (TDD)
info@vsarts.org
http://www.vsarts.org/x630.xml
Disability Served: various

This free publication offers a wide range of useful information for visual, literary, and performing artists who are disabled, and features detailed information on more than 100 job titles and mini-biographies of people with disabilities holding these jobs. Career development, vocational rehabilitation, and special education professionals will also find this to be an indispensable resource.

Quality of Life for Persons with Disabilities: International Perspectives and Issues
Brookline Books
34 University Road
Brookline, MA 02445
617-734-6772
http://www.brooklinebooks.com
Disability Served: various
This book explores the concept of quality of life as viewed by persons with disabilities in a number of settings, including work, home, and leisure.

QUEST
Muscular Dystrophy Association
3300 East Sunrise Drive
Tucson, AZ 85718
800-572-1717
publications@mdausa.org
http://www.mdausa.org/publications
Disability Served: physically disabled
This national magazine publishes articles on all aspects of living with neuromuscular disease and updates on current research.

Questions and Answers
Lowe Syndrome Association
18919 Voss Road
Dallas, TX 75287
612-869-5693
info@lowesyndrome.org
http://www.lowesyndrome.org/Lowe%20Syndrome/ Publications/index.html
Disability Served: Lowe Syndrome
This free, downloadable brochure provides basic information about Lowe Syndrome.

Questions and Answers about IDEA
National Dissemination Center for Children with Disabilities
PO Box 1492
Washington, DC 20013

800-695-0285
nichcy@aed.org
http://nichcy.org/publist.asp
Disability Served: various
This free publication describes IDEA—the United States' special education law. Core questions about the special education process, as mandated by IDEA, are asked and answered.

Questions and Answers about Stroke
National Institute of Neurological Disorders and Stroke
PO Box 5801
Bethesda, MD 20824
301-496-5751, 800-352-9424
http://www.ninds.nih.gov/disorders/stroke/stroke. htm#Publications
Disability Served: stroke
This fact sheet provides background information about stroke and contains information about signs, symptoms, and risk factors.

Questions and Answers about the Americans with Disabilities Act
Paralyzed Veterans of America
801 Eighteenth Street, NW
Washington, DC 20006-3517
301-932-7834, 888-860-7244
info@pva.org
http://www.pva.org/cgi-bin/pvastore/products.cgi?id=2
Disability Served: various
This free pamphlet answers the most frequently asked questions concerning the implications of the Americans with Disabilities Act.

Questions and Answers on Hearing Loss
Self Help for Hard of Hearing People Inc.
7910 Woodmont Avenue, Suite 1200
Bethesda, MD 20814
301-657-2248, 301-657-2249 (TTY)
bookstore@hearingloss.org
http://hearingloss.sidestreetshop.com/default.cfm
Disability Served: hearing
This brochure provides a general overview on hearing loss.

Questions for Adults to Ask the Surgeon When Being Evaluated for a Cochlear Implant
Self Help for Hard of Hearing People Inc.
7910 Woodmont Avenue, Suite 1200
Bethesda, MD 20814

301-657-2248, 301-657-2249 (TTY)
bookstore@hearingloss.org
http://hearingloss.sidestreetshop.com/default.cfm
Disability Served: hearing
This booklet provides questions that adults should ask
when being evaluated for a cochlear implant. The first
copy is free of charge.

Questions Often Asked by Parents about Special Education Services
National Dissemination Center for Children with
Disabilities
PO Box 1492
Washington, DC 20013
800-695-0285
nichcy@aed.org
http://nichcy.org/publist.asp
Disability Served: various
This free publication explains how students with
disabilities can access special education and related
services.

Quick and Easy Meals and Menus
R.A. Rapaport Publishing Inc.
PO Box 11066
Des Moines, IA 50336-1066
800-664-9269
https://www.diabetesselfmanagement.com/eds/books.
cfm
Disability Served: diabetes
This book, which contains more than 30,000 different
meal combinations, offers meal-planning advice and
a healthy-living guide for families.

Quick-Guides to Inclusion: Ideas for Educating Students with Disabilities
Paul H. Brookes Publishing Company
PO Box 10624
Baltimore, MD 21285-0624
410-337-9580, 800-638-3775
custserv@brookespublishing.com
http://www.pbrookes.com
Disability Served: various
This book provides tools and techniques that educators
can incorporate in inclusive classrooms.

Quick-Guides to Inclusion 2: Ideas for Educating Students with Disabilities
Paul H. Brookes Publishing Company
PO Box 10624

Baltimore, MD 21285-0624
410-337-9580, 800-638-3775
custserv@brookespublishing.com
http://www.pbrookes.com
Disability Served: various
This guide for educators and administrators provides
essential information and basic tips for implementing
inclusion.

Reach Out Magazine
3090 Sheridan Street, PMB# 207
Hollywood, FL 33021-3730
954-985-0319
http://reachoutmag.com
Disability Served: various
This is a free, online magazine for people with
disabilities. Its Web site also offers live chats,
personals, and message boards.

Ready, Set, Go: Helping Students with Learning Disabilities Prepare for College
Association on Higher Education and Disability
PO Box 540666
Waltham, MA 02454
781-788-0004
ahead@ahead.org
http://www.ahead.org/publications/index.htm
Disability Served: learning disabled
This brochure covers preparation for the student with
learning disabilities in the transition beyond high
school. It offers a list of 20 activities and necessary
steps (ranging from testing, to independence, to
advocacy for students with learning disabilities) to
take in preparing themselves for higher education.

A Reason for Hope
Amytrophic Lateral Sclerosis Association
27001 Agoura Road, Suite 150
Calabasas Hills, CA 91301-5104
818-880-9007
info@alsa-national.org
http://www.alsa.org/resources/magazine.cfm?CFID=104
8742&CFTOKEN=97497558
Disability Served: physically disabled
This free, online magazine provides articles of interest
to Amytrophic Lateral Sclerosis patients and their
families.

Receptive-Expressive Emergent Language Test
Pro-Ed Inc.
8700 Shoal Creek Boulevard

Austin, TX 78757-6897
800-897-3202
http://www.proedinc.com
Disability Served: communication
This test is designed for use with at-risk youngsters and assesses language skills.

Recommended Reading for Adults with Learning Disabilities
International Dyslexia Association
Chester Building, 8600 LaSalle Road, Suite 382
Baltimore, MD 21286-2044
410-296-0232
http://www.interdys.org
Disability Served: learning disabled
This online brochure lists suggested books for adults with learning disabilities.

Recommended Reading for Children and Teens with Learning Disabilities
International Dyslexia Association
8600 LaSalle Road, Chester Building, Suite 382
Baltimore, MD 21286-2044
410-296-0232
http://www.interdys.org
Disability Served: learning disabled
This online brochure lists suggested books for young people with learning disabilities.

Recommended Reading for Parents
International Dyslexia Association
8600 LaSalle Road, Chester Building, Suite 382
Baltimore, MD 21286-2044
410-296-0232
http://www.interdys.org
Disability Served: dyslexic
This online brochure lists suggested books on dyslexia for parents.

Recovering from Stroke
American Occupational Therapy Association Inc.
4720 Montgomery Lane, PO Box 31220
Bethesda, MD 20824-1220
301-652-3682, 800-377-8555
http://www.aota.org/featured/area6/links/link02.asp
Disability Served: stroke
This free tip sheet offers information on the recovery process following a stroke. It also details the services occupational therapists provide to people who have had a stroke.

Rehabilitation Nursing
Association of Rehabilitation Nurses
4700 West Lake Avenue
Glenview, IL 60025
800-229-7530
info@rehabnurse.org
http://www.rehabnurse.org/profresources/index.html
Disability Served: various
This bimonthly journal of the Association of Rehabilitation Nurses reports on medical issues and research studies.

Remedial and Special Education
Pro-Ed Inc.
8700 Shoal Creek Boulevard
Austin, TX 78757-6897
800-897-3202
http://www.proedinc.com
Disability Served: various
This bimonthly journal provides research articles and studies on special education practices.

Report on Disability Law
Business Publishers Inc.
8737 Colesville Road, 10th Floor
Silver Spring, MD 20910-3928
301-589-5103, 800-274-6737
custserv@bpinews.com
http://www.bpinews.com
Disability Served: various
The *Report on Disability Law* is a biweekly newsletter with in-depth news and analyses on policy issues and legislation related to people with disabilities.

Research and Practice for Persons with Severe Disabilities
TASH
29 West Susquehanna Avenue, Suite 210
Baltimore, MD 21204
410-828-8274
http://www.tash.org
Disability Served: developmentally disabled
This journal (formerly known as *TASH:* The Journal of the Association for Persons with Severe Handicaps) offers articles and news for members of TASH.

Resources for Adults with Disabilities
National Dissemination Center for Children with Disabilities
PO Box 1492

Washington, DC 20013
800-695-0285
nichcy@aed.org
http://nichcy.org/publist.asp
Disability Served: various
This free publication helps adults with disabilities
identify organizations and agencies designed to
assist with their specific concerns and needs, such as
employment, postsecondary education, recreation,
independent living, and assistive technology.

Resources for Elders with Disabilities
Resources for Rehabilitation
22 Bonad Road
Winchester, MA 01890
781-368-9094
info@rfr.org
http://www.rfr.org
Disability Served: elderly
This book provides information that enables elders,
family members and other caregivers, and service
providers to locate appropriate services. Published
in large print, the book includes information about
rehabilitation, laws that affect elders with disabilities,
and self-help groups.

Resources for People with Disabilities and Chronic Conditions
Resources for Rehabilitation
22 Bonad Road
Winchester, MA 01890
781-368-9094
info@rfr.org
http://www.rfr.org
Disability Served: various
This reference guide provides resources to help persons
with disabilities and chronic conditions.

Resourcing: Handbook for Special Education Resource Teachers
Council for Exceptional Children
1110 North Glebe Road, Suite 300
Arlington, VA 22201-5704
888-CEC-SPED, 866-915-5000 (TTY)
service@cec.sped.org
http://www.cec.sped.org
Disability Served: various
This handbook contains information to assist the special
education instructor in being a resource for other
teachers and staff working with special education
students.

Restructuring for Caring and Effective Education: Piecing the Puzzle Together
Paul H. Brookes Publishing Company
PO Box 10624
Baltimore, MD 21285-0624
410-337-9580, 800-638-3775
custserv@brookespublishing.com
http://www.pbrookes.com
Disability Served: various
This guide for administrators discusses school
restructuring initiatives and the measures schools
must take in order to change their organizational
structure and teaching practices to become more
inclusive for students who have disabilities.

Restructuring High Schools for All Students: Taking Inclusion to the Next Level
Paul H. Brookes Publishing Company
PO Box 10624
Baltimore, MD 21285-0624
410-337-9580, 800-638-3775
custserv@brookespublishing.com
http://www.pbrookes.com
Disability Served: various
This guide provides information on creating inclusive
classrooms at the secondary level.

Rheumatoid Arthritis
Arthritis Foundation
PO Box 7669
Atlanta, GA 30357
800-568-4045
http://www.arthritis.org/AFstore/SubCatHome.
asp?idCat=8&idSubCat=111
Disability Served: physically disabled
This free brochure details the causes and symptoms of
this common form of arthritis, including information
on exercise, treatment, and new medications.

Road to Rehabilitation Series
Brain Injury Association of America
8201 Greensboro Drive, Suite 611
McLean, VA 22102
703-761-0750, 800-444-6443
familyhelpline@biausa.org
http://www.biausa.org/Pages/road_to_rehab.html
Disability Served: traumatic brain injury
This series of free, downloadable brochures offers
a layman's guide to the process of rehabilitation
from brain injury. Topics include pain, headaches,

cognition and memory, behavior changes, speech, drug therapy, and more.

Saying No to Negative Thinking
Depressive and Bipolar Support Alliance
730 North Franklin Street, Suite 501
Chicago, IL 60610-7224
800-826-3632
bookstore@dbsalliance.org
http://www.dbsalliance.org/store
Disability Served: mental health
This free brochure discusses negative thinking as a symptom of depression and bipolar disorder.

Schizophrenia in Children
National Mental Health Association
2001 North Beauregard Street, 12th Floor
Alexandria, VA 22311
703-684-7722, 800-969-6642
http://www.nmha.org/infoctr/factsheets
Disability Served: mental health
This free fact sheet offers information regarding schizophrenia in children with the following subcategories: definition, early warning signs, treatment, and additional resources for parents.

School Psychology Review
National Association of School Psychologists
4340 East West Highway, Suite 402
Bethesda, MD 20814
301-657-0270
publications@naspweb.org
http://www.nasponline.org/publications/index.html
Disability Served: various
This professional journal is the world's second-largest psychology journal. Published four times a year, it contains theory, research, and opinion related to school psychology.

Screening for Hearing Loss and Otitis Media in Children
Alexander Graham Bell Association of the Deaf
3417 Volta Place, NW
Washington, DC 20007
866-337-5220, 202-337-5221 (TTY)
publications@agbell.org
http://www.agbell.org
Disability Served: hearing
This is a guide to hearing and middle ear screening in children.

Selected Bibliography for Parents
Cleft Palate Foundation
1504 East Franklin Street, Suite 102
Chapel Hill, NC 27514-2820
919-933-9044, 800-24CLEFT
info@cleftline.org
http://www.cleftline.org/publications
Disability Served: physically disabled
This is a list of resource publications about cleft lip/palate.

Selecting a College for Students with Learning Disabilities or Attention Deficit Hyperactivity Disorder
HEATH Resource Center, George Washington University
2121 K Street, NW, Suite 220
Washington, DC 20037
202-973-0904 (Voice/TTY), 800-544-3284
askheath@gwu.edu
http://www.heath.gwu.edu/FactSheets.htm
Disability Served: attention deficit disorder, learning disabled
This free, online resource offers tips and advice to students with learning disabilities or attention deficit hyperactivity disorder.

Selecting an ADA Consultant
6 Grant Avenue
Takoma Park, MD 20912
301-270-2470
UDandC@UniversalDesign.com
http://www.universaldesign.com/store.php
Disability Served: various
This paper provides advice on selecting an Americans with Disabilities Act consultant.

Self-Advocacy for Students Who Are Deaf or Hard of Hearing
Pro-Ed Inc.
8700 Shoal Creek Boulevard
Austin, TX 78757-6897
800-897-3202
http://www.proedinc.com
Disability Served: hearing
This book is designed to teach high school graduates who are hearing impaired to take on the role of self-advocacy.

Self-Determination: Assuming Control of Your Plans for Postsecondary Education
HEATH Resource Center
George Washington University

2121 K Street, NW, Suite 220
Washington, DC 20037
202-973-0904 (Voice/TTY), 800-544-3284
askheath@gwu.edu
http://www.heath.gwu.edu/FactSheets.htm
Disability Served: various
This is a free, online resource that offers tips to help
disabled students to become self-determined as they
explore postsecondary educational options.

Senior Step: A Guide for Adapting to Limb Loss
Amputee Coalition of America
900 East Hill Avenue, Suite 285
Knoxville, TN 37915-2568
888-267-5669, 865-525-4512 (TTY)
http://www.amputee-coalition.org
Disability Served: amputees, elderly
This guide provides support and advice to the elderly
with limb loss or who are new amputees.

Sertoman
Sertoma Foundation
1912 East Meyer Boulevard
Kansas City, MO 64132
816-333-8300
infosertoma@sertoma.org
http://www.sertoma.org
Disability Served: hearing
This publication provides information and news on the
Sertoma Foundation.

7 Principles for Controlling Your Diabetes for Life
National Diabetes Information Clearinghouse
5 Information Way
Bethesda, MD 20892-3568
800-860-8747
catalog@niddk.nih.gov
http://catalog.niddk.nih.gov/AlphaList.cfm?CH=NDIC
Disability Served: diabetes
This booklet expands on *4 Steps to Control Your
Diabetes for Life*, providing in-depth information on
comprehensive diabetes care. The first 25 copies are
free.

Severe and/or Multiple Disabilities
National Dissemination Center for Children with
Disabilities
PO Box 1492
Washington, DC 20013
800-695-0285

nichcy@aed.org
http://nichcy.org/publist.asp
Disability Served: various
This free fact sheet defines various disorders
and provides information on the incidence,
characteristics, medical implications, educational
implications, additional resources, and associated
organizations of each disease.

Sharing Solutions
Lighthouse International
111 East 59th Street
New York, NY 10022-1202
212-821-9200, 800-829-0500
http://www.lighthouse.org/scripts/newsletter
Disability Served: vision
This free, online newsletter for people with impaired
vision and their support networks can be
downloaded from Lighthouse International.

Shingles: Hope through Research
National Institute of Neurological Disorders and Stroke
PO Box 5801
Bethesda, MD 20824
301-496-5751, 800-352-9424
http://www.ninds.nih.gov/disorders/chronic_pain/
chronic_pain.htm#Publications
Disability Served: chronic pain
This is a free informational booklet on shingles.

Simple Strategies for Change
Arthritis Foundation
PO Box 7669
Atlanta, GA 30357
800-568-4045
http://www.arthritis.org/AFstore/SubCatHome.
asp?idCat=8&idSubCat=118
Disability Served: physically disabled
This free leaflet is filled with tips to improve health
and limit the impact of arthritis—one simple step
at a time.

Singular's Illustrated Dictionary of Audiology
Alexander Graham Bell Association of the Deaf
3417 Volta Place, NW
Washington, DC 20007
866-337-5220, 202-337-5221 (TTY)
publications@agbell.org
http://www.agbell.org
Disability Served: hearing

This is a dictionary of more than 3,000 terms for audiologists.

16 Famous People Who Stutter
Stuttering Foundation of America
3100 Walnut Grove Road, Suite 603, PO Box 11749
Memphis, TN 38111-0749
901-452-7342, 800-992-9392
info@stutteringhelp.org
http://www.stutteringhelp.org/Default.aspx?tabid=131
Disability Served: communication
This free, downloadable brochure features well-known and successful individuals who stutter. This brochure is especially useful to raise awareness during National Stuttering Awareness Week.

Sjögren's Syndrome Handbook
Sjogren's Syndrome Foundation Inc.
8120 Woodmont Avenue, Suite 530
Bethesda, MD 20814
301-718-0300
dbgartley@simonfoundation.org
http://www.sjogrens.org/servlet/Cart.
    catalog?categoryId=40
Disability Served: immune deficiency disorders
This revised and expanded handbook includes new articles and the latest information on Sjögren's Syndrome.

Sjögren's Syndrome Survival Guide
Sjogren's Syndrome Foundation Inc.
8120 Woodmont Avenue, Suite 530
Bethesda, MD 20814
301-718-0300
http://www.sjogrens.org/servlet/Cart.
    catalog?categoryId=40
Disability Served: immune deficiency disorders
This resource for Sjogren's sufferers provides the newest medical information, research results, and treatment methods, as well as effective and practical self-help strategies.

Social and Emotional Problems Related to Dyslexia
International Dyslexia Association
8600 LaSalle Road, Chester Building, Suite 382
Baltimore, MD 21286-2044
410-296-0232
http://www.interdys.org
Disability Served: dyslexic
This online brochure covers social and emotional problems (such as anger, anxiety, depression, etc.) of dyslexics.

Social Networks Booklets
Ablenet
2808 Fairview Avenue
Roseville, MN 55113-1308
800-322-0956
customerservice@ablenetinc.com
http://www.ablenetinc.com
Disability Served: communication
These booklets help individuals, their families, and professionals determine the most appropriate technologies and communication strategies for individuals with complex communication needs.

Social Networks Manual
Ablenet
2808 Fairview Avenue
Roseville, MN 55113-1308
800-322-0956
customerservice@ablenetinc.com
http://www.ablenetinc.com
Disability Served: communication
This manual helps practitioners guide and refine the intervention process when dealing with their patients who have complex communication needs.

Social Security Bulletin
United States Social Security Administration
4301 Connecticut Avenue, Room 209
Washington, DC 20008
http://www.ssa.gov/policy/docs/ssb
Disability Served: various
This monthly bulletin provides the latest news regarding Social Security and related programs.

Someone You Know Has Multiple Sclerosis: A Book for Families
National Multiple Sclerosis Society
733 Third Avenue
New York, NY 10017
800-344-4867
http://www.nationalmssociety.org/Newly%20Diagnosed.
    asp
Disability Served: multiple sclerosis
This free booklet for children, ages six to 12, explores children's fears and concerns while providing facts for those who have a parent with multiple sclerosis.

Sound Facts: A Guide to Noise Levels
Ear Foundation
PO Box 330867
Nashville, TN 37203

615-627-2724, 800-545-HEAR
info@earfoundation.org
http://www.earfoundation.org/articles.asp
Disability Served: hearing
This online fact sheet is illustrated with a chart that shows the decibel ratings of many common sounds.

Speaking Up and Spelling It Out: Personal Essays on Augmentative and Alternative Communication

Paul H. Brookes Publishing Company Inc.
PO Box 10624
Baltimore, MD 21285-0624
800-638-3775
custserv@brookespublishing.com
http://www.pbrookes.com
Disability Served: communication
Twenty-eight diverse individuals who use augmentative and alternative communication (AAC) provide first-person accounts of how living with AAC has affected their lives.

Special Education Law and Children Who Stutter

Stuttering Foundation of America
3100 Walnut Grove Road, Suite 603, PO Box 11749
Memphis, TN 38111-0749
901-452-7342, 800-992-9392
info@stutteringhelp.org
http://www.stutteringhelp.org/Default.aspx?tabid=131
Disability Served: communication
This free, downloadable brochure helps parents better understand special education law by providing a basic explanation of how children are identified, screened, evaluated, and determined to be eligible for speech therapy services.

Special Living

PO Box 1000
Bloomington, IL 61702-1000
309-820-9277
http://www.specialliving.com
Disability Served: physically disabled
This magazine provides useful information and articles for people with mobility impairment.

SPECIAL REPORT: Diabetes Complications— Prevention and Management

R.A. Rapaport Publishing Inc.
PO Box 11066
Des Moines, IA 50336-1066
800-664-9269

https://www.diabetesselfmanagement.com/eds/books.cfm
Disability Served: diabetes
This book will teach you, in everyday language, how complications are diagnosed, how they can be prevented, how they can be controlled, and what drugs are available to treat them.

SPECIAL REPORT: New Drug Treatments for Diabetes

R.A. Rapaport Publishing Inc.
PO Box 11066
Des Moines, IA 50336-1066
800-664-9269
https://www.diabetesselfmanagement.com/eds/books.cfm
Disability Served: diabetes
This book provides clear, easy-to-understand answers to medication questions relating to diabetes.

Special Siblings: Growing Up with Someone with a Disability

Paul H. Brookes Publishing Company Inc.
PO Box 10624
Baltimore, MD 21285-0624
800-638-3775
custserv@brookespublishing.com
http://www.pbrookes.com
Disability Served: various
Written by a woman who grew up with a brother who had cerebral palsy and mental retardation, this book offers advice to others who grow up with, and care for, disabled siblings throughout the various stages of life.

Speech-Language Delights

The Speech Bin
1965 25th Avenue
Vero Beach, FL 32960
800-477-3324
info@speechbin.com
http://www.speechbin.com
Disability Served: communication
This book provides worksheets, games, exercises, and activities to teach and reinforce speech and language skills.

Speech-Language Impairments

National Dissemination Center for Children with Disabilities
PO Box 1492
Washington, DC 20013

800-695-0285
nichcy@aed.org
http://nichcy.org/publist.asp
Disability Served: communication
This free fact sheet defines and provides information on the incidence, characteristics, educational implications of various speech-language impairments, as well as lists additional resources and associated organizations.

Spina Bifida
National Dissemination Center for Children with Disabilities
PO Box 1492
Washington, DC 20013
800-695-0285
nichcy@aed.org
http://nichcy.org/publist.asp
Disability Served: spina bifida
This free fact sheet provides information on incidence, characteristics, and educational implications of spina bifida, as well as additional resources and associated organizations.

Sports 'N Spokes
c/o PVA Publications
2111 East Highland Avenue, Suite 180
Phoenix, AZ 85016-4702
888-888-2201
http://www.pvamagazines.com/sns
Disability Served: physically disabled
This magazine covers competitive wheelchair sports and recreational opportunities.

The Spotlight
VSA arts
818 Connecticut Avenue, NW, Suite 600
Washington, DC 20006
800-933-8721, 202-737-0645 (TDD)
info@vsarts.org
http://www.vsarts.org/x621.xml
Disability Served: various
This free newsletter for performing artists features informative articles, technical assistance, and news, as well as interviews and profiles.

Staying Healthy at 50+
Federal Citizen Information Center
1800 F Street, NW
Washington, DC 20405

888-878-3256
firstgov1@mail.fedinfo.gov
http://www.pueblo.gsa.gov/results.
 tpl?id1=16&startat=1&--woSECTIONSdatarq=16&--SECTIONSword=ww
Disability Served: various
This low-cost book covers cholesterol levels, various cancers, weight control, and checkups, and provides helpful charts to keep track of medications, shots, and screening test results.

Stay Safe: Preventing Spinal Cord Injury
United Spinal Association
75-20 Astoria Boulevard
Jackson Heights, NY 11370
718-803-3782, 800-444-0120
publications@unitedspinal.org
http://www.unitedspinal.org/pages.php?catid=7
Disability Served: spinal-cord injury
This free brochure provides statistics on spinal cord injury and offers protective measures to prevent such an injury.

Straight Talk about Death for Teenagers
Centering Corporation
7230 Maple Street
Omaha, NE 68134
402-533-1200
https://www.centeringcorp.com
Disability Served: various
This book, written in a simple, direct style, discusses death and the grieving process from the first days through thinking about the future.

Stroke Connection
American Heart Association
7272 Greenville Avenue
Dallas, TX 75231
800-4-STROKE
strokeconnection@heart.org
http://www.americanheart.org/presenter.
 jhtml?identifier=3001740
Disability Served: stroke
This free, bimonthly magazine is geared toward stroke survivors and provides information and resources.

Stroke: Hope through Research
National Institute of Neurological Disorders and Stroke
PO Box 5801
Bethesda, MD 20824

301-496-5751, 800-352-9424
http://www.ninds.nih.gov/disorders/stroke/stroke.
    htm#Publications
Disability Served: stroke
This free informational booklet about stroke provides
    current data about available therapies, current
    research, and clinical trials.

Stroke Rehabilitation Information
National Institute of Neurological Disorders and Stroke
PO Box 5801
Bethesda, MD 20824
301-496-5751, 800-352-9424
http://www.ninds.nih.gov/disorders/stroke/stroke.
    htm#Publications
Disability Served: stroke
This free fact sheet offers information about stroke
    including effects, types of rehabilitation, and
    prevention.

Stroke Risk Factors and Symptoms
National Institute of Neurological Disorders and Stroke
PO Box 5801
Bethesda, MD 20824
301-496-5751, 800-352-9424
http://www.ninds.nih.gov/disorders/stroke/stroke.
    htm#Publications
Disability Served: stroke
This free fact sheet describes the risk factors and
    symptoms associated with stroke.

Student Slate
National Federation of the Blind
1800 Johnson Street
Baltimore, MD 21230
410-659-9314
nfbstore@nfb.org
http://www.nfb.org/publications.html
Disability Served: vision
This publication, published on cassette and on the
    Internet by the National Association of Blind
    Students, is the voice of organized blind students.

Students with Disabilities and Access to Community College
HEATH Resource Center, George Washington University
2121 K Street, NW, Suite 220
Washington, DC 20037
202-973-0904 (Voice/TTY), 800-544-3284
askheath@gwu.edu

http://www.heath.gwu.edu/FactSheets.htm
Disability Served: various
This is a free, online resource that lists suggested
    questions for disabled students who are considering
    enrollment at a community college.

Students with Learning Disabilities
Prentice Hall/Pearson Education
One Lake Street
Upper Saddle River, NJ 07458
http://www.pearsoned.com
Disability Served: learning disabled
This textbook provides an introduction to learning
    disabilities.

Stutter Buddies: Newsletter for Children Who Stutter
National Stuttering Association
119 West 40th Street, 14th Floor
New York, NY 10018
800-937-8888
info@westutter.org
http://www.nsastutter.org/material/index.
    php?matid=116
Disability Served: communication
This quarterly newsletter, for kids in the six to 12 age
    group who stutter, contains articles contributed by
    children from all over the country who also stutter.

Suicide Prevention and Mood Disorders
Depressive and Bipolar Support Alliance
730 North Franklin Street, Suite 501
Chicago, IL 60610-7224
800-826-3632
bookstore@dbsalliance.org
http://www.dbsalliance.org/store
Disability Served: mental health
This free brochure includes sections covering topics such
    as recognizing risk factors, how to help someone who is
    considering suicide, and how to create a "Plan for Life."

Suicide Prevention Card
Depressive and Bipolar Support Alliance
730 North Franklin Street, Suite 501
Chicago, IL 60610-7224
800-826-3632
bookstore@dbsalliance.org
http://www.dbsalliance.org/store
Disability Served: mental health
This free card will easily fit in a wallet or pocket, and
    includes tips for coping with suicidal thoughts,

a hotline number, and space to write names and numbers of people you can call for help.

Support Group News

Multiple Sclerosis Foundation Inc.
6350 North Andrews Avenue
Fort Lauderdale, FL 33309-2130
954-776-6805, 888-MSFOCUS
support@msfocus.org
http://www.msfacts.org/publications/pub_subscriptions.
html
Disability Served: multiple sclerosis
This free bimonthly publication provides information on
the positive aspects of belonging to a support group
and how to start a support group.

Survival Strategies for Going Abroad: A Guide
for People with Disabilities

Mobility International USA
PO Box 10767
Eugene, OR 97440
541-343-1284 (Voice/TTY)
http://www.miusa.org/publications
Disability Served: various
More than 20 experienced disabled travelers offer tips
on participating in international programs.

Tackling Low Back Pain

American Occupational Therapy Association Inc.
4720 Montgomery Lane, PO Box 31220
Bethesda, MD 20824-1220
301-652-2682, 800-377-8555
http://www.aota.org/featured/area6/links/link02.asp
Disability Served: back injury, chronic pain
This free tip sheet offers information on how to help
people with low back pain cope with specific
situations. It also provides an overview of how
occupational therapists can help.

Taking Care of Both of You: Understanding Mood
Changes after the Birth of Your Baby

Depressive and Bipolar Support Alliance
730 North Franklin Street, Suite 501
Chicago, IL 60610-7224
800-826-3632
bookstore@dbsalliance.org
http://www.dbsalliance.org/store
Disability Served: mental health
This free brochure will help prospective and new
mothers recognize the symptoms and risk factors

of postpartum depression, provide tips for talking to
health care providers, and give suggestions on how
to stay healthy.

Taking Diabetes to School

Juvenile Diabetes Foundation
120 Wall Street
New York, NY 10005-4001
800-533-2873
info@jdrf.org
http://www.jdrf.org/index.cfm?page_id=100250
Disability Served: diabetes
This book helps elementary school students teach their
classmates about diabetes.

Talking Book Topics

National Library Service for the Blind and Physically
Handicapped
1291 Taylor Street, NW
Washington, DC 20011
202-707-5100, 202-707-0744 (TDD)
nls@loc.gov
http://www.loc.gov/nls
Disability Served: vision
This bimonthly publication provides reviews and
synopses of recorded books and publications
available at cooperating libraries.

A Teacher's Guide to Duchenne Muscular Dystrophy

Muscular Dystrophy Association
3300 East Sunrise Drive
Tucson, AZ 85718
800-572-1717
publications@mdausa.org
http://www.mdausa.org/publications
Disability Served: physically disabled
This free booklet for teachers helps explain Duchenne
muscular dystrophy and offers practical information
on how to cope with school problems faced by
youngsters with the disease.

Teaching Conversation to Children with Autism

Woodbine House
6510 Bells Mill Road
Bethesda, MD 20817
800-843-7323
http://www.woodbinehouse.com/Communication.
45.0.0.2.htm
Disability Served: autism

This book for parents and professionals describes a method to help children with autism initiate and sustain conversation through the use of written and audiotape scripts.

The Ten Keys to Helping Your Child Grow Up with Diabetes

Juvenile Diabetes Foundation
120 Wall Street
New York, NY 10005-4001
800-533-2873
info@jdrf.org
http://www.jdrf.org/index.cfm?page_id=100250
Disability Served: diabetes
This book for parents and caregivers of children with diabetes addresses the psychological, social and emotional hurdles that often complicate the lives of youngsters with diabetes.

Test Critiques

Pro-Ed Inc.
8700 Shoal Creek Boulevard
Austin, TX 78757-6897
800-897-3202
http://www.proedinc.com
Disability Served: various
This text provides studies of more than 800 tests and assessment tools.

Testing for Dyslexia

International Dyslexia Association
8600 LaSalle Road, Chester Building, Suite 382
Baltimore, MD 21286-2044
410-296-0232
http://www.interdys.org
Disability Served: dyslexic
This online brochure provides an overview of testing options to diagnose dyslexia. A Spanish-language version is also available.

Test of Language Development

Pro-Ed Inc.
8700 Shoal Creek Boulevard
Austin, TX 78757-6897
800-897-3202
http://www.proedinc.com
Disability Served: communication
This test is designed to identify and evaluate language disorders in children.

Test of Mathematical Abilities

Pro-Ed Inc.
8700 Shoal Creek Boulevard
Austin, TX 78757-6897
800-897-3202
http://www.proedinc.com
Disability Served: learning disabled
This test is designed to assess the math skills of students in grades three through 12.

Test of Nonverbal Intelligence

Pro-Ed Inc.
8700 Shoal Creek Boulevard
Austin, TX 78757-6897
800-897-3202
http://www.proedinc.com
Disability Served: learning disabled
This test is designed to assess intelligence, aptitude, and reasoning skills through problem-solving tasks.

Test of Phonological Awareness

Pro-Ed Inc.
8700 Shoal Creek Boulevard
Austin, TX 78757-6897
800-897-3202
http://www.proedinc.com
Disability Served: communication
This test is designed to assess phonological awareness of individual sounds.

Test of Written Spelling

Pro-Ed Inc.
8700 Shoal Creek Boulevard
Austin, TX 78757-6897
800-897-3202
http://www.proedinc.com
Disability Served: learning disabled
This test measures the spelling skills of students.

That's Life! Literature Series

Ablenet
2808 Fairview Avenue
Roseville, MN 55113-1308
800-322-0956
customerservice@ablenetinc.com
http://www.ablenetinc.com
Disability Served: various
This literature series fills the gap in age-appropriate literature for secondary students with disabilities.

They are developed in themed sets with low-vocabulary paperbacks and optional prerecorded modules.

360: The Accessible Lifestyle
PO Box 922
Clifton, NJ 07014
917-568-4077
http://www.360-mag.com/home.cfm
Disability Served: physically disabled
This is an e-zine for the people who are in wheelchairs.

Tinnitus: A Self-Management Guide for the Ringing in Your Ears
American Tinnitus Association
PO Box 5
Portland, OR 97207-0005
503-248-9985, 800-634-8978
dan@ata.org
http://www.ata.org/resources/order.html
Disability Served: hearing
This self-management guide includes workbook exercises so readers can assess the nature and extent of their problem with tinnitus.

Tinnitus: Questions and Answers
American Tinnitus Association
PO Box 5
Portland, OR 97207-0005
503-248-9985, 800-634-8978
dan@ata.org
http://www.ata.org/resources/order.html
Disability Served: hearing
This book answers hundreds of questions clearly and accurately on topics of interest to people with tinnitus.

Tinnitus Today
American Tinnitus Association
PO Box 5
Portland, OR 97207-0005
503-248-9985, 800-634-8978
dan@ata.org
http://www.ata.org/resources
Disability Served: hearing
This quarterly journal for patients and healthcare professionals contains up-to-date medical and research news, feature articles on urgent tinnitus issues, questions and answers, self-help suggestions, and feedback from people with tinnitus.

Tips for Helping a Person with Diabetes
National Diabetes Information Clearinghouse
5 Information Way
Bethesda, MD 20892-3568
800-860-8747
catalog@niddk.nih.gov
http://catalog.niddk.nih.gov/AlphaList.cfm?CH=NDIC
Disability Served: diabetes
This fact sheet provides practical tips and suggestions for helping loved ones with diabetes. The first 25 copies are free.

Tips for Kids: What Is Diabetes?
National Diabetes Information Clearinghouse
5 Information Way
Bethesda, MD 20892-3568
800-860-8747
catalog@niddk.nih.gov
http://catalog.niddk.nih.gov/AlphaList.cfm?CH=NDIC
Disability Served: diabetes
This publication, one in a series of colorful, reproducible tip sheets, contains the basics about managing diabetes for children and their families. The first 25 copies are free.

Toilet Training for Individuals with Autism and Related Disorders
Future Horizons
721 West Abram Street
Arlington, TX 76013
800-489-0727
info@futurehorizons-autism.com
http://www.futurehorizons-autism.com
Disability Served: autism
This provides 200 toilet training tips, 50 case examples, and 40 cautions..

The Toolbox
c/o Breaking New Ground
Purdue University, 1146 ABE Building
West Lafayette, IN 47907-1146
765-494-5088, 800-825-4264
http://pasture.ecn.purdue.edu/ABE/Extension/BNG/Resource%20Center/printed.html
Disability Served: physically disabled
This annual publication targets farmers with physical disabilities and provides news and helpful information.

Topics in Early Childhood Special Education
Pro-Ed Inc.
8700 Shoal Creek Boulevard

Austin, TX 78757-6897
800-897-3202
http://www.proedinc.com
Disability Served: various
This quarterly publication provides articles relating
to special education, including research studies,
professional papers, curriculum descriptions, and
more.

To Teach a Dyslexic
AVKO Educational Research Foundation
3084 West Willard Road
Clio, MI 48420
866-AVKO-612
sales@avko.org
http://www.avko.org/bookstore.htm
Disability Served: dyslexic, learning disabled
This text provides a dyslexic's account of how he learned
to read and in turn taught other dyslexics how to read.

Tourette Syndrome: Questions and Answers
Tourette Syndrome Association
42-40 Bell Boulevard
Bayside, NY 11361
718-224-2999
http://tsa-usa.org/Merchant2/merchant.
mvc?Screen=CTGY&Store_Code=TOS&
Category_Code=BFPW
Disability Served: Tourette Syndrome
This brochure covers commonly asked questions and
provides succinct and accurate answers.

**Transition from Two-Year to Four-Year Institutions
for Students with Disabilities**
DO-IT (Disabilities, Opportunities, Internetworking
and Technology)
PO Box 355670
Seattle, WA 98195-5670
206-685-3648, 800-972-3648
doit@u.washington.edu
http://www.washington.edu/doit/Brochures/Academics
Disability Served: various
This free publication offers advice for the disabled
student on the transition from a two-year to a four-
year institution.

**Transition to Adulthood: A Resource for Assisting Young
People with Emotional or Behavioral Difficulties**
Paul H. Brookes Publishing Company
PO Box 10624

Baltimore, MD 21285-0624
410-337-9580, 800-638-3775
custserv@brookespublishing.com
http://www.pbrookes.com
*Disability Served: behavioral disorders, emotionally
disabled adolescents*
This guide provides strategies for designing and
implementing transition programs for students
with emotional or behavioral disabilities.

Transliterating: Show Me the English
Registry of the Interpreters for the Deaf
333 Commerce Street
Alexandria, VA 22314
703-838-0030, 703-838-0459 (TTY)
info@rid.org
http://www.rid.org/pubs.html
Disability Served: hearing
This book is commonly used in curriculum for
currently enrolled students who have taken
at least one semester of interpreting skills. It
provides a comprehensive overview of the task of
transliterating.

Traumatic Brain Injury
American Occupational Therapy Association Inc.
4720 Montgomery Lane, PO Box 31220
Bethesda, MD 20824-1220
301-652-2682, 800-377-8555
http://www.aota.org/featured/area6/links/link02.asp
Disability Served: traumatic brain injury
This free tip sheet offers information to help people
overcoming traumatic brain injury cope with specific
situations. It also provides an overview of how
occupational therapists can help.

Traumatic Brain Injury
National Dissemination Center for Children with
Disabilities
PO Box 1492
Washington, DC 20013
800-695-0285
nichcy@aed.org
http://nichcy.org/publist.asp
Disability Served: traumatic brain injury
This free fact sheet provides information on the signs,
symptoms, and characteristics of traumatic brain
injury. It also provides tips for parents, teachers, and
schools, and lists additional resources and associated
organizations.

Traumatic Brain Injury: Hope through Research
National Institute of Neurological Disorders and Stroke
PO Box 5801
Bethesda, MD 20824
301-496-5751, 800-352-9424
http://www.ninds.nih.gov/disorders/tbi/tbi.
htm#Publications
Disability Served: traumatic brain injury
This free booklet, prepared by the National Institute of
Neurological Disorders and Stroke, defines traumatic
brain injury and describes the signs, symptoms, and
rehabilitation processes.

**Treatment Experiences and Preferences of Patients
with Primary Immune Deficiency Diseases:
National Survey**
Immune Deficiency Foundation
40 West Chesapeake Avenue, Suite 308
Towson, MD 21204
800-296-4433
idf@primaryimmune.org
http://www.primaryimmune.org/pubs/pubs.htm
Disability Served: immune deficiency disorders
This free, downloadable report outlines the results
of a national survey on treatment experiences
and preferences of patients with primary immune
deficiency diseases.

12 QUESTIONS
R.A. Bloch Cancer Foundation Inc.
4400 Main Street
Kansas City, MO 64111
816-932-8453, 800-433-0464
http://www.blochcancer.org
Disability Served: cancer patients and survivors
This free, online list contains 12 questions for a newly
diagnosed cancer patient to ask their physician.

25 Things To Do
Centering Corporation
7230 Maple Street
Omaha, NE 68134
402-533-1200
https://www.centeringcorp.com
Disability Served: various
This book provides healing activities for children who
have suffered loss or change in their lives.

Understanding and Controlling Your High Blood Pressure
American Heart Association
7272 Greenville Avenue

Dallas, TX 75231
800-242-8721
http://www.americanheart.org/presenter.
jhtml?identifier=3001740
Disability Served: physically disabled
This free brochure provides information to help people
understand and treat high blood pressure.

**Understanding and Teaching Emotionally Disturbed
Children and Adolescents**
Pro-Ed Inc.
8700 Shoal Creek Boulevard
Austin, TX 78757-6897
800-897-3202
http://www.proedinc.com
Disability Served: emotionally disabled adolescents
This teacher's guide offers teaching methods, strategies,
and background information on students who are
diagnosed as emotionally disturbed.

Understanding Mood Disorders
American Occupational Therapy Association Inc.
4720 Montgomery Lane, PO Box 31220
Bethesda, MD 20824-1220
301-652-2682, 800-377-8555
http://www.aota.org/featured/area6/links/link02.asp
Disability Served: mental health
This free tip sheet offers information on how to help
people with mood disorders cope with specific
situations, and also provides an overview of how
occupational therapists can help.

Understanding Treatment Choices for Prostate Cancer
Federal Citizen Information Center
1800 F Street, NW
Washington, DC 20405
888-878-3256
firstgov1@mail.fedinfo.gov
http://www.pueblo.gsa.gov/results.
tpl?id1=16&startat=1&--woSECTIONS
datarq=16&--SECTIONSword=ww
Disability Served: cancer patients and survivors
This free booklet describes how prostate cancer is
diagnosed, lists available treatment options, and
discusses follow-up care.

United States Association for Blind Athletes Newsletter
United States Association for Blind Athletes
33 North Institute Street
Colorado Springs, CO 80909
719-630-0422

http://www.usaba.org
Disability Served: vision
This newsletter provides news on the association's activities.

United States Hemophilia Treatment Centers Directory
National Hemophilia Foundation
116 West 32nd Street, 11th Floor
New York, NY 10001
212-328-3700, 800-42-HANDI
handi@hemophilia.org
http://www.hemophilia.org/resources/handi_pubs.htm
Disability Served: inherited bleeding disorders
This free directory, updated biannually by the Centers for Disease Control and Prevention, provides primary contact information for hemophilia treatment centers in the United States.

Universal Design: A Guide for Students
Association on Higher Education and Disability
PO Box 540666
Waltham, MA 02454
781-788-0004
ahead@ahead.org
http://www.ahead.org/publications/index.htm
Disability Served: various
This brochure explains how universal design principles are applied to learning. It encourages students to think about their educational experience in a new way.

Universal Design in Higher Education
Association on Higher Education and Disability
PO Box 540666
Waltham, MA 02454
781-788-0003
ahead@ahead.org
http://www.ahead.org/publications/index.htm
Disability Served: various
This brochure explains universal design (UD) principles in a straightforward manner. The concepts and applications of UD are presented for faculty, administrators, and other campus staff.

Unlocking Potential
Woodbine House
6510 Bells Mill Road
Bethesda, MD 20817
800-843-7323
http://www.woodbinehouse.com/Learning-Disabilities.17.0.0.2.htm

Disability Served: attention deficit disorder, learning disabled
This book is a guide to postsecondary school options—college, technical school, apprenticeship, remedial life skills programs, and employment—for young people with learning disabilities and attention deficit/hyperactivity disorder.

Use Your Home to Stay at Home: Expanding the Use of Reverse Mortgages to Pay for Long Term Care
National Council on the Aging
300 D Street, SW, Suite 801
Washington, DC 20024
202-479-1200
info@ncoa.org
http://www.ncoa.org/content.cfm?sectionID=30
Disability Served: various
This free, online resource explores the potential of using home equity to pay for in-home services and support.

Using the Telephone: A Guide for Those Who Stutter
Stuttering Foundation of America
3100 Walnut Grove Road, Suite 603, PO Box 11749
Memphis, TN 38111-0749
901-452-7342, 800-992-9392
info@stutteringhelp.org
http://www.stutteringhelp.org/Default.aspx?tabid=131
Disability Served: communication
This free, downloadable brochure serves as a helpful guide for those who have difficulty speaking on the telephone.

Ventilator-Assisted Living
Post-Polio Health International
4207 Lindell Boulevard, #110
St Louis, MO 63108-2915
314-534-0475
info@post-polio.org
http://www.post-polio.org
Disability Served: physically disabled
This newsletter focuses on news pertinent to ventilator users.

Videos About Dyslexia and Other Learning Disabilities
International Dyslexia Association
8600 LaSalle Road, Chester Building, Suite 382
Baltimore, MD 21286-2044
410-296-0232
http://www.interdys.org
Disability Served: dyslexic, learning disabled

This online brochure provides a list of videos about dyslexia from a variety of companies and organizations.

VIEWS
Registry of the Interpreters for the Deaf
333 Commerce Street
Alexandria, VA 22314
703-838-0030, 703-838-0459 (TTY)
http://www.rid.org/views.html
Disability Served: hearing
This monthly publication provides news on interpreting issues.

Vision
National Catholic Office for the Deaf
7202 Buchanan Street
Landover Hills, MD 20784-2236
301-577-1684, 301-577-4184 (TTY)
ncod@erols.com
http://www.ncod.org/vision.html
Disability Served: hearing
This publication is designed for Catholics who are deaf or hard of hearing.

Visual Impairments
National Dissemination Center for Children with Disabilities
PO Box 1492
Washington, DC 20013
800-695-0285
nichcy@aed.org
http://nichcy.org/publist.asp
Disability Served: vision
This free fact sheet defines various visual impairments and provides information on their incidence, characteristics, and educational implications, as well as provides additional resources and associated organizations.

Voice of the Diabetic
National Federation of the Blind
1800 Johnson Street
Baltimore, MD 21230
410-659-9314
nfbstore@nfb.org
http://www.nfb.org/publications.html
Disability Served: diabetes, vision
This publication, published four times per year, focuses on living with the diabetes and vision difficulties.

Articles discuss research, coping tools and strategies, success stories, and individuals whose attitude and achievements can serve as inspiration.

Voice of the Nations Blind
National Federation of the Blind
1800 Johnson Street
Baltimore, MD 21230
410-659-9414
nfbstore@nfb.org
http://www.nfb.org/publications.html
Disability Served: vision
This online publication of the National Federation of the Blind offers news and updates on issues and events of interest to the blind.

Von Willebrand Disease: Just the FAQs
National Hemophilia Foundation
116 West 32nd Street, 11th Floor
New York, NY 10001
212-328-3700, 800-42-HANDI
handi@hemophilia.org
http://www.hemophilia.org/resources/handi_pubs.htm
Disability Served: inherited bleeding disorders
This booklet for both males and females with von Willebrand Disease describes the signs and symptoms of the disorder, explains its inheritance, provides a summary of the classification system for von Willebrand Disease, explains treatment options and products, and discusses lifestyle concerns. Single copies are free to members.

Walking Guide
Arthritis Foundation
PO Box 7669
Atlanta, GA 30357
800-568-4045
http://www.arthritis.org/AFstore/CategoryHome.asp?idCat=8
Disability Served: physically disabled
Order one free copy of this brochure to discover information on a walking program, from what you need to get started to the elements that are crucial.

Walking Tomorrow
Christopher Reeve Paralysis Foundation
500 Morris Avenue
Springfield, NJ 07081
800-225-0292
http://www.christopherreeve.org

Disability Served: spinal-cord injury
This publication provides medical updates regarding research on spinal-cord injury.

Washington Watch
United Cerebral Palsy
1660 L Street, NW, Suite 700
Washington, DC 20036
202-776-0406, 202-973-7197 (TTY)
http://www.ucp.org/ucp_general.cfm/1/12591
Disability Served: various
This weekly publication provides current news regarding legislative issues concerning persons with cerebral palsy and other disabilities.

What Does a Kid with Tourette Syndrome Look Like? Just Like Any Other Kid!
Tourette Syndrome Association
42-40 Bell Boulevard
Bayside, NY 11361
718-224-2999
http://tsa-usa.org/Merchant2/merchant.
    mvc?Screen=CTGY&Store_Code=TOS&Category_
    Code=E
Disability Served: Tourette Syndrome
This publication will help layman and professionals understand the complexities and the unique characteristics of Tourette Syndrome.

What Every Child Needs for Good Mental Health
National Mental Health Association
2001 North Beauregard Street, 12th Floor
Alexandria, VA 22311
703-684-7722, 800-969-6642
http://www.nmha.org/infoctr/factsheets
Disability Served: mental health
This free fact sheet offers information regarding what every child needs for good mental health. Subject headings include unconditional love, confidence, self-esteem, and play time.

What Everyone Should Know about Epilepsy
Epilepsy Foundation
4351 Garden City Drive
Landover, MD 20785-7223
800-332-1000
http://www.epilepsyfoundation.org
Disability Served: epilepsy
This booklet contains brief descriptions of causes, seizure types, and available treatments as well as information about living with epilepsy, the reactions of others, and where to get help.

What Helps and What Hurts
Depressive and Bipolar Support Alliance
730 North Franklin Street, Suite 501
Chicago, IL 60610-7224
800-826-3632
bookstore@dbsalliance.org
http://www.dbsalliance.org/store
Disability Served: mental health
This free brochure offers advice on how to talk to your loved ones who are dealing with symptoms of depression or bipolar disorder.

What I Need To Know about Hepatitis A
National Digestive Diseases Information Clearinghouse
2 Information Way
Bethesda, MD 20892-3570
800-891-5389
nddic@info.niddk.nih.gov
http://catalog.niddk.nih.gov/PubType.
    cfm?Type=174&CH=NDDIC
Disability Served: physically disabled
This free brochure defines Hepatitis A and lists the signs, symptoms, and treatment options associated with the disease.

What I Need To Know about Hepatitis B
National Digestive Diseases Information Clearinghouse
2 Information Way
Bethesda, MD 20892-3570
800-891-5389
nddic@info.niddk.nih.gov
http://catalog.niddk.nih.gov/PubType.
    cfm?Type=174&CH=NDDIC
Disability Served: physically disabled
This free brochure defines Hepatitis B and lists the signs, symptoms, and treatment options associated with the disease.

What I Need To Know about Hepatitis C
National Digestive Diseases Information Clearinghouse
2 Information Way
Bethesda, MD 20892-3570
800-891-5389
nddic@info.niddk.nih.gov
http://catalog.niddk.nih.gov/PubType.
    cfm?Type=174&CH=NDDIC
Disability Served: physically disabled

This free brochure defines Hepatitis C and lists the signs, symptoms, and treatment options associated with the disease.

What Is Multiple Sclerosis?

National Multiple Sclerosis Society
733 Third Avenue
New York, NY 10017
800-344-4867
http://www.nationalmssociety.org/Newly%20Diagnosed.asp
Disability Served: multiple sclerosis
This free brochure defines multiple sclerosis (MS) and covers the symptoms, treatment options, general disease patterns, and diagnosis of MS.

What Is Vocal Hoarseness?

The Speech Bin
1965 25th Avenue
Vero Beach, FL 32960
800-477-3324
info@speechbin.com
http://www.speechbin.com
Disability Served: communication
These brochures are designed to provide information about voice disorders to educators, parents, and others.

What's Wrong/Hidden Pictures

Pro-Ed Inc.
8700 Shoal Creek Boulevard
Austin, TX 78757-6897
800-897-3202
http://www.proedinc.com
Disability Served: learning disabled
These three humorous game boards of hidden pictures are designed to teach consonant blend sounds.

What You Need to Know about Skin Cancer

Federal Citizen Information Center
1800 F Street, NW
Washington, DC 20405
888-878-3256
firstgov1@mail.fedinfo.gov
http://www.pueblo.gsa.gov/results.tpl?id1=16&startat=1&--woSECTIONS
datarq=16&--SECTIONSword=ww
Disability Served: cancer patients and survivors
This free booklet explains that the most common cancer in the United States—skin cancer—is among the

most curable, if caught in time. It offers tips on what to watch for and how to do skin self-exams.

What You Need to Know about Stroke

National Institute of Neurological Disorders and Stroke
PO Box 5801
Bethesda, MD 20824
301-496-5751, 800-352-9424
http://www.ninds.nih.gov/disorders/stroke/stroke.htm#Publications
Disability Served: stroke
This free, educational booklet gives advice on how to act quickly to save a life when someone is having a stroke, and provides detailed information on stroke prevention.

When a Loved One Has ALS: A Caregiver's Guide

Muscular Dystrophy Association
3300 East Sunrise Drive
Tucson, AZ 85718
800-572-1717
publications@mdausa.org
http://www.mdausa.org/publications
Disability Served: physically disabled
This comprehensive guide to caring for a person with Amytrophic Lateral Sclerosis at home covers everything from physical care, to psychological and emotional concerns, to getting financial assistance.

When Hearing Aids Aren't Enough

Self Help for Hard of Hearing People Inc.
7910 Woodmont Avenue, Suite 1200
Bethesda, MD 20814
301-657-2248, 301-657-2249 (TTY)
bookstore@hearingloss.org
http://hearingloss.sidestreetshop.com/default.cfm
Disability Served: elderly, hearing
This booklet summarizes the current research on cochlear implants and the elderly and answers questions about cochlear implants.

When Pre-Schoolers Are Not "On-Target"

Learning Disabilities Association of New York State
4156 Library Road
Pittsburgh, PA 15234-1349
412-341-1515
http://www.ldanatl.org/aboutld/resources/guide.asp
Disability Served: learning disabled
This guidebook is a valuable resource for parents, early childhood educators, and child care providers.

When Your Child Has a Disability: The Complete Sourcebook of Daily and Medical Care
Paul H. Brookes Publishing Company Inc.
PO Box 10624
Baltimore, MD 21285-0624
800-638-3775
custserv@brookespublishing.com
http://www.pbrookes.com
Disability Served: various
This is a comprehensive resource for parents with children who have disabilities. It covers a variety of disabilities, including mental retardation, autism, hearing impairment, Down Syndrome, visual impairment, communication disorders, seizure disorders, spina bifida, attention deficit disorder, cerebral palsy, and genetic syndromes.

When Your Child Is Deaf: A Guide for Parents
Pro-Ed Inc.
8700 Shoal Creek Boulevard
Austin, TX 78757-6897
800-897-3202
http://www.proedinc.com
Disability Served: hearing
This is a useful guide for parents with children who are deaf.

Where to Turn . . . Your Guide to Federal Disability Policies and Programs
Brain Injury Association of America
8201 Greensboro Drive, Suite 611
McLean, VA 22102
703-761-0750, 800-444-6443
familyhelpline@biausa.org
http://www.biausa.org/Pages/where_to_turn.html
Disability Served: various
This free, downloadable 426-page informative document was supported by the U.S. Department of Health and Human Services Administration and the Brain Injury Association of America.

Who Is at Risk for Spina Bifida?
Spina Bifida Association of America
4590 MacArthur Boulevard, NW, Suite 250
Washington, DC 20007-4226
202-944-3285, 800-621-3141
sbaa@sbaa.org
http://www.sbaa.org/site/PageServer?pagename=asb_facts
Disability Served: spina bifida

This free fact sheet describes increased risk factors for spina bifida.

Why Are You So Sad? A Child's Book about Parental Depression
Magination Press
750 First Street, NE
Washington, DC 20002-4242
800-374-2721
magination@apa.org
http://www.maginationpress.com
Disability Served: mental health
This book helps children understand and cope with parents who are suffering from depression.

Why Speech Therapy?
Stuttering Foundation of America
3100 Walnut Grove Road, Suite 603, PO Box 11749
Memphis, TN 38111-0749
901-452-7342, 800-992-9392
info@stutteringhelp.org
http://www.stutteringhelp.org/Default.aspx?tabid=131
Disability Served: communication
This free, downloadable brochure explains what to look for and what to expect from therapy, and serves as an important tool for finding a therapist and setting realistic goals.

Wide Range Achievement Test
Pro-Ed Inc.
8700 Shoal Creek Boulevard
Austin, TX 78757-6897
800-897-3202
http://www.proedinc.com
Disability Served: various
This kit provides test forms and information for the Wide Range Achievement Test.

A Woman's Guide to Coping with Disability
Resources for Rehabilitation
22 Bonad Road
Winchester, MA 01890
781-368-9094
info@rfr.org
http://www.rfr.org
Disability Served: various
This book addresses the special needs of women with disabilities and chronic conditions. Topics include social relationships, sexual functioning, pregnancy, childrearing, caregiving, and employment. Special

attention is paid to ways in which women can advocate for their rights with the health care and rehabilitation systems.

Women with Disabilities Aging Well: A Global View
Paul H. Brookes Publishing Company
PO Box 10624
Baltimore, MD 21285-0624
410-337-9580, 800-638-3775
custserv@brookespublishing.com
http://www.pbrookes.com
Disability Served: developmentally disabled
This guide discusses health and well-being issues of women with developmental disabilities as they age.

Working Relationships: Creating Career Opportunities for Job Seekers with Disabilities Through Employer Partnerships
Paul H. Brookes Publishing Company Inc.
PO Box 10624
Baltimore, MD 21285-0624
800-638-3775
custserv@brookespublishing.com
http://www.pbrookes.com
Disability Served: various
A useful tool for educators and other professionals helping the disabled find employment.

Young Children with Special Needs
Thomson Delmar Learning
Attn: Order Fulfillment, PO Box 6904
Florence, KY 41022
800-347-7707
http://www.delmarlearning.com
Disability Served: developmentally disabled
This book outlines developmental levels of motor skills, cognitive skills, language skills, social skills, and more.

You've Just Been Diagnosed . . . What Now?
Depressive and Bipolar Support Alliance
730 North Franklin Street, Suite 501
Chicago, IL 60610-7224
800-826-3632
bookstore@dbsalliance.org
http://www.dbsalliance.org/store
Disability Served: mental health
This free brochure provides basic facts about mood disorders and helps those who have been diagnosed live with their diagnosis.

PUBLISHERS

The following publishing companies provide books, magazines, and other materials of interest to persons with disabilities, their families, caregivers, and others who work with the disabled.

Ablenet

2808 Fairview Avenue
Roseville, MN 55113-1308
800-322-0956
customerservice@ablenetinc.com
http://www.ablenetinc.com
Disability Served: various
This organization provides a variety of publications and other tools to help teach children with disabilities.

Alexander Graham Bell Association of the Deaf

3417 Volta Place, NW
Washington, DC 20007
866-337-5220, 202-337-5221 (TTY)
publications@agbell.org
http://www.agbell.org
Disability Served: hearing
This association offers books and journals for those who are deaf or hard of hearing. It also offers a selection of audio-visual materials.

American Cancer Society

1599 Clifton Road, PO Box 49528
Atlanta, GA 30359-0528
800-ACS-2346
http://www.cancer.org
Disability Served: cancer patients and survivors
This association offers a variety of publications for people with cancer, their families, and medical professionals.

American Diabetes Association

1701 North Beauregard Street
Alexandria, VA 22311
800-342-2383
AskADA@diabetes.org
http://www.diabetes.org
Disability Served: diabetes
This organization offers a wealth of information resources to people with diabetes, as well as to professionals.

American Foundation for the Blind

11 Penn Plaza, Suite 300
New York, NY 10001
212-502-7600, 800-232-5463
afbinfo@afb.net
http://www.afb.org
Disability Served: hearing, vision
The American Foundation for the Blind publishes a wide selection of books, textbooks, and videos for the visually impaired and for the deaf-blind.

American Heart Association

7272 Greenville Avenue
Dallas, TX 75231
800-242-8721
http://www.americanheart.org
Disability Served: physically disabled
This association offers publications about preventing and treating heart disease.

American Physical Therapy Association

1111 North Fairfax Street
Alexandria, VA 22314-1488
703-684-2782, 800-999-2782, 703-683-6748 (TDD)
http://www.apta.org
Disability Served: various
This association offers publications for consumers a
nd professionals.

American Psychiatric Association

1000 Wilson Boulevard, Suite 1825
Arlington, VA 22209
703-907-7300, 888-35-PSYCH
apa@psych.org
http://www.healthyminds.org/letstalkfacts.cfm
Disability Served: mental health
This organization offers the Let's Talk Series, publications on mental disorders and how to improve mental health. Its publishing arm, American Psychiatric Publishing, offers resources for mental health professionals.

Association on Higher Education and Disability

PO Box 540666
Waltham, MA 02454
781-788-0004
ahead@ahead.org
http://www.ahead.org/publications/index.htm
Disability Served: various

This association publishes resources for the layman and professionals regarding students with disabilities who pursue higher education.

Brain Injury Association of America

8201 Greensboro Drive, Suite 611
McLean, VA 22102
703-761-0750, 800-444-6443
familyhelpline@biausa.org
http://www.biausa.org
Disability Served: traumatic brain injury
The Brain Injury Association of America offers a wealth of resources, including books, brochures, and journals.

Brookline Books

34 University Road
Brookline, MA 02445
617-734-6772
http://www.brooklinebooks.com
Disability Served: various
This company offers books dealing with disability issues, particularly for educators. It also publishes children's books.

Centering Corporation

7230 Maple Street
Omaha, NE 68134
402-533-1200
https://www.centeringcorp.com
Disability Served: various
This organization offers publications that help people, especially children, deal with grief and loss.

Cleft Palate Foundation

1504 East Franklin Street, Suite 102
Chapel Hill, NC 27514-2820
919-933-9044, 800-24CLEFT
info@cleftline.org
http://www.cleftline.org/publications
Disability Served: physically disabled
The foundation offers resources for people with cleft palates.

Council for Exceptional Children (CEC)

1110 North Glebe Road, Suite 300
Arlington, VA 22201-5704
888-CEC-SPED, 866-915-5000 (TTY)
service@cec.sped.org
http://www.cec.sped.org

Disability Served: various
The CEC publishes journals and other materials for parents and educators of exceptional children.

Depressive and Bipolar Support Alliance

730 North Franklin Street, Suite 501
Chicago, IL 60610-7224
800-826-3632
bookstore@dbsalliance.org
http://www.dbsalliance.org/store
Disability Served: mental health
The alliance offers books, brochures, and videos on mental health issues. All of the alliance's resources are reviewed by its scientific advisory board for scientific and medical accuracy.

DO-IT (Disabilities, Opportunities, Internetworking and Technology)

PO Box 355670
Seattle, WA 98195-5670
206-685-3648, 800-972-3648
doit@u.washington.edu
http://www.washington.edu/doit/Brochures/Academics
Disability Served: various
DO-IT provides resources for students who are disabled and their teachers, at the secondary and postsecondary levels.

Elsevier Inc.

655 Avenue of the Americas
New York, NY 10010
212-989-5800
http://www.sciencedirect.com
Disability Served: various
Elsevier Inc. publishes a variety of professional journals on disability-related topics.

Epilepsy Foundation

4351 Garden City Drive
Landover, MD 20785-7223
800-332-1000
http://www.epilepsyfoundation.org
Disability Served: epilepsy
The foundation offers books, pamphlets, manuals, and videos on epilepsy.

Federal Citizen Information Center

1800 F Street, NW
Washington, DC 20405

888-878-3256
firstgov1@mail.fedinfo.gov
http://www.pueblo.gsa.gov
Disability Served: various
The Federal Citizen Information Center is a government organization that provides an eclectic mix of free publications to consumers interested in health-related issues and other topics.

Future Horizons

721 West Abram Street
Arlington, TX 76013
800-489-0727
info@futurehorizons-autism.com
http://www.futurehorizons-autism.com
Disability Served: Asperger Syndrome, autism
This is one of the leading publishers of books, videos, and newsletters about autism/Asperger Syndrome.

Gallaudet University Press

800 Florida Avenue, NE
Washington, DC 20002
202-651-5488 (Voice/TTY)
valencia.simmons@gallaudet.edu
http://gupress.gallaudet.edu
Disability Served: hearing
This university press offers a variety of books and other materials of interest to the hearing impaired and the professionals who work with them. Specialties include sign language and children's resources.

Greenwood Publishing Group Inc.

88 Post Road West
Westport, CT 06881
203-226-3571
http://www.greenwood.com
Disability Served: various
This publisher offers reference and professional books, including some educational handbooks regarding disabilities.

Grey House Publishing

185 Millerton Road, PO Box 860
Millerton, NY 12546
518-789-8700, 800-562-2139
http://www.greyhouse.com
Disability Served: various
This company publishes a variety of disability-related directories.

The Haworth Press

10 Alice Street
Binghamton, NY 13904
607-722-5857, 800-342-9678
http://www.haworthpressinc.com
Disability Served: various
This company publishes materials on a variety of disabilities and related topics such as occupational therapy.

HEATH Resource Center

2121 K Street, NW, Suite 220
Washington, DC 20037
202-973-0904 (Voice/TTY), 800-544-3284
askheath@gwu.edu
http://www.heath.gwu.edu
Disability Served: various
The HEATH Resource Center at George Washington University publishes resources on postsecondary education for students who are disabled.

Immune Deficiency Foundation

40 West Chesapeake Avenue, Suite 308
Towson, MD 21204
800-296-4433
idf@primaryimmune.org
http://www.primaryimmune.org/pubs/pubs.htm
Disability Served: immune deficiency disorders
This organization publishes a variety of educational materials for people with immune deficiency disorders, as well as for health care professionals.

International Dyslexia Association

Chester Building, 8600 LaSalle Road, Suite 382
Baltimore, MD 21286-2044
410-296-0232
http://www.interdys.org
Disability Served: dyslexic
This association offers dyslexia-related publications and videos for educators, adults, college students, parents, and teens.

Juvenile Diabetes Foundation

120 Wall Street
New York, NY 10005-4001
800-533-2873
info@jdrf.org
http://www.jdrf.org/index.cfm?page_id=100250
Disability Served: diabetes

This foundation offers a variety of resources on childhood diabetes.

Learning Disabilities Association of America
4156 Library Road
Pittsburgh, PA 15234-1349
412-341-1515
http://www.ldanatl.org/aboutld/resources/index.asp
Disability Served: learning disabled
This organization provides a wealth of resources on learning disabilities.

L'Institut Roeher
York University, 4700 Keele Street
Toronto, ON M3J 1P3
Canada
416-661-9611, 800-856-2207
info@roeher.ca
http://www.roeher.ca
Disability Served: mentally disabled
This institute publishes all of its research findings (books, bibliographies, etc.) in English and French. Most of its research is on various topics of interest to people with disabilities.

Love Publishing Company
9101 East Kenyon Avenue, Suite 2200
Denver, CO 80237
303-221-7333
lpc@lovepublishing.com
http://www.lovepublishing.com
Disability Served: various
This company's titles include professional books in counseling and special education.

LRP Publications
747 Dresher Road, Suite 500, PO Box 980
Horsham, PA 19044
800-341-7874, 215-658-0938 (TTY)
http://www.shoplrp.com/disability/cat-Books_Pamphlets.html
Disability Served: various
This company offers brochures, newsletters, pamphlets, books, CD-ROMs, and tipsheets on disability-related topics.

Magination Press
750 First Street, NE
Washington, DC 20002-4242
800-374-2721
magination@apa.org
http://www.maginationpress.com
Disability Served: various
This company publishes books that help children ages four through 18 address the challenges of growing up.

Multiple Sclerosis Foundation Inc.
6350 North Andrews Avenue
Fort Lauderdale, FL 33309-2130
954-776-6805, 888-MSFOCUS
support@msfocus.org
http://www.msfacts.org
Disability Served: multiple sclerosis
This association offers booklets and other publications on multiple sclerosis.

Muscular Dystrophy Association
3300 East Sunrise Drive
Tucson, AZ 85718
800-572-1717
publications@mdausa.org
http://www.mdausa.org/publications
Disability Served: physically disabled
The association offers a variety of informational and educational publications on muscular dystrophy.

National Association for Parents of the Visually Impaired Inc.
PO Box 317
Watertown, MA 02471
admin@spedex.com
http://www.spedex.com/napvi/order.html
Disability Served: vision
This advocacy organization for parents of children with vision difficulties offers books, magazines, and other resources, some of which are available in Spanish.

National Association for the Visually Handicapped
22 West 21st Street, 6th Floor
New York, NY 10010
212-889-3141
navh@navh.org
http://www.navh.org/faq.html#large
Disability Served: vision
The National Association for the Visually Handicapped offers the large-print loan library, a free-by-mail library of more than 7,000 titles in large print. It is available to anyone in the United States.

National Center for Learning Disabilities
381 Park Avenue South, Suite 1401
New York, NY 10016

212-545-7510
http://www.ld.org/LDInfoZone
Disability Served: learning disabled
This association offers a wealth of publications on
learning disabilities.

National Council on the Aging

300 D Street, SW, Suite 801
Washington, DC 20024
202-479-1200
info@ncoa.org
http://www.ncoa.org/content.cfm?sectionID=30
*Disability Served: chemical dependency, elderly, mental
health*
The council provides legal, medical, and caregiving
resources for the elderly and their caregivers.

National Diabetes Information Clearinghouse

5 Information Way
Bethesda, MD 20892-3568
800-860-8747
catalog@niddk.nih.gov
http://catalog.niddk.nih.gov/AlphaList.cfm?CH=NDIC
Disability Served: diabetes
The clearinghouse offers more than 60 publications
on diabetes, some of which are available in several
languages.

National Digestive Diseases Information
Clearinghouse

2 Information Way
Bethesda, MD 20892-3570
800-891-5389
nddic@info.niddk.nih.gov
http://digestive.niddk.nih.gov
Disability Served: physically disabled
The clearinghouse provides a plethora of publications on
digestive disorders.

National Dissemination Center for Children with
Disabilities

PO Box 1492
Washington, DC 20013
800-695-0285
nichcy@aed.org
http://nichcy.org/publist.asp
Disability Served: various
The National Dissemination Center for Children with
Disabilities offers more than 100 publications on
disability-related topics.

National Down Syndrome Society

666 Broadway
New York, NY 10012
800-221-4602
info@ndss.org
http://www.ndss.org/content.cfm?fuseaction=InfoRes.
SrchResMat
Disability Served: Down Syndrome
The society offers articles and publications on Down
Syndrome at its Web site.

National Federation of the Blind

1800 Johnson Street
Baltimore, MD 21230
410-659-9314
nfbstore@nfb.org
http://www.nfb.org/publications.html
Disability Served: vision
This organization offers large print, Braille, and tape
publications for people with vision impairments.

National Hemophilia Foundation

116 West 32nd Street, 11th Floor
New York, NY 10001
212-328-3700, 800-42-HANDI
handi@hemophilia.org
http://www.hemophilia.org/resources/handi_pubs.htm
Disability Served: inherited bleeding disorders
This organization offers publications for people with
bleeding disorders, and their families, as well as
healthcare providers, educators, librarians, and
healthcare organizations.

National Institute of Child Health and Human
Development

PO Box 2006
Rockville, MD 20847
800-370-2943
NICHDInformationResourceCenter@mail.nih.gov
http://www.nichd.nih.gov/publications/pubs.cfm
Disability Served: various
The National Institute of Child Health and Human
Development offers health publications that focus on
disabilities that affect children.

National Institute of Neurological Disorders and Stroke

PO Box 5801
Bethesda, MD 20824
301-496-5751, 800-352-9424
http://www.ninds.nih.gov/disorders/stroke/stroke.
htm#Publications
Disability Served: various

The institute publishes a wealth of information on disorders of the brain and nervous system.

National Mental Health Association

2001 North Beauregard Street, 12th Floor
Alexandria, VA 22311
703-684-7722, 800-969-6642
http://www.nmha.org/infoctr/factsheets
Disability Served: mental health
This organization offers brochures, booklets, videos, and other materials on mental health.

National Multiple Sclerosis Society

733 Third Avenue
New York, NY 10017
800-344-4867
http://www.nationalmssociety.org
Disability Served: multiple sclerosis
The society publishes magazines and booklets on multiple sclerosis.

National Parkinson Foundation

1501 Northwest Ninth Avenue/Bob Hope Road
Miami, FL 33136-1454
305-243-6666, 800-327-4545
contact@parkinson.org
http://www.parkinson.org/site/pp.asp?c=9dJFJLPwB&b
=116364
Disability Served: Parkinson's Disease
This organization offers print publications for Parkinson patients and caregivers in English and Spanish, a quarterly magazine for medical practitioners, and a list of video or other media resources about Parkinson's Disease.

Paralyzed Veterans of America

801 Eighteenth Street, NW
Washington, DC 20006-3517
301-932-7834, 888-860-7244
info@pva.org
http://www.pva.org
Disability Served: spinal-cord injury
This organization offers publications to help paralyzed veterans avoid discrimination in the workplace and in other settings.

Paul H. Brookes Publishing Company

PO Box 10624
Baltimore, MD 21285-0624
410-337-9580, 800-638-3775
custserv@brookespublishing.com
http://www.pbrookes.com
Disability Served: various
This publisher offers books concerned with a wide range of disabilities and related concerns, including developmental disabilities, mental health, and special education.

Pro-Ed Inc.

8700 Shoal Creek Boulevard
Austin, TX 78757-6897
800-897-3202
http://www.proedinc.com
Disability Served: various
This company offers books, journals, and other materials on many topics, including special education and developmental disabilities.

R.A. Bloch Cancer Foundation Inc.

4400 Main Street
Kansas City, MO 64111
816-932-8453, 800-433-0464
http://www.blochcancer.org
Disability Served: cancer patients and survivors
The foundation provides a variety of resources to people with cancer and their caregivers.

R.A. Rapaport Publishing Inc.

PO Box 11066
Des Moines, IA 50336-1066
800-664-9269
https://www.diabetesselfmanagement.com/eds/books.
cfm
Disability Served: diabetes
This organization publishes resources to help people control and manage their diabetes.

Reference Service Press

5000 Windplay Drive, Suite 4
El Dorado Hills, CA 95762
916-939-9620
findaid@aol.com
http://www.rspfunding.com
Disability Served: various
This company publishes *Financial Aid for the Disabled and Their Families,* a popular resource for disabled students who are seeking financial aid.

Resources for Rehabilitation

22 Bonad Road
Winchester, MA 01890

781-368-9094
info@rfr.org
http://www.rfr.org
Disability Served: various
This publisher specializes in resources for rehabilitation.

Self Help for Hard of Hearing People Inc.
7910 Woodmont Avenue, Suite 1200
Bethesda, MD 20814
301-657-2248, 301-657-2249 (TTY)
bookstore@hearingloss.org
http://hearingloss.sidestreetshop.com/default.cfm
Disability Served: hearing
This organization publishes books and brochures for
    people with hearing-related disorders.

The Speech Bin
1965 25th Avenue
Vero Beach, FL 32960
800-477-3324
info@speechbin.com
http://www.speechbin.com
Disability Served: various
This company offers books, tests, software, and other
    materials for rehabilitation professionals, therapists,
    and educators.

Spina Bifida Association of America
4590 MacArthur Boulevard, NW, Suite 250
Washington, DC 20007-4226
202-944-3285, 800-621-3141
sbaa@sbaa.org
http://www.sbaa.org
Disability Served: spina bifida
This organization publishes a wealth of information
    on spina bifida.

Springer Publishing Company
11 West 42nd Street
New York, NY 10036
877-687-7476
http://www.springerpub.com
Disability Served: various
This publisher offers educational books and textbooks
    in such areas as rehabilitation, public health,
    psychology, and geriatrics.

Stuttering Foundation of America
3100 Walnut Grove Road, Suite 603, PO Box 11749
Memphis, TN 38111-0749

901-452-7342, 800-992-9392
info@stutteringhelp.org
http://www.stutteringhelp.org
Disability Served: communication
This organization publishes useful information for
    people who stutter and their families. Its Web site
    provides a listing of state libraries that feature
    resources on stuttering.

Tourette Syndrome Association
42-40 Bell Boulevard
Bayside, NY 11361
718-224-2999
http://tsa-usa.org
Disability Served: Tourette Syndrome
The Tourette Syndrome Association offers brochures,
    flyers, videos and other materials for people
    with Tourette Syndrome, their families, and their
    caregivers.

United Spinal Association
75-20 Astoria Boulevard
Jackson Heights, NY 11370
718-803-3782, 800-444-0120
publications@unitedspinal.org
http://www.unitedspinal.org
Disability Served: spinal-cord injury
This organization offers free publications about
    spinal-cord injury at its Web site.

Wiley Inc.
111 River Street
Hoboken, NJ 07030
800-825-7550
http://www3.interscience.wiley.com/cgi-bin/home
Disability Served: various
This company offers a variety of journals, books, and
    other publications on disabilities.

Woodbine House
6510 Bells Mill Road
Bethesda, MD 20817
800-843-7323
http://www.woodbinehouse.com/ADD-&-
    ADHD.9.0.0.2.htm
Disability Served: various
This company publishes books on a variety
    of disabilities.

SPORTS PROGRAMS

These organizations promote the participation of people with disabilities in sports and athletic events. Services may include training, competitions, and adapted equipment and facilities.

AbilityPlus Inc.
PO Box 253
Waterville Valley, NH 03215
603-236-8311
http://www.abilityplus.org
Disability Served: various
This is a nonprofit adaptive skiing and recreation organization for individuals with disabilities.

AccessSportAmerica
119 High Street
Acton, MA 01720
978-264-0985, 866-45SPORT
info@AccesSportAmerica.org
http://www.windsurf.org
Disability Served: various
This organization is dedicated to the discovery of higher function, fitness, and fun for children and adults of all disabilities, through high-challenge sports, individual training, and building community.

America Deaf Recreational Club
c/o Fleener Enterprises
6742 Western Avenue, Suite 14
Buena Park, CA 90621
president@adrclub.org
http://www.adrclub.org
Disability Served: hearing
This group provides nationwide recreational opportunities for people with hearing disabilities, their friends, and relatives.

Annual Santa Barbara Sports Festival
PO Box 50001
Santa Barbara, CA 93150
805-897-2680
RHanna@SantaBarbaraCA.gov
http://www.semananautica.com
Disability Served: various
The festival offers sporting events for persons with disabilities. Contact the organization for dates.

Canadian Deaf Sports Association
4545, Avenue Pierre-de-Courbertin, C.P. 1000, Succ. "M"
Montreal, QC H1V 3R2
Canada
800-855-0511, 514-252-3069 (TDD)
office@assc-cdsa.com
http://www.assc-cdsa.com
Disability Served: hearing
This organization promotes and facilitates fitness, amateur sports, and recreation among deaf Canadians of all ages from local recreation to Olympics level sports.

Canadian Wheelchair Basketball Association
2211 Riverside Drive, Suite B2
Ottawa, ON K1H 7X5
Canada
613-260-1296
cwba@cwba.ca
http://www.cwba.ca
Disability Served: various
The Canadian Wheelchair Basketball Association is the national sports governing body responsible for the organization of wheelchair basketball in Canada.

Disabled Sports USA
451 Hungerford Drive, Suite 100
Rockville, MD 20850
301-217-0960, 301-217-0963 (TDD)
http://www.dsusa.org
Disability Served: various
Disabled Sports USA offers nationwide sports rehabilitation programs to anyone with a permanent disability. Activities include winter skiing, water sports, summer and winter competitions, fitness, and special sports events. Participants include those with visual impairments, amputations, spinal cord injury, dwarfism, multiple sclerosis, head injury, cerebral palsy, and other neuromuscular and orthopedic conditions.

Dream Catchers, USA
PO Box 701
Killen, AL 35645
256-272-0286
DreamCatcherMail@aol.com
http://www.dreamcatchersusa.org
Disability Served: various

The purpose of this organization is to help advance independence, productivity, and confidence in people with disabilities and the terminally ill. It offers fishing trips, hunting trips, shooting competitions, and other outdoor adventures.

Extreme Adaptive Sports
504 Brett Place
South Plainfield, NJ 07080
908-313-5590
tom@sitski.com
http://www.sitski.com
Disability Served: various
This organization helps people with different disabilities enjoy the sport of skiing by using adapted ski equipment.

Handicapped Scuba International
1104 El Prado
San Clemente, CA 92672-4637
949-498-4540
hsa@hsascuba.com
http://www.hsascuba.com
Disability Served: various
This organization offers recreational diving instruction to people with various disabilities.

International Paralympic Committee (IPC)
Adenauerallee 212-214
Bonn 53113
Germany
49-228-2097-200
info@paralympic.org
http://www.paralympic.org
Disability Served: hearing
The International Paralympic Committee (IPC) is the international governing body of sports for athletes with a disability. The IPC supervises and coordinates the organization of the Paralympic Summer and Winter Games and other multi-disability competitions.

National Sports Center for the Disabled
PO Box 1290
Winter Park, CO 80482
970-726-1540, 303-316-1540
info@nscd.org
http://www.nscd.org
Disability Served: various

This organization provides therapeutic recreation and competitive opportunities for children and adults with disabilities.

National Veterans Wheelchair Games
Paralyzed Veterans of America
801 18th Street, NW
Washington, DC 20006-3517
202-872-1300, 800-424-8200
info@pva.org
http://www.pva.org/sports/games/gameindex.htm
Disability Served: physically disabled
This athletic event for physically disabled veterans takes place every summer.

Skating Association for the Blind and Handicapped
1200 East and West Road
West Seneca, NY 14224
716-675-7222
sabah@sabahinc.org
http://www.sabahinc.org
Disability Served: various
The Skating Association for the Blind and Handicapped provides weekly adaptive ice skating lessons, adaptive skating equipment, intense volunteer support, and the opportunity to perform in an annual ice-skating spectacular. Its services are available to children and adults of varying disabilities.

Special Olympics Inc.
1133 19th Street, NW
Washington, DC 20036
202-628-3630
info@specialolympics.org
http://www.specialolympics.org
Disability Served: various
The Special Olympics offers children and adults with intellectual disabilities year-round training and competition in 26 Olympic-type summer and winter sports. There is no charge to participate in Special Olympics.

United States Association of Blind Athletes
33 North Institute Street
Colorado Springs, CO 80903
719-630-0422
media@usaba.org
http://www.usaba.org
Disability Served: vision

The mission of the United States Association of Blind Athletes is to increase the number and quality of grassroots-through-competitive, world-class athletic opportunities for Americans who are blind or visually impaired. It provides athlete and coach identification and support, program and event management, and national and international representation.

United States Cerebral Palsy Athletic Association

25 West Independence Way
Kingston, RI 02881
401-874-7465
info@ndsaonline.org
http://www.uscpaa.org
Disability Served: cerebral palsy, stroke, traumatic brain injury
This association provides both individualized sports training and competitive opportunities for athletes with cerebral palsy, or other related challenges, such as traumatic brain injuries or strokes.

USA Deaf Sports Federation (USADSF)

102 North Krohn Place
Sioux Falls, SD 57103-1800
605-367-5760, 605-367-5761
HomeOffice@usdeafsports.org
http://www.usdeafsports.org
Disability Served: hearing
This organization promotes sports for deaf athletes in the United States. The USADSF is also affiliated with the United States Olympic Committee.

PART IV
INDEXES

DISABILITIES INDEX

GEOGRAPHIC LOCATION INDEX

ORGANIZATION NAME INDEX